P9-AFI-674

Validated by
THE INTERNATIONAL
FIRE SERVICE TRAINING
ASSOCIATION

Published By
FIRE PROTECTION
PUBLICATIONS
Oklahoma State University

Cover Photo Courtesy of:
Kern F. Braswell — Tulsa, Oklahoma

Second Edition

Self-Contained
Breathing Apparatus

Dedication

This manual is dedicated to the members of that unselfish organization of men and women who hold devotion to duty above personal risk, who count on sincerity of service above personal comfort and convenience, who strive unceasingly to find better ways of protecting the lives, homes and property of their fellow citizens from the ravages of fire and other disasters ... The Firefighters of All Nations.

Dear Firefighter:

The International Fire Service Training Association (IFSTA) is an organization that exists for the purpose of serving firefighters' training needs. Fire Protection Publications is the publisher of IFSTA materials. Fire Protection Publications staff members participate in the National Fire Protection Association, International Association of Fire Chiefs, and the International Society of Fire Service Instructors.

If you need additional information concerning our organization or assistance with manual orders, contact:

Customer Services
Fire Protection Publications
Oklahoma State University
Stillwater, OK 74078-0118
(800) 654-4055

For assistance with training materials, recommended material for inclusion in a manual or questions on manual content, contact:

Technical Services
Fire Protection Publications
Oklahoma State University
Stillwater, OK 74078-0118
(405) 744-5723

First Printing, July 1991
Second Printing, August 1992

© 1991 by the Board of Regents, Oklahoma State University
All rights reserved
ISBN 0-87939-093-X
Library of Congress 91-71902
Second Edition
Printed in the United States of America

Table of Contents

PREFACE XI
GLOSSARY XIV
INTRODUCTION 1
Breathing Apparatus: Yesterday And Today 1
Purpose And Scope 2

1   THE BODY 7
Introduction 7
The Respiratory System 7
    Anatomy 8
    External Respiration 9
    Internal Respiration 10
    Defense Mechanisms 11
Cardiovascular System 12
The Body's Reaction While Wearing SCBA 14
    Mental Fitness 15
    Emotional Stability Of The User 15
    Controlled Breathing 16
    Degree Of Physical Exertion 16
Physical Fitness 17
Summary 20
Review 21

2   RESPIRATORY HAZARDS 27
Introduction 27
Oxygen Deficiency 28
Elevated Temperatures 28
Flashover And Backdraft 29
    Flashover 29
    Backdraft 29
Smoke 30
Toxic Gases 30
    Carbon Monoxide (CO) 34
    Hydrogen Chloride (HCl) 37
    Hydrogen Cyanide (HCN) 37
    Carbon Dioxide (CO_2) 38
    Phosgene ($COCl_2$) 39
    Oxides of Nitrogen (NO_2, NO) 39
    Acrolein (CH_2CHCHO) 40
    Formaldehyde (HCHO) 41
    Hydrogen Sulfide (H_2S) 41
    Sulfur Dioxide (SO_2) 41
    Benzene (C_6H_6) 42
    Asbestos 42

Respiratory Hazards Not Associated With Fire 42
    Oxygen-Deficient Atmospheres 42
    Hazardous Materials Incidents 43
Summary 45
Review 46

3   TYPES OF SCBA **53**
Introduction 54
Duration Of Air Supply 55
    Condition Of SCBA 56
    Cylinder Pressure 56
Open-Circuit Breathing Apparatus 56
Components 56
    Backpack And Harness Assembly 58
    Air Cylinder Assembly 58
    Regulator Assembly 59
    Facepiece Assembly 63
Accessories 65
    Improving Communication 65
    Reducing Facepiece Fogging 66
    Aiding Vision 66
Airline Equipment 66
Closed-Circuit Breathing Apparatus 67
    Operation 68
    Positive Pressure 69
    Maintenance 69
    Advantages And Disadvantages 70
Selection Of SCBA 70
    Geographical Area And Climate 70
    Response Hazards Typically Encountered 70
    Economic Factors 71
    Operational Considerations 71
    Desired Features And Accessories 71
    Manufacturer's Reliability 71
    Meeting Standards 71
Summary 72
Review 73

4   SAFETY AND TRAINING **81**
Introduction 81
General Safety 82
    Facial And Long Hair 82
    Protective Clothing 83
    Donning 84
    Eyeglasses And Contact Lenses 84
    Use In High Or Low Temperatures 85
    Accidental Submersion 85
    Communication 85

Working In Teams 86
Personal Alert Safety Systems (PASS) 86
Doffing 86
Physical Conditioning 86
The Firefighter's Safety Responsibilities 87
Knowing SCBA Protection Limits And Safety Features 87
Knowing Air Supply Duration 88
Calculating Point Of No Return 88
Ensuring Facepiece Fit 90
Following Basic Safety Guidelines 90
The Department's Responsibilities At The Station 91
Testing Facepiece Fit 91
Record Keeping 94
Following General Safety Guidelines 95
The Department's Safety Responsibilities At The Emergency Scene 97
Entry Control 97
Guide Line System 99
Monitoring Systems In The United States And Canada 100
SCBA Training 102
Training Sequence 104
Facilities 107
Advanced Training (Smoke Diver School) 113
Keeping Training Records 115
Summary 116
Review 117

5   DONNING AND DOFFING 125
Introduction 125
Donning The Open-Circuit SCBA 125
Donning The Backpack 125
Donning The Facepiece 138
Doffing The Open-Circuit SCBA 148
Doffing With Harness-Mounted Regulator 148
Doffing With Facepiece-Mounted Regulator 151
Donning The Closed-Circuit SCBA 152
Doffing The Closed-Circuit SCBA 158
Changing Cylinders 160
Open-Circuit SCBA 160
Closed-Circuit SCBA 162
Summary 163
Review 164

6   INSPECTION, CARE, AND TESTING OF SCBA 173
Introduction 173
Department Responsibility 174
Daily Or Weekly Inspection 174
Facepiece Assembly 175
Cylinder Assembly 177

Regulator Assembly 178

Harness And Backpack Assembly 180

Storage 181

Inspection And Care After Each Use 181

Monthly Inspection 183

Records And Maintenance 186

Records 186

Storage 187

Repair And Reconditioning 188

Rebuilding 189

Cylinder Testing 189

SCBA Advisories 190

Modification 190

Summary 191

Review 192

7   AIR CYLINDER RECHARGING SYSTEMS **199**

Introduction 199

Compressors 200

Location Of Compressor 202

Safety Factors 204

Shop-Built Compressors 207

Air Purification Systems 207

Recommended Dew Point Levels 209

Computing Air Purification Cartridge Life 210

Testing Air Quality 212

Mobile Air Cascade And/Or Compressor Units 215

Recharging SCBA Cylinders 217

Filling From A Cascade System 218

Filling From A Compressor/Purifier 220

Rapid Refilling Of Cylinder While Wearing SCBA 221

Summary Of Breathing-Air Compressor and Purifier Guidelines 222

Equipment And Operating Safety 222

Equipment Setup 222

Operation And Charging 222

Maintenance 222

Summary 223

Review 224

8   USING SCBA **233**

Introduction 233

Fireground Uses Of SCBA 234

Engine Company Operations 234

Truck Company Operations 234

Rescue Company Operations 235

Special Situations Involving Fireground Operations 237

Temperature Extremes 237

Structure Types 238

Special Situations Involving Nonfireground Operations 240
    Hazardous Materials Incidents 240
    Special Protective Clothing 240
    Air Duration 241
    Changing Air Cylinders 243
    Emergency Escape 243
    Confined Space Entry 243
Summary 251
Review 252

9   EMERGENCY CONDITIONS BREATHING **257**
Introduction 257
Department Responsibility 258
Firefighter Responsibility 259
SCBA Teams 260
Emergency Conditions Breathing 261
    Skip Breathing 261
    Using The Bypass Valve 261
    Using A Cylinder Transfilling System 261
    Using Other Types Of Emergency Escape Breathing Support Systems 264
    Using A Common Regulator 264
    Using The Low-Pressure Hose-To-Facepiece Method 265
    Using The Filter Method 266
    Using A 5-Minute Escape Device 267
Accidental Submersion 267
    SCBA Operation 267
    Firefighter Guidelines 269
Summary 270
Review 271

APPENDIX A — SCBA—Past, Present, And Future 277
APPENDIX B — Regulating Agencies, Organizations, And Other Sources Of Information 281
APPENDIX C — Tulsa Fire Department Self-Contained Breathing Apparatus Program 285
APPENDIX D — Example Of A Standard Operating Procedure (SOP) 295
APPENDIX E — Manufacturers Of SCBA 299
APPENDIX F — SCBA Inspection And Maintenance Checklist 345
REVIEW ANSWERS **347**
INDEX **353**

List Of Tables

1.1 Air Consumption Caused By Various Activities 17

1.2 Target Pulse Rates During Exercise, Ages 20-60 19

2.1 Physiological Effects Of Reduced Oxygen (Hypoxia) 28

2.2 Chart Of Common Fire Gases 33

2.3 Effects Of Carboxyhemoglobin 35

2.4 Toxic Effects Of Carbon Monoxide 36

2.5 Effects Of Carbon Dioxide 38

2.6 Concentrations Of Oxygen And Their Effects 43

3.1 Air Volume Of 30-Minute Cylinder At Various Pressures 56

7.1 Number Of 45 ft^3 (1 275 L) Cylinders Filled In One Hour
     By Compressors Of Different Output 202

7.2 Air Quality Standards 210

7.3 Moisture Conversion Data 211

7.4 Allowable Breathing-Air Contamination Levels
     (Canadian Standards Association) 213

7.5   Allowable Breathing-Air Contamination Levels (OSHA And
     U.S. Navy Standards) 214

9.1 Lifeline Signals 259

THE INTERNATIONAL FIRE SERVICE TRAINING ASSOCIATION

The International Fire Service Training Association (IFSTA) was established as a "nonprofit educational association of fire fighting personnel who are dedicated to upgrading fire fighting techniques and safety through training."

This training association was formed in November 1934, when the Western Actuarial Bureau sponsored a conference in Kansas City, Missouri. The meeting was held to determine how all the agencies interested in publishing fire service training material could coordinate their efforts. Four states were represented at this initial conference. It was decided that, since the representatives from Oklahoma had done some pioneering in fire training manual development, other interested states should join forces with them. This merger made it possible to develop training materials broader in scope than those published by individual agencies. This merger further made possible a reduction in publication costs, since it enabled each state or agency to benefit from the economy of relatively large printing orders. These savings would not be possible if each individual state or department developed and published its own training material.

To carry out the mission of IFSTA, Fire Protection Publications was established as an entity of Oklahoma State University. Fire Protection Publications' primary function is to publish and disseminate training texts as proposed and validated by IFSTA. As a secondary function, Fire Protection Publications researches, acquires, produces, and markets high-quality learning and teaching aids as consistent with IFSTA's mission. The IFSTA Executive Director is officed at Fire Protection Publications.

IFSTA's purpose is to validate training materials for publication, develop training materials for publication, check proposed rough drafts for errors, add new techniques and developments, and delete obsolete and outmoded methods. This work is carried out at the annual Validation Conference.

The IFSTA Validation Conference is held the second full week in July, at Oklahoma State University or in the vicinity. Fire Protection Publications, the IFSTA publisher, establishes the revision schedule for manuals and introduces new manuscripts. Manual committee members are selected for technical input by Fire Protection Publications and the IFSTA Executive Secretary. Committees meet and work at the conference addressing the current standards of the National Fire Protection Association and other standard-making groups as applicable.

Most of the committee members are affiliated with other international fire protection organizations. The Validation Conference brings together individuals from several related and allied fields, such as

— key fire department executives and training officers,
— educators from colleges and universities
— representatives from governmental agencies,
— delegates of firefighter associations and industrial organizations, and
— engineers from the fire insurance industry.

Committee members are not paid, nor are they reimbursed for their expenses by IFSTA or Fire Protection Publications. They come because of commitment to the fire service and its future through training. Being on a committee is prestigious in the fire service community, and committee members are acknowledged leaders in their fields.

This unique feature provides a close relationship between the International Fire Service Training Association and other fire protection agencies, which helps to correlate the efforts of all concerned.

IFSTA manuals are now the official teaching texts of most of the states and provinces of North America. Additionally, numerous U.S. and Canadian government agencies as well as other English-speaking countries have officially accepted the IFSTA manuals.

COPYRIGHT LAW
AN EDUCATOR'S RESPONSIBILITIES

The law limits what you may copy, under what conditions you may copy, and for what purpose you may copy. Authors and publishers have specific rights under the law. However, the law permits educators access to information and to copy materials under clearly defined guidelines.

These guidelines include:

- The purpose and character of use: whether the purpose is commercial or nonprofit educational
- The nature of the copyrighted work (example: Is the work a textbook meant for classroom use?)
- The amount and substantiality copied in relation to the copyrighted work as a whole
- Whether the copied material will affect the potential sales or value of the copyrighted work

A single copy may be made by a teacher, by request, for research or teaching of a chapter from a book; an article from a periodical; short stories or essays; or a chart, diagram, or drawing. Multiple copies for the classroom must not exceed one copy per student and must meet the test of "brevity, spontaneity, and cumulative effect," which are defined as follows:

- Brevity is either a complete article, story, or essay of less than 2,500 words or an excerpt from any work of not more than 1,000 words or 10 percent of the work, whichever is less for example, (one chart, graph, diagram, drawing, cartoon, or picture per book or periodical issue).
- Spontaneity is (if permission is not sought prior to use) the decision to use the article or excerpt so close in time that it would be unreasonable to expect a timely reply to a request for permission.
- Cumulative Effect is no more than one piece copied from the same author nor no more than three articles from the same periodical volume during one classroom term. There can be no more than nine instances of multiple copying per course, per class term.

Under no circumstances can there be copying of or from works intended to be consumable in the course. These include workbooks, answer sheets, and the like. Copying shall not substitute for the purchase of books, publisher's reprints, or periodicals.

The copyright law specifies a monetary penalty for legal damages for each violation. Even a defendant (individual and/or the organization) not found in violation must bear court costs and attorney's fees.

Permission to copy is obtained by writing to the publisher with the following information:

- Title, author(s), and editor(s)
- Edition and/or issue
- Exact amount of material to be copied
- Nature of use, including if it is for resale
- How material will be reproduced
- Number of copies to be made

Copies of copyrighted materials must include a credit line to the original work, author or editor, and the publisher with copyright notice or reprint permission.

Preface

This second edition of **Self-Contained Breathing Apparatus** would not be possible without the assistance of many people. First, acknowledgement and grateful thanks are extended to the members of the IFSTA Validating Committee who contributed their time and wisdom to this manual:

Chairman
Glenn A. Boughton
Broken Arrow, Oklahoma

Secretary
Robert Higgs
Battalion Chief
Topeka Fire Department
Topeka, Kansas

Jack Bennett
Chief
Menlow Park Fire District
Menlo Park, California

Joe McDonagh
Maryland Fire and Rescue Institute
University of Maryland
College Park, Maryland

Paul C. Smith
Director, Fire Academy
Justice Institute of B.C.
Vancouver, British Columbia

Brud Gorman
Assistant Chief
Concord Fire Department
Concord, New Hampshire

Vice-Chairman
Ralph Dunbar
Chief of Budget and Personnel
Norfolk Fire Department
Norfolk, Virginia

Darrel J. Begnaud
Program Coordinator
LSU Firemen Training Program
Baton Rouge, Louisiana

Kent W. Koelz
Palm Beach Fire-Rescue Department
Palm Beach, Florida

Jerry Cortor
Vice President
McDonnell Douglas Corporation
Clearwater, Florida

Clell West
Fire Chief
Las Vegas Fire Department
Las Vegas, Nevada

Ray Simpson
Maryland Fire and Rescue Institute
University of Maryland
College Park, Maryland

A special thank-you to Chief Bill Markgraf, Columbia (Missouri) Fire Department, and to Jack Vanchuk, RPD/Hazmat Support Services, Inc. of Canada. Thank-you goes also to Kevin M. Roche, Fire Protection Engineer; Ken Simmons, Captain, City of Phoenix Fire Department; and Scott Kerwood, Fire Protection Safety Engineer, Tulsa Fire Department, who provided a careful technical review. Andrew J. Carlson, Instructor, Connecticut State Fire School and Lt. Ron Mullen, Training Officer, Branford (Connecticut) Fire Department, also reviewed the manuscript and offered valuable comments. We are grateful to everyone who shared their time and expertise.

Also assisting with photography, equipment, or advice were:

Jess Andrews, Fire Service Training Program Coordinator, Oklahoma State University

Kevin Smith, Fire Service Training, Oklahoma State University
Michael Hegedus, Interspiro USA, Inc.
Martin Grantham, MSA
Edmond (Oklahoma) Fire Department
Henrico County (Virginia) Fire Department
Hanover County (Virginia) Fire Department
Richmond City (Virginia) Fire Department
Chesterfield County (Virginia) Fire Department
Virginia Department of Fire Programs

The following individuals and organizations generously granted permission to reprint copyrighted materials or provided photographs and illustrations:

Survivair
National Draeger, Inc.
Interspiro USA, Inc.
Racal Panorama, Inc.
Mine Safety Appliances Company (MSA)
International Safety Instruments (ISI)
Scott Aviation
Biomarine, Inc.
North Safety Equipment
Lynx - S.T.O.P., Lafayette, Louisiana
(**NOTE:** See Appendix E for further information about these companies.)
Cover photo courtesy of:
Kern F. Braswell, Visual Communications, Tulsa Fire Department

Many new photographs of various types of SCBA and related equipment are used in this manual. The use of these photographs must not be construed as any special endorsement by IFSTA or by the editors of Fire Protection Publications.

Gratitude is also extended to the following members of the Fire Protection Publications staff whose editing, coordination, production, artwork, and photography make this publication both grammatically correct and visually appealing.

Lynne C. Murnane, Senior Editor
William Westhoff, Senior Editor
Mike Wieder, Senior Editor
John Hoss, Associate Editor
Carol Smith, Associate Editor
Barbara Adams, Publications Specialist
Marsha Sneed, Publications Specialist
Cynthia Brakhage, Publications Specialist
Beth Ann Chlouber, Publications Specialist
Robert Fleischner, Publications Specialist
Susan S. Walker, Instructional Development Coordinator
Don Davis, Coordinator, Publications Production
Ann Moffat, Senior Graphic Designer
Desa Porter, Graphic Designer
Lori Schoonover, Graphic Designer
Karen Murphy, Phototypesetting Technician

Research Technicians
Ward Barnett
Tommy Hicks
Gordon Earhart
Ed McManus
Rick Windham
Kevin Kolb

Photography
Gordon Earhart
Robert Fleischner
Christian Jaehrling
Robbie Kaale
Bill Westhoff
Rick Windham
Tommy Hicks

Gene P. Carlson
Assistant Director
Fire Protection Publications

Glossary

A

ABSORBENT — A substance which allows another substance to penetrate into the interior of its structure.

ACROLEIN (CH₂ CHC HO) — A toxic gas produced when wood, paper, cotton, plastic materials, and oils and fats burn; inhaled, acrolein can cause nose and throat irritation, nausea, shortness of breath, pulmonary edema, lung damage, and can eventually lead to death.

ADMISSION VALVE — The pressure regulator valve that lets the air flow to the user.

ADRENALINE — A chemical released by the body that causes the breathing rate to increase and the body to prepare for "fight or flight."

ADSORBENT — A material, such as activated carbon, that has the ability to condense or hold molecules of other substances on its surface.

AEROBIC CAPACITY — Oxygen capacity and efficiency of the lungs and blood in the cardiovascular and respiratory systems.

AFTERCOOLER — The air compressor component that cools the air that has been heated during compression.

AIR CYLINDER — The metal or composite cylinder that contains compressed air for the breathing apparatus.

AIR PURIFIER — An air-filtration system for compressed breathing air.

AIRLINE SYSTEM — System in which breathing air is supplied to the SCBA wearer from a remote source of air.

ALVEOLI — Air sacs of the lungs; place where oxygen is passed to the blood.

ANSI — American National Standards Institute; a voluntary standards-setting organization that examines and certifies existing standards and creates new standards.

ANTIFOGGING CHEMICAL — Chemical used to prohibit fogging inside the facepiece.

AORTA — The largest artery coming directly from the heart; carries oxygenated blood.

ASBESTOS — Carcinogenic substance used for insulation and ceiling materials in older buildings; inhaled asbestos fibers travel to the lungs, causing scaring, reduced lung capacity, and cancer.

ASPHYXIA — Death from insufficient oxygen.

ASPHYXIANT — Any substance that prevents oxygen from combining in sufficient quantities with the blood or being used by body tissues.

AUDIBLE ALARM — A bell, whistle, or other sound-producing alerting device.

B

B.A. — Abbreviation for breathing apparatus.

BACKDRAFT — An explosion caused by the ignition and burning of heated gases within a confined area, usually after a sudden inrush of air, as when a door is opened.

BACKPACK — The assembly that holds the air cylinder and regulator of the SCBA to the wearer.

BENZENE (C₆H₆) — Highly toxic carcinogen produced when PVC plastics and gasoline burn; inhalation of high levels can cause unconsciousness and death from respiratory paralysis.

BLEED — Process of releasing a liquid or gas under pressure. In this text, the release of air from the regulator or cylinder.

BRANCH GUIDE LINE — A line branching from the main guide line; identified with a plastic tally containing one, two, three, or four holes to indicate the branch.

BREATHING AIR — Compressed air that is filtered and contains no more contaminants than are allowed by standards; Grade D is the level required by NIOSH. (See also *Grade D breathing air*.)

BREATHING-AIR COMPRESSOR — An air compressor specially designed to produce pure air for human consumption; not to be confused with high-pressure, unpurified air or shop air.

BREATHING TUBE — Low-pressure hose that extends from the regulator to the facepiece on SCBA.

BUDDY BREATHING — A method of sharing another person's SCBA. (See also *Team emergency conditions breathing*.)

BUDDY SYSTEM — Safety system in which users of SCBA always work in teams of two or three.

BYPASS BREATHING — An emergency procedure in which the SCBA wearer closes the mainline valve and opens the bypass valve for air when a regulator malfunctions.

BYPASS VALVE — A valve that when opened lets air bypass its normal route through the regulator; used when a regulator malfunctions.

C

CAISSON — A watertight structure within which construction work is carried out under water; also a large box used to hold ammunition.

CANISTER APPARATUS — A type of breathing apparatus that uses filtration, adsorption, or absorption to remove toxic substances from the air. Generally referred to as *gas masks*, canister apparatus are not acceptable for use in fire fighting operations or IDLH atmospheres.

CARBON DIOXIDE (CO$_2$) — A gas produced by complete combustion or "clean burning" of a fire or through decomposition of organic products. Can be dangerous at high levels as it causes increased respiratory rates that increase levels of smoke and toxic gases entering the body.

CARBON DIOXIDE SCRUBBER — A chemical that removes carbon dioxide from exhaled breath so that the exhalation can be combined with oxygen and reinhaled as with closed-circuit breathing apparatus.

CARBON MONOXIDE (CO) — A colorless, odorless, highly toxic gas formed by the incomplete combustion of most fuels, specifically carbon or a carbonaceous material, including gasoline.

CARBOXYHEMOGLOBIN — Hemoglobin saturated with carbon monoxide and therefore unable to absorb needed oxygen.

CARCINOGEN — Cancer-producing substance.

CARDIOPULMONARY SYSTEM — The heart and lungs.

CARDIOVASCULAR SYSTEM — The heart and blood vessels.

CASCADE SYSTEM — Three or more large air cylinders, each usually with a capacity of 300 cubic feet (8 490 L), from which SCBA cylinders are recharged. Also called an *air bank*.

CATALYST — A substance that modifies (usually increases) the rate of a chemical reaction without being consumed in the process.

CFM (cfm) — Cubic Feet Per Minute; a volume of material flowing past or through a specified measuring point.

CHARGING STATION — A unit where compressed air cylinders are filled. Consists of a container in which SCBA cylinders rest while being charged, usually shielded to prevent injury to personnel if the cylinder ruptures, and a control panel that allows the operator to monitor and control the filling process.

CHEMICAL ENTRY SUIT — Protective apparel designed to protect the firefighter's body from certain liquid or gaseous chemicals. May be used to describe both Level A and Level B protection.

CHEMICAL SCRUBBER — (See *Carbon Dioxide Scrubber*.)

CILIA — Tiny hairlike projections that help move mucus from the lungs.

CLAUSTROPHOBIA — A pathological fear of confined spaces.

CLOSED-CIRCUIT APPARATUS — Breathing apparatus in which the wearer's exhalations are recycled after carbon dioxide and moisture are removed and some oxygen is added. Usually a long-duration device.

COMPOSITE CYLINDER — A lightweight air cylinder made of more than one material; often aluminum wrapped with fiberglass.

COMPRESSED AIR — Air under greater than atmospheric pressure; used as a portable supply of breathing air for SCBA.

COMPRESSED GAS ASSOCIATION (CGA) — An association that promulgates standards relating to compressed gases.

COMPRESSOR — Machine designed to compress air or any gas.

CONFINED SPACE — Any space not intended for continuous occupation, having limited openings for entry or exit, and providing unfavorable natural ventilation.

CONTROLLED BREATHING — Technique for consciously reducing air consumption by forcing exhalation from the mouth and allowing natural inhalation through the nose.

CORRUGATED HOSE — Hose shaped into folds or parallel, alternating ridges and grooves to improve flexibility.

CYLINDER PRESSURE GAUGE — A device, attached to the air cylinder outlet, that indicates the air pressure in the cylinder.

D

DEFENSE MECHANISM — System such as nasal hair, mucus, or cilia that protects the body from invasion by foreign particles and injury.

DEMAND APPARATUS — Breathing apparatus with a regulator that supplies air to the facepiece only when the wearer inhales or when the bypass valve has been opened; hence "demand." Also, a negative-pressure apparatus. Not to be used for fire fighting or IDLH atmospheres.

DEMAND VALVE — The valve within the regulator that lets breathing air pass to the wearer when the wearer inhales.

DERMATITIS — Inflammation of the skin.

DESICCANT — A substance that has a high affinity for water and is used as a drying agent.

DEW POINT — The temperature at which the water vapor in air precipitates as droplets of liquid.

DIASTOLE — The normal, rhythmic relaxation and dilatation of the heart during which the cavities fill with blood; the "relaxed" portion of a heartbeat. (See also *systole*.)

DIFFUSION — Process by which oxygen moves from alveoli to the blood cells in the thin-walled capillaries. Also, the process by which hazardous materials pass through protective clothing.

DIGESTER — A large, circular container used at sewage treatment plants to clean raw sewage.

DISINFECT — To destroy, neutralize, or inhibit the growth of harmful microorganisms.

DONNING MODE — State of positive-pressure SCBA when the donning switch is activated.

DONNING SWITCH — Device on a positive-pressure regulator that when activated stops airflow while the unit is being donned. Airflow is resumed with the user's first inhalation.

DOT — Department of Transportation; a government agency that regulates the use, labeling, maintenance, and transportation of compressed gas cylinders.

DOT 3AA — The DOT specification of type and material of cylinder construction; specifically, steel.

DOWNSTREAM — Direction of airflow from a high-pressure source to a low-pressure source. For example, the facepiece is downstream from the air cylinder.

E

E.C.O. — Entry Control Officer.

EDEMA — Excessive accumulation of body fluid in the tissues, causing swelling.

EEBSS — Emergency Escape Breathing Support System; formerly called *buddy breathing*.

ELASTOMER — The generic term for the rubber, neoprene, silicone, or plastic resin material of the facepiece seal, low-pressure hose, and similar SCBA components.

ELECTROLYSIS — Chemical change; especially decomposition produced in an electrolyte by an electric current. Also a form of corrosion found in aluminum.

ELECTROLYTE — A substance that dissociates into ions in solution or when fused, thereby becoming electrically conducting. A component within the human body that can be lost to sweating.

EMPHYSEMA — Dilation of the alveoli, resulting in labored breathing and increased susceptibility to infection. A chronic obstructive pulmonary disease.

ENTRY CONTROL BOARD — A record keeping clipboard equipped with a clock, tables, and slots for tallies; used by entry control officers in the United Kingdom, Australia, and New Zealand to keep track of all firefighters wearing SCBA.

EPIGLOTTIS — Thin, leaf-shaped muscle that closes off the trachea during eating and opens to allow air into the trachea during respiration.

ESOPHAGUS — The tube that allows food to pass into the stomach; referred to as the *food pipe* or *gullet*.

ETIOLOGIC AGENT — A biologically hazardous material.

EXCELSIOR — Slender, curved wood shavings used for starting fires.

EXHALATION VALVE — A one-way valve that lets exhaled air out of the facepiece.

EXPLOSIVE BREATHING TECHNIQUE — Individual emergency conditions breathing technique used by a firefighter wearing SCBA during accidental submersion; the firefighter holds his or her breath, rapidly inhales and exhales, and then holds breath again.

EXPLOSIVE LIMITS — The percentage of gas that must mix with air in order to support an explosion; gases with wide explosive ranges are the most dangerous. Commonly abbreviated as *LEL* and *UEL* for lower and upper explosive limits, respectively.

EXTERNAL RESPIRATION — The inhalation and exhalation of air into and from the lungs.

F

FACEPIECE — That part of an SCBA that fits over the face and includes the head harness, facepiece lens, exhalation valve, and connection for either a regulator or a low-pressure hose.

FACTORY CERTIFIED — Qualification of fire department personnel who attend special manufacturers' repair schools to become formally qualified in certain testing and maintenance procedures.

FILTER BREATHING — Individual emergency conditions breathing technique used by a firefighter with a depleted air supply. The firefighter inserts the regulator end of the low-pressure hose into a pocket or glove or inside the turnout coat to help filter smoke particles and to protect the firefighter from inhaling superheated air.

FILTER CANISTER — A filtration device containing chemicals to filter out harmful substances through adsorption or absorption on negative-pressure respirators. Not to be used for fire fighting or IDLH atmospheres.

FIRE ENTRY SUIT — A type of protective apparel that enables a firefighter to contact flames for a short time. Due to their weight and expense, they are seldom used.

FIVE-MINUTE ESCAPE CYLINDER — Small cylinder used as a backup air source with airline respirators.

FLASHOVER — The simultaneous ignition of highly heated combustible gases in a confined area.

FORMALDEHYDE (HCHO) — A colorless gas with a characteristic pungent odor produced when wood, cotton, and newspaper burn; an eye, nose, and throat irritant.

FREE-BURNING STAGE — The second stage of burning; the fire burns rapidly using up oxygen and building up heat that accumulates in upper areas at temperatures that may exceed 1,300°F (700°C).

FREEFLOW — The continuous flow of air from the regulator, usually venting into the atmosphere.

FUME TEST — A qualitative test of facepiece fit in which a smoke tube is used to check for leakage around the facepiece.

G

GASKETS — Rubber seals or packings used at joints to prevent the escape or inflow of gases.

GRADE D BREATHING AIR — A classification of allowable contamination levels in breathing air (CGA Grade D allows no more than 20 ppm carbon monoxide, 1,000 ppm carbon dioxide, and 5 mg/m^3 oil vapor).

H

HAZARDOUS ATMOSPHERE — Any of the following that can harm an unprotected firefighter: heat, flame, smoke, toxic gases, and radioactive particles.

HAZARDOUS MATERIAL — Any substance or form that may pose an unreasonable risk to health, safety, or property; may range from chemicals in liquid or gas form to radioactive materials to etiologic agents.

HEAD HARNESS — The straps that hold the facepiece in place. Also referred to as a *spider strap*.

HEMOGLOBIN — The oxygen-carrying component of red blood cells.

HIGH-PRESSURE AIR — Air pressurized to 3,000 to 5,000 psi (21 000 kPa to 35 000 kPa). Used to differentiate from older air cylinders using a pressure range from 1,800 to 2,200 psi (12 600 kPa to 15 400 kPa).

HIGH-PRESSURE HOSE — The hose leading from the air cylinder to the regulator; may be at cylinder pressure or reduced to some lower pressure.

HOPCALITE™ — A catalytic chemical that converts carbon monoxide to carbon dioxide.

HYDROGEN CHLORIDE (HCl) — Gas produced by the combustion of polyvinyl chlorides; when inhaled, it mixes with the moisture in the respiratory tract and forms hydrochloric acid.

HYDROGEN CYANIDE (HCN) — A colorless, toxic gas with a faint odor similar to bitter almonds; produced by the combustion of nitrogen-bearing substances.

HYDROGEN SULFIDE (H₂S) — A colorless gas with a strong rotten egg odor produced when rubber insulation, tires, and woolen materials burn and by the decomposition of sulfur-bearing organic material; dangerous because it quickly deactivates the sense of smell.

HYDROSTATIC TEST — A periodic test of breathing-air cylinders to determine whether they can safely contain compressed air.

HYPOXIA — Condition caused by a deficiency in the amount of oxygen reaching body tissues.

I

IDLH (Immediately Dangerous to Life and Health) — Any atmosphere that poses an immediate hazard to life or produces immediate irreversible, debilitating effects on health. A companion measurement to the PEL, IDLH concentrations represent concentrations above which respiratory protection should be required. IDLHs are expressed in ppm or mg/m³.

IGNITION TEMPERATURE — The minimum temperature to which a fuel in air must be heated in order to start self-sustained combustion independent of the heating source.

INDIVIDUAL EMERGENCY CONDITIONS BREATHING — Procedures or techniques performed by an individual during emergencies where SCBA malfunctions, remaining air supply is inadequate for escape, or air supply is depleted.

INERTING — Introducing a nonflammable gas, e.g., nitrogen or carbon dioxide, to a flammable atmosphere in order to remove the oxygen and prevent an explosion.

INHALATION TUBE — (See *Low-Pressure Hose.*)

INTERCOSTAL — ᴠ space between the ribs.

INTERNAL RESPIRATION — The exchange of oxygen and carbon dioxide in the bloodstream at the cellular level.

ISOAMYL ACETATE — Banana oil; used for an odor test of facepiece fit.

L

LEL (Lower Explosive Limit) — The lowest percentage of fuel/oxygen mixture required to support combustion. Any mixture with a lower percentage would be considered "too lean."

LENS FOGGING — Condensation on the inside of the facepiece lens caused by moisture in the wearer's exhalations.

LEVEL A PROTECTION — The highest level of skin, respiratory, and eye protection that can be afforded by personal protective equipment. Consists of positive-pressure, self-contained breathing apparatus, totally encapsulating chemical-protective suit, inner and outer gloves, and chemical-resistant boots.

LEVEL B PROTECTION — Personal protective equipment that affords the highest level of respiratory protection, but a lesser level of skin protection. Consists of positive-pressure, self-contained breathing apparatus, hooded chemical-resistant suit, inner and outer gloves, and chemical-resistant boots.

LIPID PNEUMONIA — Pneumonia that may follow the aspiration of an oily substance such as mineral oil or other oils.

LONG-DURATION APPARATUS — A breathing apparatus that supplies the wearer with air for more than 30 minutes.

LOW-PRESSURE ALARM — A bell, whistle, or other audible alarm that warns the wearer when the SCBA air supply is low and needs replacement — usually 25 percent of full container pressure.

LOW-PRESSURE HOSE — Generally, the hose containing pressure slightly above atmospheric leading from the regulator to the facepiece; also called a *breathing tube.*

M

MAIN GUIDE LINE — A special rope used in the United Kingdom, Australia, and New Zealand as a safety guide line to indicate a route between the entry control point and the scene of operations.

MAINLINE VALVE — The valve that when opened lets air from the cylinder travel its normal route through the regulator to the facepiece.

MAZE — A training facility — with or without smoke, lighted or unlighted — in which firefighters wearing SCBAs must negotiate obstacles to perform certain tasks.

MECHANICAL FILTER — An air-purification component that physically separates the greatest part of water, oil, and other contaminants from compressed air. Also may refer to the filter on a negative-pressure respirator that performs the same task.

MEDIUM-PRESSURE AIR — Air pressurized from 2,000 to 3,000 psi (14 000 kPa to 21 000 kPa). Used to distinguish specific types of breathing air cylinders: 2,200 psi (15 400 kPa) from 4,500 psi (31 500 kPa) cylinders.

MICRON — A unit of length equal to one-millionth of a meter.

MOLECULAR SIEVE — The air-purification component that chemically absorbs water from compressed air.

MSHA — (U.S.) Mine Safety and Health Administration; the government organization that regulates mine safety.

N

NEGATIVE BUOYANCY — Tendency to sink.

NEGATIVE PRESSURE — Air pressure less than that of the surrounding atmosphere; a partial vacuum.

NFPA — National Fire Protection Association; a nonprofit organization that promotes fire safety and issues standards for the fire service.

NFPA 704 PLACARD — Color-coded, symbol-specific placard affixed to facilities to inform of fire hazards, life hazards, special hazards, and reactivity potential.

NIOSH — (U.S.) National Institute for Occupational Safety and Health; government agency that helps ensure the safety of breathing apparatus through investigation and recommendation.

NITROGEN-BEARING SUBSTANCES — Substances that produce hydrogen cyanide: synthetic fibers such as nylon, some plastics (particularly in aircraft), natural fibers such as wool, polyurethane foam, rubber, and paper.

NOSECUP — A device inside a facepiece that directs the wearer's exhalations away from the facepiece lens and thus prevents internal fogging of the lens.

O

O-RING — A circular gasket with rounded edges used for sealing between two machined surfaces; usually made of rubber or silicone.

OBJECTIVE TEST — Test in which the results are scientifically accurate or correct and cannot be influenced by outside factors.

ODOR TEST — A qualitative test of facepiece fit.

OLFACTORY FATIGUE — The gradual inability of a person to detect odors after initial exposure. May be extremely rapid in the case of some toxins such as hydrogen sulfide.

OPEN-CIRCUIT APPARATUS — Breathing apparatus in which the wearer's exhalations are vented to the surrounding atmosphere.

OSHA — (U.S.) Occupational Safety and Health Administration; regulatory agency mandated by Congress to enforce safety and health standards through fines and citations.

OXIDES OF NITROGEN — Nitrogen oxide (NO_2) and nitric oxide (NO); can mix with moisture in the air and respiratory tract and form nitric and nitrous acids that can burn the lungs.

xx

OXYGEN (O₂) — A colorless, odorless, tasteless gas constituting 21 percent of the atmosphere.

OXYGEN DEFICIENCY — Inadequate oxygen in the air breathed; causes hypoxia.

OXYGEN-GENERATING APPARATUS — An SCBA that chemically generates oxygen for breathing by the wearer; this apparatus is no longer acceptable by the fire service.

OXYHEMOGLOBIN — The combination of oxygen and hemoglobin.

P

PARTICULATE — A very small solid, such as dust, suspended in the atmosphere.

PASS (Personal Alert Safety System) — A motion detector worn by firefighters to alert others in the event that the firefighter becomes incapacitated.

PEL (Permissible Exposure Limit) — The amount of a substance a worker may be exposed to without injury, measured in parts per million, ppm, or milligrams per cubic meter, mg/m³.

PERSONAL LINE — A short 20-foot (6-m) rope, used in the United Kingdom, Australia, and New Zealand by an SCBA team member to maintain contact with another team member or the main guide line.

PERSONAL PROTECTIVE EQUIPMENT — A generic term referring to any equipment or apparel designed to protect a human from a specific injury: gloves, boots, SCBA, hard hats, turnout coats, and ear plugs.

PHARYNX — Throat; the area behind the tongue and mouth where the esophagus and the trachea originate.

PHOSGENE (COCl₂) — Toxic gas produced when refrigerants such as freon, plastics containing polyvinyl chloride (PVC), or electrical wiring insulation contact flames. May be absorbed through the skin as well as through the lungs.

PNEUMOCONIOSIS — A lung disease resulting from chronic inhalation of irritant particles.

POINT OF NO RETURN — That time at which the remaining operation time of the SCBA is equal to the time necessary to return safely to a nonhazardous atmosphere.

POSITIVE BUOYANCY — Tendency to float.

POSITIVE PRESSURE — Air pressure greater than that of the surrounding atmosphere.

POSITIVE-PRESSURE APPARATUS — Breathing apparatus that supplies air to the facepiece under a pressure greater than the surrounding atmosphere.

POSITIVE-PRESSURE TEST — A test to verify that there is positive pressure within a facepiece. After donning the facepiece, the wearer pulls the sealing surface of the facepiece away from the skin, allowing air to escape.

PPM (ppm) — Parts Per Million; a ratio of the volume of contaminants (parts) compared to the volume of air (million parts).

PRESSURE-DEMAND DEVICE — An SCBA that may be operated in either positive-pressure or demand mode. This type of SCBA is presently being phased out and replaced with positive-pressure-only apparatus.

PREVENTIVE MAINTENANCE — Ongoing inspection and upkeep intended to prolong the life of the SCBA and to prevent breakdown.

PROPER SEAL — The result of the facepiece fitting snugly against the bare skin and preventing entry of smoke, fumes, or gases.

PROTECTION FACTOR — The ratio of contaminants in the atmosphere outside the facepiece to the contaminants inside the facepiece. Determined by quantitative fit testing from the manufacturer.

PROXIMITY SUIT — Protective apparel that allows the wearer to get closer to heat and flame than possible when wearing common protective clothing. Used for fighting very intense fires.

PSI (psi) — Pounds Per Square Inch; a ratio of force divided by a given area; a measurement of pressure.

PULMONARY EDEMA — The accumulation of fluids in the lungs.

PURGING — Freeing from impurities, such as ventilating a contaminated space by introducing fresh air.

PURIFICATION SYSTEM — A series of mechanical and chemical filters through which compressed breathing air is passed to remove moisture, oil, carbon monoxide, and other contaminants.

PVC (Polyvinyl Chloride) — A synthetic chemical used in the manufacture of plastics.

Q

QUALITATIVE TEST (FACEPIECE FIT) — A test in which the wearer's sense of smell or taste is used to determine whether a facepiece fits properly. Examples are the irritant fume test, the odor test, and the taste test.

QUANTITATIVE TEST (FACEPIECE FIT) — A test in which the amount of contaminants inside the facepiece is determined with instruments.

QUICK-FILL™ SYSTEM — Mine Safety Appliances Company (MSA) system that can be used as an EEBSS or that can be used to refill SCBA cylinders during nonemergency conditions.

R

REBREATHER — Closed-circuit breathing apparatus.

REGULATOR — A device between the facepiece and air cylinder that reduces the pressure of the air coming from the cylinder.

REGULATOR BREATHING — An emergency procedure in which the firefighter breathes directly from the regulator outlet if the low-pressure hose or facepiece is damaged.

REGULATOR GAUGE — A gauge, connected to the regulator, that indicates the pressure of the air reaching the regulator; used as an indication of the air pressure in the air cylinder.

REMOTE PRESSURE GAUGE — A pressure gauge that is not mounted on the regulator but can be seen by the SCBA wearer; commonly found on SCBAs that have facepiece-mounted regulators.

RESPIRATORY SYSTEM — The organs involved in the intake and exchange of gases between an organism and the environment.

ROLLOVER — A phenomenon — often mistaken for flashover — in which the flame quickly travels across the ceiling of a room.

S

SANITIZE — To make free from dirt or micro-organisms that endanger health.

SCBA — Self-contained breathing apparatus.

SCF (scf) — Standard Cubic Foot; the amount of air in a cubic foot at sea level and at 70°F.

SCFM (scfm) — Standard Cubic Feet per Minute; a volume of material based on the Standard Cubic Foot flowing past or through a specified measuring point.

SEQUENTIAL TRAINING — Preferred training method in which the student is taken step by step from simple to complex exercises when learning to use an SCBA.

SKIP BREATHING — An emergency procedure in which the firefighter inhales normally, holds the inhalation for as long as it would take to exhale, takes another breath, and then exhales; used only when the firefighter is stationary and must wait for help.

SMOKE DIVER — Highly trained user of an SCBA.

SMOKE DIVER SCHOOL — School that provides the firefighter with 25 to 30 hours of sequential training in SCBA use.

SMOKE ROOM — Enclosed area into which mechanically generated smoke is introduced and in which firefighters perform training exercises while wearing SCBA.

SMOKE TUBE — Device containing stannic or titanium tetrachloride used to produce nontoxic smoke for testing facepiece seal.

SMOLDERING STAGE — The third stage of fire in which oxygen is below 15 percent, flame may cease to exist, the temperature throughout is high, and high fuel vapors may cause a backdraft.

SODIUM SACCHARIN — Chemical substance used in qualitative facepiece fit taste tests.

SOP (Standard Operating Procedure) — Written procedures by which the fire department operates under normal conditions.

SPEAKING DIAPHRAGM — Device on some facepieces that aids oral communication.

STEL (Short-Term Exposure Limit) — A 15-minute time-weighted average that should not be exceeded at any time during a work day. Exposures at the STEL should not last longer than 15 minutes and should not be repeated more than four times per day with at least 60 minutes between exposures.

STRESS TEST — A test in which a person's vital functions are monitored while the person labors.

SUBJECTIVE TEST — Test in which the results may be influenced by the subject being tested, by the test itself, by the tester, or by other outside factors.

SULFUR DIOXIDE (SO₂) — A colorless gas with a highly irritating rotten egg odor produced when sulfur-containing materials burn; its pervasive odor makes it detectable below its IDLH level of 100 ppm.

SUMP — An area in the air-purification system that receives drainage.

SWEETENER — The component (generally charcoal) in an air-purification system that removes odors and tastes from the compressed breathing air.

SWITCHABLE REGULATOR — A positive-pressure breathing apparatus regulator that has a switch to accommodate donning.

SYNERGISTIC EFFECT — The phenomenon in which the combined properties of substances have an effect greater than their simple arithmetical sum of effects.

SYSTOLE — The rhythmic contraction of the heart by which blood is pumped throughout the body. (See also *diastole.*)

T

TALLY — A rectangular plastic identification tag used for entry control in the United Kingdom, Australia, and New Zealand.

TEAM EMERGENCY CONDITIONS BREATHING (buddy breathing) — Procedures or techniques performed by a team of two individuals during emergencies when the SCBA of one person malfunctions or no longer has adequate air supply.

TLV (Threshold Limit Value) — A time-weighted average concentration under which most people can work consistently for 8 hours a day, day after day, with no harmful effects.

TOXIC ATMOSPHERE — Any area inside or outside a structure where inhaled air contains substances harmful to human life or health.

TRACHEA — The windpipe or tube that conducts air to and from the lungs.

TRANSFILLING SYSTEM — SCBA designed so that two SCBAs can be connected by a hose, allowing the air pressure of the two SCBA cylinders to equalize; used as an EEBSS to equalize air pressure of one cylinder with an adequate air supply and another cylinder with depleted or inadequate air supply.

TURNAROUND MAINTENANCE TAG — A tag — generally attached to the valve on the oxygen tank of closed-circuit SCBA — that tells when the unit was last serviced, lists what services were performed, and indicates that the unit is ready to perform.

U

UPSTREAM — The direction opposite the airflow; the regulator is upstream from the facepiece.

V

VAPOR DENSITY — The weight of a volume of pure vapor or gas (with no air present) compared to the weight of an equal volume of dry air at the same temperature and pressure.

Introduction

BREATHING APPARATUS: YESTERDAY AND TODAY

During the nine years that have elapsed between the publication of the first edition of **Self-Contained Breathing Apparatus** and this second edition of the book, there have been many changes. Equipment and self-contained breathing apparatus (SCBA) have been technically updated and new equipment invented; new standards have been written and old ones revised. New safety concerns have been addressed in this edition, and procedures once thought to be most efficient have been reconsidered and revised. Even the uses of SCBA have been expanded. Yesterday SCBA was used primarily on the fireground; today it is used with equal frequency in rescue and emergency incidents involving hazardous materials.

Not too long ago, as explained in Appendix A, SCBA was in its infancy. Twenty years ago, for instance, the technology was not available to determine what was in smoke; furthermore, new synthetic materials that are in heavy use today did not exist then. Today, however, there is no doubt that the smoke and toxic gases present at fires and hazardous materials incidents can cause respiratory injuries and even death. Many *preventable* firefighter deaths have been attributed to inhalation of smoke or toxic fumes. A direct relationship has also been established between smoke inhalation and heart diseases and cancer. Therefore, the emphasis today is on *mandatory* SCBA use.

Today it is considered foolhardy rather than courageous when a firefighter literally attempts to be a "smoke eater." The classic picture of a firefighter leaning out of a window for air should no longer be tolerated. Some veterans say, "We didn't use breathing apparatus 20 years ago, why should I use one now?" Others add, "I'm still here. I've got lungs of leather. Smoke won't hurt you."

This attitude must change. To effectively perform their jobs and to ensure their own safety, firefighters *must* wear SCBA in hazardous atmospheres. The best attitude for the firefighter to have is to assume that *any* unknown atmosphere is hazardous. All firefighters should be taught: **WHEN IN DOUBT, WEAR SCBA.**

Because of these safety and health concerns — and because of the ongoing technological advances in respiratory protection — government and private agencies have recognized the need for regulations governing SCBA training, use, and maintenance. Those primary government agencies involved in respiratory regulations for the fire service in the United States today are the National Institute for Occupational Safety and Health (NIOSH) and the Occupational Safety and Health Administration (OSHA); in Canada, the Canadian Standards Association. Voluntary organizations such as the National Fire Protection Association (NFPA) and the American National Standards Institute (ANSI) also publish standards that address respiratory protection for the fire service. These agencies and organizations are discussed in more detail in Appendix B.

Each fire department should have an SCBA program and ongoing SCBA training that meet NIOSH, OSHA, ANSI, and NFPA standards. A sample SCBA program is given in Appendix C. In addition, each department should create its own written policies and procedures — standard operating procedures (SOPs) — based on these standards. Most important, the department SOPs should make SCBA use *mandatory* for all personnel on the fireground or for anyone likely to encounter a hazardous atmosphere. A sample set of SOPs is given in Appendix D. Firefighters must be equipped with SCBA and be trained in its use and maintenance. The safety provided by SCBA can be attained only through proper training and mandatory use.

PURPOSE AND SCOPE

The purpose of this second edition of **Self-Contained Breathing Apparatus** is to make available information needed by the firefighter for safe and effective SCBA use and by the fire department for developing an SCBA program that includes comprehensive, ongoing, sequential SCBA training. This manual stresses the need for mandatory use of SCBA and references current standards and regulations that have been developed requiring its use, whether the situation be structural fire fighting, industrial fire fighting, hazardous materials incidents, or rescue.

There are two types of self-contained breathing apparatus used in the fire service today: open-circuit and closed-circuit. Open-circuit SCBA uses compressed air, while closed-circuit SCBA uses compressed or liquid oxygen. All open-circuit and closed-circuit SCBA used in the fire service today must be positive pressure as required by ANSI and NFPA standards. Both types of systems are covered in detail in this manual.

The initial chapters in this book introduce the reader to the physiology of the body as it relates to SCBA protection, define and discuss respiratory hazards, and familiarize the student with various types of SCBA presently on the market. Appendix E provides more detailed information on the features, accessories, and donning and doffing procedures for specific SCBA manufacturers. Subsequent chapters outline the firefighter's and the department's responsibilities concerning safety and training; provide approved methods for donning and doffing; provide procedures for inspecting, maintaining, and testing SCBA; and describe SCBA use, both on the fireground and in special emergency situations.

The material in **Self-Contained Breathing Apparatus** provides the information necessary to meet the minimum SCBA knowledge and skill levels required by the following standards:

- NFPA 1404, *Standard for a Fire Department Self-Contained Breathing Apparatus Program*
- NFPA 1500, *Standard on Fire Department Occupational Safety and Health Program*
- NFPA 1981, *Standard on Open-Circuit Self-Contained Breathing Apparatus for Fire Fighters*
- NFPA 1403, *Standard on Live Fire Training Evolutions in Structures*
- NFPA 1001, *Standard for Fire Fighter Professional Qualifications*
- NFPA 1982, *Standard on Personal Alert Safety Systems (PASS) for Fire Fighters*
- NFPA 1904, *Standard for Aerial Ladder and Elevating Platform Fire Apparatus*
- ANSI Z88.2-1980, *Practices for Respiratory Protection*
- ANSI Z88.5-1981, *Practices for Respiratory Protection for the Fire Service*
- ANSI Z88.6-1984, *For Respiratory Protection—Respirator Use—Physical Qualifications for Personnel*

This second edition of **Self-Contained Breathing Apparatus** has been completely revised through the IFSTA Validating Committee and replaces the material in the first edition. Because of the rapidly changing technology in the area of SCBA, new procedures, standards, and technology have been incorporated into the text. In addition, all photographs and illustrations have been updated to reflect approved apparatus and procedures of the 90s. Included are sections on the history of SCBA, why SCBA is necessary, how to don them, how to use them safely, how to train firefighters to use them safely, how to maintain and test them, and how to recharge air cylinders.

This text covers all the information called for by NFPA 1404, *Standard for a Fire Department Self-Contained Breathing Apparatus Program*, 1989. The reader is aided by a glossary; comprehensive appendices containing a history of SCBA, donning and doffing procedures for various makes of SCBA, SCBA programs and SOPs, and other pertinent technical information; step-by-step procedures; and end-of-chapter review questions and answers.

Written with both the instructor and student in mind, this new edition places special emphasis on mandatory SCBA use. Also, information has been organized and presented to facilitate sequential learning and training. Time and the experience of hundreds of instructors and firefighters have proven beyond any doubt that sequential training is the only way to ensure that a firefighter will use SCBA properly, with confidence, and safely.

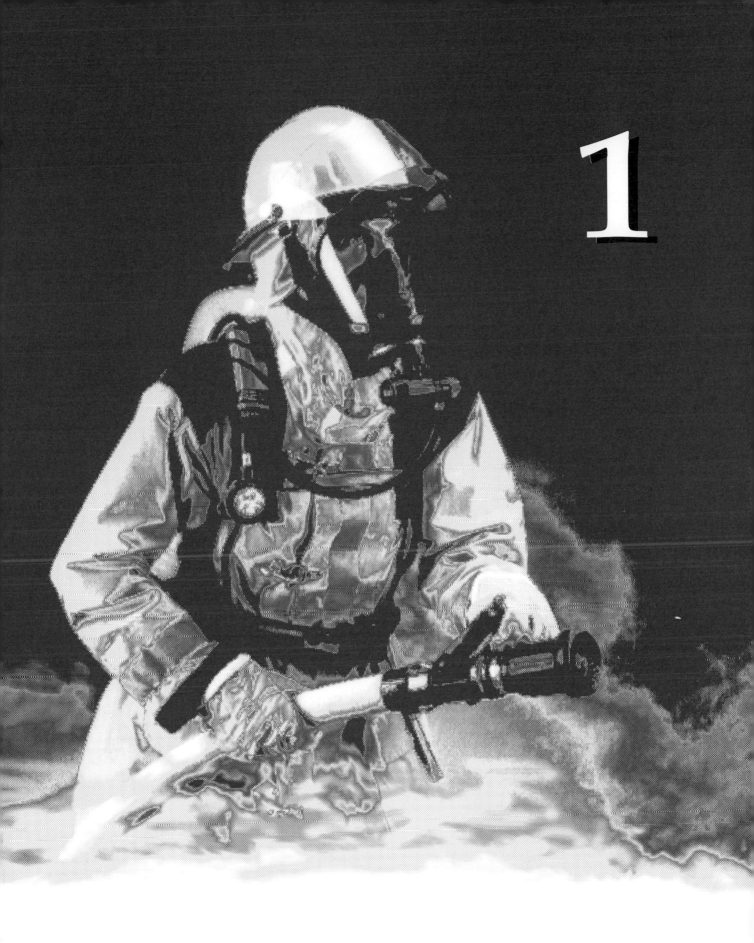

The Body

This chapter provides information that addresses the following standards:

NFPA STANDARD 1404
Fire Department Self-Contained Breathing Apparatus Program
1989 Edition

Emergency Scene Use
3-1.5

Chapter 4—SCBA Training
4-2.1
4-2.1.1
4-2.2
4-2.5
4-2.6

NFPA STANDARD 1500
Fire Department Occupational Safety and Health Program
1987 Edition

Chapter 5—Protective Clothing and Protective Equipment
5-3.3
5-3.6

Chapter 8—Medical
8-1.1
8-1.2
8-1.3
8-2.1
8-2.2
8-5.1
8-5.2
8-5.3

ANSI STANDARD Z88.5-1981
Practices for Respiratory Protection for the Fire Service

Section 3—SCBA Program
3.3
Section 10—Program Evaluation

ANSI STANDARD Z88.2-1980
Practices for Respiratory Protection

Section 3—Respirator Program Requirements
3.5.3

Chapter 1
The Body

INTRODUCTION

The body is a remarkable system with great capabilities; however, it obviously has its limitations. Our bodies can be adversely affected by injury, disease, age, exposure to hazardous materials, and inactivity or lack of physical conditioning. Because fire fighting involves physical stress and exertion, and because firefighters depend on their physical abilities to perform their duties, they must have a basic understanding of how the body functions. They must also have a complete understanding of the importance of maintaining their bodies in good physical condition. This knowledge will also help firefighters realize the importance of wearing self-contained breathing apparatus and taking other safety precautions to protect their bodies—in particular, their respiratory and cardiovascular systems.

To help the firefighter understand the body's physical abilities and limitations, this chapter focuses on the respiratory system, the cardiovascular system, the body's reaction to wearing self-contained breathing apparatus (SCBA), and physical fitness.

THE RESPIRATORY SYSTEM

Body cells need a continuous supply of oxygen to live and to convert food to energy. Oxygen is supplied to the body by the respiratory system. The respiratory system enables gas exchange to occur: Oxygen is delivered to body cells, and carbon dioxide is removed from body cells. The body takes in oxygen and removes carbon dioxide by breathing, or external respiration. Inhalation provides oxygen, and exhalation removes carbon dioxide. Internal respiration refers to the exchange of oxygen and carbon dioxide between the blood and body cells and to the use of oxygen by the cells. Oxygen, supplied through the respiratory system, is passed to the circulatory system and then is delivered to the cells. To enable body cells to exchange gases, the respiratory system first exchanges gases with blood, the blood circulates, and then blood cells and body cells exchange gases.

Anatomy

The organs of the respiratory system are the nose, pharynx, larynx, trachea, bronchi, and lungs (Figure 1.1). Each of the organs of the respiratory system plays a part in enabling body cells to receive oxygen and exchange gases. Air can enter the system through the nose or mouth. If air enters through the nose, it will pass through small, scroll-like bones called turbinates. The turbinates are covered by mucous membranes, which help to warm and humidify the air as the air travels towards the lungs. Air then enters the pharynx (throat). There are two tubes through

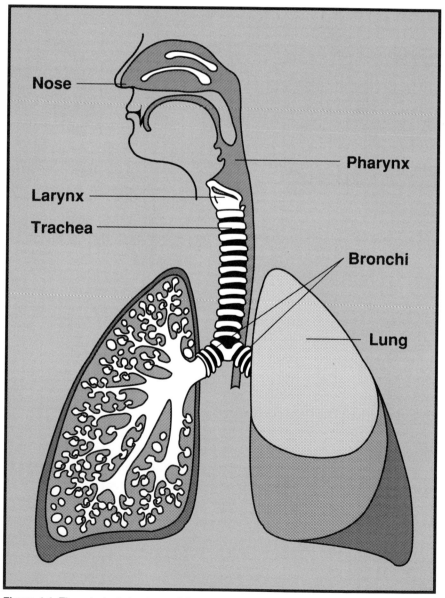

Figure 1.1 The principal structures of the upper and lower airways in the respiratory system are shown.

which air can travel: one is the trachea (windpipe), and the other is the esophagus (food pipe), which is situated behind the trachea. When a person swallows, the epiglottis — a thin, leaf-shaped muscle — closes off the trachea. When a person breathes, the epiglottis relaxes and allows air into the trachea.

Traveling further, air passes through the larynx, or voice box. The vocal cords of the voice box regulate the amount of airflow. From the larynx, air enters the trachea. The trachea then branches into two main bronchi, which continue to branch into many bronchioles. The bronchioles subdivide into smaller tubes, finally ending in microscopic branches that divide into alveolar ducts. The alveolar ducts end in several alveolar sacs, the walls of which contain numerous alveoli. It is estimated that some 300 million alveoli are present in the lungs. It is in the alveoli where the actual exchange of oxygen and carbon dioxide occurs (Figures 1.2 and 1.3).

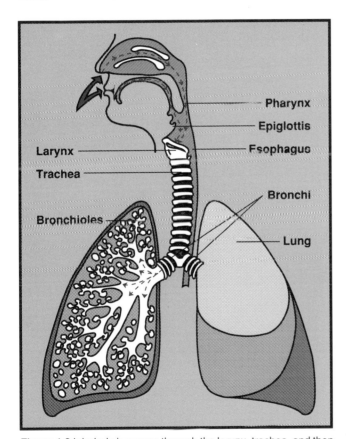

Figure 1.2 Inhaled air passes through the larynx, trachea, and then moves into the bronchi and bronchioles.

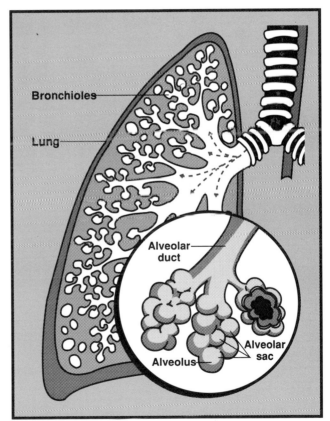

Figure 1.3 From the bronchioles, air moves through the alveolar ducts and into the alveolar sacs.

External Respiration

The body takes in oxygen and removes carbon dioxide by external respiration, which is the transfer of oxygen and carbon dioxide in the lungs. Ordinarily, respiratory action is an involuntary effort. However, respiration can be voluntarily controlled by sighing, coughing, and other similar body reactions.

Normally, when the blood's carbon dioxide level rises, receptors in the brain stem and aorta stimulate breathing. The brain stem sends signals to the respiratory muscles: the diaphragm and the intercostal rib muscles (the muscles between the ribs). The contraction and relaxation of these muscles causes pressure changes inside the chest, which in turn cause air to move in and out (an operation similar to that of the regulator diaphragm). The contraction of the diaphragm and the intercostal muscles causes an increase in the chest's capacity for air and causes a decrease in pressure inside the chest. During inspiration, the pressure in the chest, which is less than atmospheric pressure, allows air to move into the lungs. When these muscles relax, the pressure in the lungs increases and causes the air to flow out (Figure 1.4).

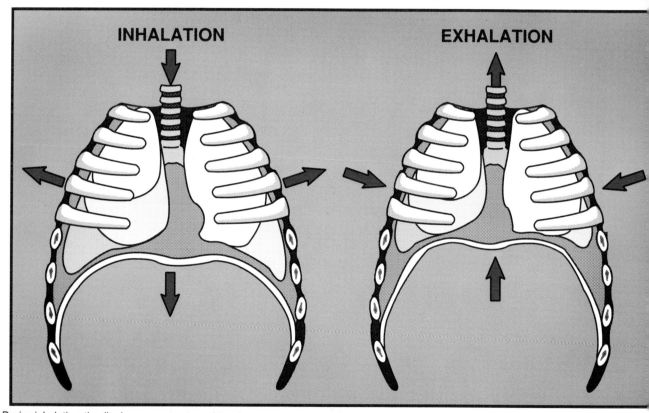

Figure 1.4 During inhalation, the diaphragm contracts and the chest expands as the lungs fill with air. During exhalation, the diaphragm relaxes, the chest contracts, and air moves out of the lungs.

Internal Respiration

Internal respiration is the actual exchange of oxygen and carbon dioxide between the blood and body cells. This process of gas exchange occurs by diffusion, that is, movement from an area of higher concentration to an area of lower concentration. Inhalation enables air to make its way to the alveoli. The thin-walled alveoli are surrounded by capillaries, and it is in these capillaries that gas exchange takes place. The oxygen content in the alveoli is high due to the breath of air taken in. Blood that has returned from the body cells—and that in the capillaries— is low in oxygen but high in carbon dioxide. By diffusion, the oxygen moves from the alveoli to the blood cells in the thin-walled capillaries.

Carbon dioxide (CO_2) moves from the blood cells to the alveoli by diffusion, also. The carbon dioxide is exhaled, and oxygen is brought in on the next breath. The oxygen-rich blood cells lose their oxygen to the oxygen-poor body cells, and carbon dioxide diffuses from the body cells (high concentration of CO_2) to the blood cells (low concentration of CO_2). Then, again by diffusion, carbon dioxide moves from the blood cells in the capillaries to the alveoli (Figure 1.5). The carbon dioxide is exhaled, and oxygen is brought in with the next breath.

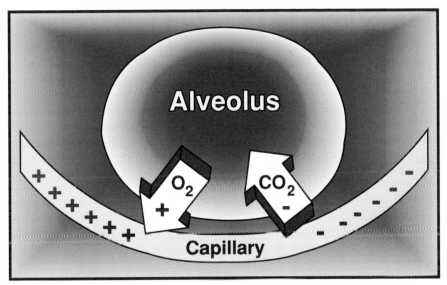

Figure 1.5 It is within the tiny alveoli that the exchange of carbon dioxide and oxygen takes place.

Exposure to smoke and/or toxic gases can result in serious injury or death because the body cannot live for more than four to six minutes without a constant supply of oxygen. By learning how the body functions, the firefighter should have a better understanding of the consequences of *not* wearing SCBA. Entering a hazardous atmosphere without SCBA exposes the body to smoke and/or toxic gases. Toxic gases that reach the alveoli can damage them, preventing normal gas exchange from occurring. If toxic gases burn the lung tissue, the alveoli fill with fluids, and gas exchange cannot occur. Undamaged alveoli exposed to high concentrations of toxic gases pass these gases, through diffusion, to the blood cells. Once in the blood cells, these toxic gases go on to destroy the body cells. Toxic substances capable of passing through the alveoli and into the bloodstream have the quickest effect on the body.

Defense Mechanisms

The body has defense mechanisms to help protect it and the respiratory system from invasion by foreign particles and injury.

An important factor in these protection systems is the size of the particle entering the body. The smaller the particle, the more easily it can penetrate the body's defenses.

One of the body's defense mechanisms is the nose. Large particles are caught in the nasal hairs; and air is warmed and humidified as it passes by the turbinates, which serve to increase the surface area of the mucous membranes in the nasal passage. The whole respiratory tract is lined with mucus, which is produced in the bronchi. Mucus traps the particles that do not get filtered by the nose. Mucus is constantly being moved up the throat toward the nose by tiny, hairlike projections called cilia. Foreign particles trapped in the bronchi may take a few hours to be dislodged. Too, smoking and inhaling vapors can destroy and paralyze the cilia, thus eliminating one of the body's natural defenses. If the particle is an irritant and is able to make it to the bronchi, it may cause the bronchi to constrict to minimize the amount of airflow. The result is a characteristic wheezing sound.

Very small particles, vapors, and gases will reach the alveoli. Like other parts of the respiratory system, the alveoli have their own special defenses. The alveolar lining is different from the mucous lining of the respiratory tract, but it serves the same function. This defense can be quickly overpowered, however, if large amounts of vapor or particles are present. Damaged alveoli are not replaced and cannot exchange oxygen. In addition, certain vapors cause the damaged alveoli—and soon the lungs—to fill with fluid. This accumulation of fluid in the lungs is called pulmonary edema. Pulmonary edema also affects healthy alveoli, filling them with fluid and preventing gas exchange.

Gases that have reached the alveoli generally pass into the bloodstream. Once in the bloodstream, they may attack other parts of the body such as the liver, heart, nervous system, or brain. Obviously, wearing SCBA is necessary to protect the body from airborne toxins.

CARDIOVASCULAR SYSTEM

The cardiovascular, or circulatory, system serves as the body's transportation system. One function of the cardiovascular system is to transport oxygen-rich blood from the respiratory system and deliver it to cells. Included in the cardiovascular system are the heart, the blood, and the blood vessels. (**NOTE:** The cardiovascular system has other components and functions, such as the lymphatic system and the transport of food from the digestive system. This manual focuses on the cardiovascular system only as it relates to the transportation of oxygen and removal of wastes from the blood.)

The heart is a double pump that beats between 60 and 100 times a minute (Figure 1.6). It is about the size of a man's closed fist and lies under the sternum (breastbone) slightly toward the left. The septum divides the heart into right and left cavities. Each cavity has an atrium (receiving chamber) and a ventricle (pumping chamber). The left ventricle is the largest chamber and is made of very thick muscle. The right side of the heart receives blood that has come from the body after delivering nutrients and oxygen to body cells. It sends this blood to the lungs, where carbon dioxide is exchanged for oxygen. The left side of the heart receives this oxygenated blood from the lungs and pumps it out to the body (Figure 1.7).

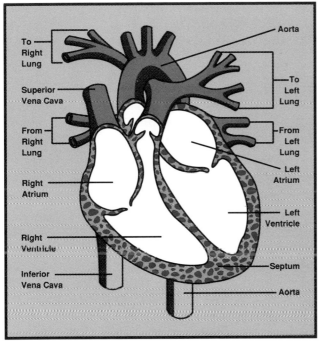

Figure 1.6 A front sectional view of the human heart, displaying the four chambers, valves, openings, and major vessels, is shown.

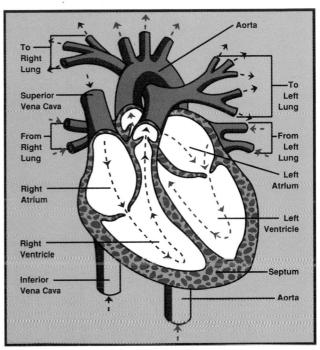

Figure 1.7 Oxygen-poor blood is pumped from the right ventricle through the pulmonary artery to the lungs. Oxygen-rich blood from the lungs travels back to the heart where it is pumped out to the body through the aorta.

The heart muscle, called the myocardium, has a unique property that other muscles do not have: the ability to generate its own impulse. Thus, the heart does not require a signal from the brain to beat. A special area of the right atrium, called the sinoatrial node (SA node), initiates an impulse 60 to 100 times a minute to cause the heart muscle to contract. The heart's contracting and pumping blood is called systole. The heart's relaxing and filling with blood is called diastole.

The blood vessels transport the blood pumped from the heart throughout the body. There are three types of vessels: arteries, veins, and capillaries. Arteries carry blood *away* from the heart, and veins carry blood *to* the heart. In general, arteries carry oxygenated blood, and veins carry deoxygenated blood. The exceptions to this rule are the pulmonary arteries and veins. The pulmonary artery carries deoxygenated blood from the right atrium to the lung. The pulmonary vein carries oxygenated blood from the lungs to the heart.

Capillaries are the smallest blood vessels; they connect the smallest veins with the smallest arteries. Capillaries are very small, thin-walled vessels that surround the alveoli and tissue cells, allowing gases and nutrients to be exchanged.

The blood, which travels through the heart, arteries, and veins, carries oxygen to all the cells. Blood cells carry out other functions as well, including carrying nutrients to cells and carrying waste from cells. In terms of respiration, the most important cells are the red blood cells. Red blood cells contain hemoglobin. The hemoglobin carries the oxygen, which becomes chemically bonded to the hemoglobin. An important note about hemoglobin is that it has a great affinity for carbon monoxide. This means that the blood would rather carry carbon monoxide than oxygen, and carbon monoxide is present in large quantities at fires. Therefore, a firefighter not wearing SCBA can very rapidly develop problems because of carbon monoxide poisoning.

THE BODY'S REACTION WHILE WEARING SCBA

Fire fighting is strenuous work that requires using great amounts of energy during short periods of time. A firefighter needs both physical and mental preparation and training (Figure 1.8).

How does wearing SCBA affect the firefighter? When a positive-pressure mask is worn, there is positive pressure throughout the lungs, not just in the mask. The positive pressure in the facepiece keeps out the toxic atmosphere. The positive pressure in the lungs causes the lungs to become hyperinflated; that is, the amount of air left in the lungs is greater than normal due to breathing out against resistance. With more air in the lungs, the alveoli exchange gases more efficiently.

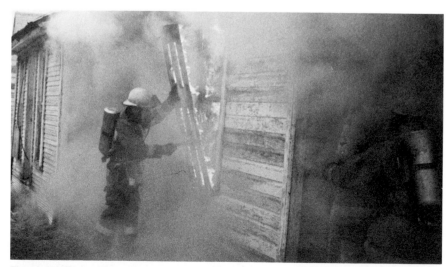

Figure 1.8 Firefighters must be in excellent physical condition to perform the strenuous duties necessary on the fireground.

However, wearing SCBA has some negative effects on the body. No matter how physically fit the firefighter, using SCBA generally causes a 20 percent decrease in physical performance. Also, in open-circuit SCBA, when the firefighter exhales into the mask, some of that air is brought in on the next inhalation. This inhaled air contains more carbon dioxide than normal; increased levels of carbon dioxide cause respirations to increase. In the past, a problem developed when the respiratory cycle increased beyond a certain flow rate. Older positive-pressure regulators could not meet the wearer's peak flow demands when the inhalation rate exceeded 40 L/min. When this flow rate was exceeded, it caused negative pressure within the facepiece. However, newer performance standards require a minimum flow rate of 100 L/min. As of 1987, positive-pressure regulators have all been manufactured to meet National Fire Protection Association (NFPA) standards and to sustain a flow of 100 L/min, with maximum capabilities of 400 to 500 L/min. Some models designed for buddy breathing are capable of even higher flow rates. Today, then, SCBA that comply with the current NFPA 1981, *Standard on Open-Circuit Self-Contained Breathing Apparatus for Fire Fighters*, provide enough flow to maintain a positive pressure within the facepiece even under extreme increased breathing.

Mental Fitness

A firefighter's body and mind must be prepared to deal with almost any situation when the firefighter arrives on the scene. When a firefighter responds to an emergency, the body automatically gears itself for fighting or fleeing the situation. This primitive response to fear or danger is known as a "fight or flight" response and is an automatic process. The brain increases the heart rate and respiration rate. Anticipating increased work levels, the brain also causes the liver to release extra sugar for energy.

Emotional Stability Of The User

Fire fighting can be a frightening experience. Fear in a firefighter can trigger the same responses as in anyone else — sweating, dry mouth, and increased breathing rate. The body reacts by releasing adrenaline, which chemically causes the breathing rate to increase. Tense or fearful firefighters use their air supplies faster than those firefighters who remain calm. However, a trained firefighter in good physical condition should be able to override some of the increased breathing rates through controlled breathing.

Also, many people feel "closed in" or claustrophobic when they first put on a breathing apparatus facepiece. This feeling increases the mental stress and "fight or flight" response. However, greater confidence in equipment and in fire fighting skills comes from ongoing training. For instance, realistic simulations as described in Chapter 4, Safety and Training, provide firefighters with practice in entering dark, smoky atmospheres with little or no visibility. They can also practice communicating through masks, which muffle the voice.

Controlled Breathing

Controlled breathing is the technique used for most efficient air use while working. It is a conscious effort to reduce air consumption by forcing exhalation from the mouth and allowing natural inhalation through the nose. Firefighters should practice and perfect controlled breathing methods in training sessions until using such methods becomes second nature (Figure 1.9).

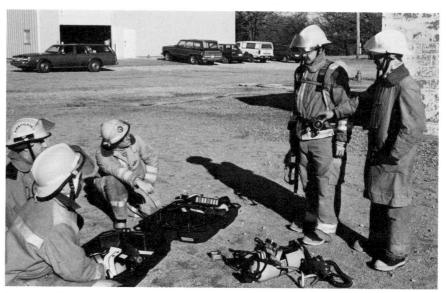

Figure 1.9 Practicing controlled breathing techniques during training sessions will enable the firefighter to perform more calmly and efficiently during an actual incident.

Training the firefighter to be conscious of breathing usually causes an immediate drop in the firefighter's breathing rate. Hearing another person breathing may cause an untrained breather to increase his or her breathing rate. However, firefighters should *not* hold their breath. Due to the body's release of adrenaline, oxygen is being consumed at a high rate, and holding the breath may cause unconsciousness.

As the firefighter's level of exertion increases, the body generates more carbon dioxide. Using a nosecup increases the efficiency of carbon dioxide and oxygen exchange by forcing exhalation directly out the exhalation valve. Forcing out exhalation allows an inrush of air from the tank. This air, which is low in carbon dioxide, permits the firefighter to breathe more slowly.

Degree Of Physical Exertion

The oxygen needs of any individual, physically fit or not, increase when exertion levels increase. Table 1.1 describes some activities and their corresponding rates of air consumption. For purposes of comparison, the 45-cubic-foot (30-minute) cylinder holds 1,275 liters of air when filled to its normal operating pressure.

TABLE 1.1
AIR CONSUMPTION CAUSED BY VARIOUS ACTIVITIES

Activity	Oxygen Consumed		Air Breathed		Respirations per Minute
	ft³/min	L/min	ft³/min	L/min	
Rest Reclining	0.0084	0.237	0.2721	7.7	16.8
Rest Standing	0.0116	0.328	0.3675	10.4	17.1
Walking at 2 mph	0.0276	0.780	0.6572	18.6	14.7
Walking at 3 mph	0.0376	1.065	0.8763	24.8	16.2
Walking at 4 mph	0.0564	1.595	1.318	37.3	18.2
Walking at 5 mph	0.0899	2.543	2.152	60.9	19.5
Running	0.106	3.0	3.5	100.0	>20.0

Table adapted from p. 47 in Southern Australian Country Fire Services *Fire Fighters Training Notes*.

PHYSICAL FITNESS

Physical fitness is an increasing concern in the fire service. Fire fighting tasks may tax a firefighter to his or her physical limits; therefore, above-average strength and endurance are required. Being in good physical condition lessens the chances of fatigue, and thus the firefighter will be less likely to make mental errors or be injured.

Extra physical work requires extra oxygen for the muscles. Depending on their physical condition, individuals performing the same work may require different levels of exertion and oxygen use. A firefighter in poor physical condition will have to work harder and thus will consume a supply of air faster than a firefighter in good physical condition. Duration rating tests do not fully take into account the extra oxygen needed by the overweight or otherwise physically unfit firefighter.

The two greatest risks to firefighter fitness and performance are being overweight and smoking cigarettes. Excessive body weight strains the body's cardiovascular system. During extreme exertion, this strain can lead to heart failure. Cigarette smoking greatly compounds the effects of fire fighting by reducing lung capacity and by leading to the development of chronic lung diseases.

Standards established by NFPA and the American National Standards Institute (ANSI) address the physical fitness issue. ANSI Standard Z88.5, *Practices for Respiratory Protection for the*

Fire Service, recommends that firefighters be physically fit. ANSI Z88.6, *For Respiratory Protection—Respirator Use—Physical Qualifications for Personnel*, gives guidelines for departments and physicians to use in determining whether a firefighter is physically qualified to use a respirator. Both NFPA 1500, *Standard on Fire Department Occupational Safety and Health Program*, and NFPA 1404, *Standard for a Fire Department Self-Contained Breathing Apparatus Program*, require that firefighters be checked annually by a physician before they are allowed to use SCBA. Therefore, accurate records of physical fitness and medical examinations of each firefighter need to be kept. NFPA 1500 also lists guidelines for departments to follow in regard to health programs.

A physical training program should aim at improving the aerobic capacity of the cardiovascular system. Aerobic exercises such as swimming, jogging, and bicycling are good for cardiovascular conditioning. Firefighters should exercise for 30 to 45 minutes at least two to three times a week. It is important to take 5 to 10 minutes at the beginning and end of the workout for a warm-up and cool-down. For the workout to be of greatest value, 70 to 85 percent of the maximum heart rate must be reached and maintained.

To find your maximum heart rate without using the table, subtract your age from 220, then multiply by 0.70 and 0.85 to determine the 70 to 85 percent target range. For example, to compute a healthy 20-year-old's target heart rate, take the following steps:

Step 1: Subtract 20 (the age) from 220.

$$220 - 20 = 200$$

Step 2: Multiply 200 by 0.70 and 0.85 to determine the 70 and 85 percent ranges.

$$200 \times 0.70 = 140$$

$$200 \times 0.85 = 170$$

This firefighter should strive to maintain a pulse of 140 to 170 during the workout.

A 32-year-old using the same formula would strive to maintain a heart rate of 131 to 160 during the workout. Beginners, those over 35, and individuals who are overweight should start at a lower rate—60 to 65 percent—and work their way up to a higher range as their cardiovascular conditioning improves. Table 1.2 shows 10-second pulse rates from which a 1-minute heart rate can be calculated. *All firefighters should be examined by a physician before beginning a physical fitness program.*

Muscle-toning exercises such as pushups, situps, and weight lifting will increase muscular conditioning (Figure 1.10). Aerobic

TABLE 1.2 TARGET PULSE RATES DURING EXERCISE AGES 20-60			
	Target Pulse Rate*		
Age	60%	85%	Max
20 - 22	20	28	33
23 - 25	20	28	33
26 - 28	19	27	32
29 - 31	19	27	32
32 - 34	19	26	31
35 - 37	18	26	31
38 - 40	18	26	30
41 - 43	18	25	30
44 - 46	18	25	29
47 - 49	17	24	29
50 - 52	17	24	28
53 - 55	17	24	28
56 - 58	16	23	27
59 - 61	16	23	27

*Taken for 10 seconds

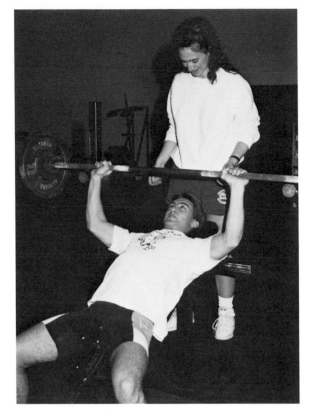

Figure 1.10 Muscle-toning exercises are an important part of a complete physical fitness program.

exercise will increase cardiovascular conditioning. A good physical conditioning program will include both cardiovascular conditioning and muscular conditioning.

In order for a conditioning program to be successful, the following points must be considered:

- Firefighters must understand their physical needs. Occasional strenuous activity on the job cannot be considered sufficient to maintain fitness.

- The program must include efforts to reduce the risks that seriously affect the health and performance of firefighters. The two biggest risks are being overweight and smoking cigarettes.

- The program must have the full cooperation of all fire department personnel, including management and labor.

- The program must provide for periodic evaluation of all fire department members.

It is important to remember that a high level of physical fitness cannot be accomplished overnight. It takes time for a fitness program to upgrade the performance of a fire department. Therefore, it is important that a good, well-supported, long-range program be instituted under the supervision of physicians and qualified exercise instructors.

SUMMARY

Fire fighting is a physically demanding profession, and firefighters depend upon their physical capabilities to perform their duties. For this reason, firefighters should have some understanding of how the body functions. Knowing the capabilities and limitations of the respiratory system is especially important because this system is particularly vulnerable to injury. Wearing SCBA in hazardous atmospheres will help lessen the chance of respiratory injuries.

The organs that comprise the respiratory system include the nose, pharynx, larynx, trachea, bronchi, and lungs. Respiration occurs both externally and internally. External respiration refers to the exchange of oxygen and carbon dioxide in the lungs. Internal respiration refers to the exchange of oxygen and carbon dioxide between the blood and body cells and to the use of oxygen by body cells. The circulatory system plays a vital role in internal respiration because the blood carries oxygen to the cells and picks up carbon dioxide from them.

Developing and following a physical fitness program is an important part of helping firefighters get into good physical condition. A fitness program must include both cardiovascular and muscular conditioning. If firefighters are in good physical condition, are well trained, and are comfortable wearing breathing apparatus, they are less likely to sustain respiratory injuries.

Chapter 1 Review

Answers on page 347

TRUE-FALSE: Mark each statement true or false. If false, explain why.

1. Air can enter the respiratory system through either the nose or the mouth.

   ☐ T ☐ F _____

   _____

2. The two tubes in the body through which air can travel are the trachea and the epiglottis.

   ☐ T ☐ F _____

   _____

3. Alveoli undamaged by the presence of toxic gases can pass the toxic gases to the blood cells.

   ☐ T ☐ F _____

   _____

4. Veins carry oxygenated blood away from the heart, and arteries carry deoxygenated blood to the heart.

   ☐ T ☐ F _____

   _____

5. During a certain period of time, a tense or fearful firefighter will use approximately the same quantity of air that a calm firefighter will use.

   ☐ T ☐ F _____

   _____

6. Duration rating tests of oxygen supplies take into account the extra oxygen needed by those individuals who are not physically fit.

   ☐ T ☐ F _____

   _____

LISTING

7. What are the two major functions of the respiratory system?

   A. _____

   B. _____

8. List the organs of the respiratory system.

   A. _____

   B. _____

C. _____

D. _____

E. _____

F. _____

9. What are the two greatest risks to the firefighter's fitness and performance?

A. _____

B. _____

10. List the three types of blood vessels.

A. _____

B. _____

C. _____

FILL IN THE BLANK: Fill in the blanks with the correct response.

11. _____ changes inside the chest cause air to move in and out.

12. The heart is divided into the left and right sides. Each side has a(n) _____ (receiving chamber) and a(n) _____ (pumping chamber).

13. The physical and mental stress experienced by a firefighter responding to an alarm can cause elevation in _____ and _____.

14. Red blood cells contain _____, which carries the oxygen.

SHORT ANSWER: Answer each item briefly.

15. Define external respiration.

_____

_____

_____

16. Define internal respiration.

_____

_____

_____

17. What is controlled breathing?

_____

_____

_____

18. The exchange of carbon dioxide and oxygen within the body occurs by diffusion. What is diffusion?

_____

_____

_____

19. How do toxic gases affect the lung tissue?

_____

_____

_____

_____

20. What are some of the negative effects on the body caused by wearing self-contained breathing apparatus?

_____

_____

_____

_____

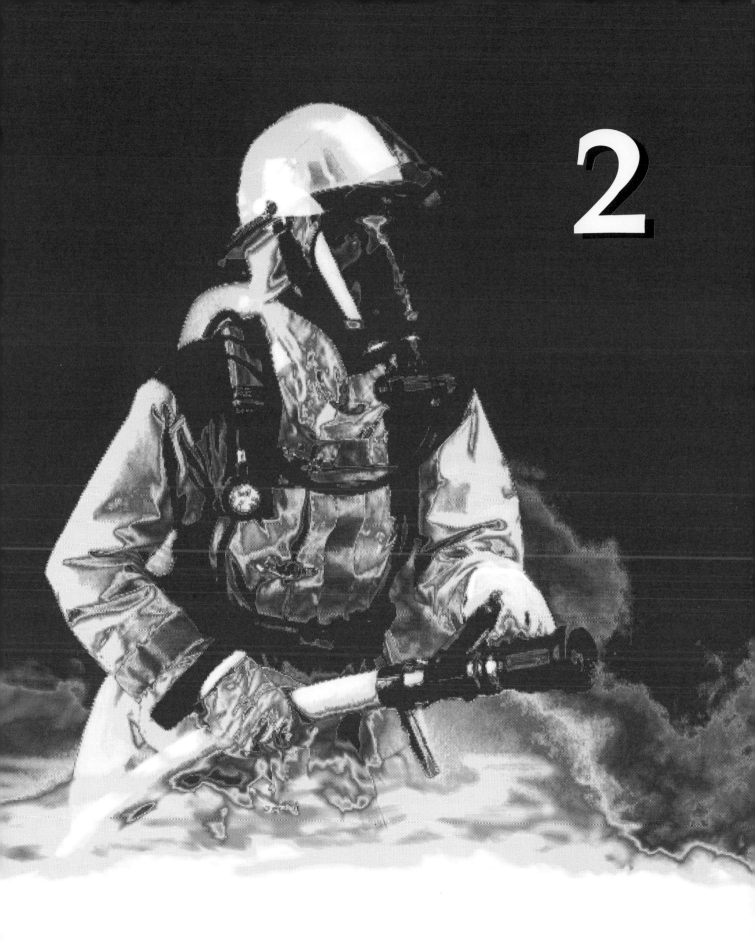

Respiratory Hazards

This chapter provides information that addresses the following standards:

NFPA STANDARD 1001
Fire Fighter Professional Qualifications
1987 Edition

Chapter 3—Fire Fighter I
3-6.1

NFPA STANDARD 1404
Fire Department Self-Contained Breathing Apparatus Program
1989 Edition

Chapter 3—Emergency Scene Use
3-1.2
3-1.3
3-1.5

Chapter 4—SCBA Training
4-8

NFPA STANDARD 1500
Fire Department Occupational Safety and Health Program
1987 Edition

Chapter 5—Protective Clothing and Protective Equipment
5-1.1
5-1.2
5-3.1

ANSI STANDARD Z88.5-1981
Practices for Respiratory Protection for the Fire Service

Section 9—Special Problems
9.5
9.8
9.9

ANSI STANDARD Z88.2-1980
Practices for Respiratory Protection

Section 4—Classification of Respiratory Hazards
4.1

CSA STANDARD Z94.4-M1982
Selection, Care, and Use of Respirators

9. Use of Respirators
9.2.1
9.2.1.2
9.3
9.3.3

Chapter 2
Respiratory Hazards

INTRODUCTION

Firefighters must be familiar with the different types of respiratory hazards they will encounter. Although the body is amazing in its scope of possible activities, its adaptation to environmental change is limited by the narrow range of permissible oxygen concentration in the air breathed. This limitation is clearly demonstrated by the body's extremely low tolerance to a variety of foreign substances in the air. Firefighters routinely encounter situations that tax or even exceed this adaptive capacity. Without protective breathing apparatus, the body can sustain fatal injuries when exposed to respiratory hazards. Wearing SCBA is the surest way to protect the body from these hazards (Figure 2.1).

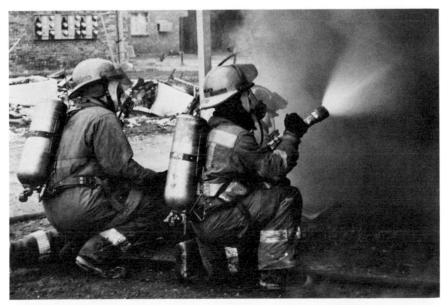

Figure 2.1 Wearing full protective clothing and SCBA is the surest way to protect the body from respiratory hazards.

This chapter covers hazards from fires and from nonfire incidents. Respiratory hazards from fires are separated into oxygen-deficient atmospheres, elevated temperatures, flashover, backdraft, smoke, and toxic gases. Other hazardous atmospheres not associated with structural fire fighting are also discussed.

OXYGEN DEFICIENCY

Because the combustion process requires oxygen, fires remove large amounts of oxygen from the air. Fires also produce toxic gases in large quantities. Table 2.1 shows the physiological effects of hypoxia (lack of oxygen) due to reduced percentages of oxygen in the atmosphere.

TABLE 2.1
PHYSIOLOGICAL EFFECTS OF REDUCED OXYGEN (HYPOXIA)

Oxygen in Air (Percent)	Symptoms
21	None — normal conditions
17	Some impairment of muscular coordination; increase in respiratory rate to compensate for lower oxygen content
12	Dizziness, headache, rapid fatigue
9	Unconsciousness
6	Death within a few minutes from respiratory failure and concurrent heart failure

NOTE: These data cannot be considered absolute because they do not account for differences in breathing rate or length of time exposed.
These symptoms occur only from reduced oxygen. If the atmosphere is contaminated with toxic gases, other symptoms may develop.

ELEVATED TEMPERATURES

Fire brings elevated temperatures. Ceiling temperatures in a burning room can reach over 1,000°F (538°C). Inhaling superheated air, especially moist superheated air (such as happens after water is applied to a fire), will cause intense burns of the respiratory tract. Pulmonary edema, which can completely block the airways, results quickly. When this condition occurs, the alveoli fill with liquid and normal gas exchange cannot occur.

WARNING
Inhaling superheated air can cause serious injury or death.

Excessive heat conducted to the lungs very quickly can also result in a serious drop in blood pressure. This situation can lead to cardiovascular collapse through shock. Inhalation injuries are often fatal, so prompt medical attention is essential. It is vital that the firefighter remember that wearing SCBA not only keeps out toxic gases, but also protects the respiratory system from temperatures that the body cannot withstand.

FLASHOVER AND BACKDRAFT

Two very dangerous situations firefighters can encounter during a fire are flashover and backdraft. Both conditions have characteristic warning signs, and the likelihood of their occurrence can be reduced by using good ventilation techniques and tactics.

Flashover

Flashover is caused by excessive accumulation of heat from a fire. As the fire burns, all the combustible contents in the area are heated and give off flammable gases. As the heat becomes more intense, the flammable gases are raised to their ignition temperatures. When the ignition temperatures are reached, all the combustibles ignite simultaneously and the area is suddenly fully involved in fire. The fire spreads rapidly, producing greater amounts of toxic gases. SCBA must be used to protect against the intense heat and toxic gases associated with flashover.

A phenomenon often confused with flashover is called "rollover." The flames of a fire, like smoke or water, seek the path of least resistance. When obstructed in their vertical movement, they will try to proceed by moving horizontally; thus they will "roll" across the ceiling.

Backdraft

A backdraft can occur in the late free-burning or smoldering stage of a fire. When the fire has reached the smoldering stage, most of the available oxygen in the room has been used, but heat and fuels are still present in large quantities. All that is necessary to create a backdraft is the introduction of oxygen into the area without proper ventilation. The result is very rapid oxidation, resulting in an explosion known as a backdraft (Figure 2.2). Full protective gear, including SCBA, helps lessen the possibility of injuries.

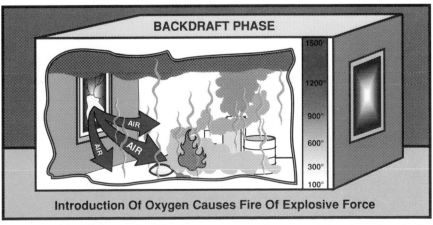

Figure 2.2 A backdraft can occur with explosive force when oxygen is introduced into the fire area.

The following conditions indicate the possibility of a backdraft:

- Black smoke becoming dense gray-yellow
- Confinement and excessive heat in a windowless structure
- Little or no visible flame
- Smoke leaving the building in puffs or at intervals
- Smoke-stained windows with heat-induced cracking of glass

SMOKE

The smoke encountered at most fires consists of a mixture of oxygen, nitrogen, carbon dioxide, carbon monoxide, finely divided carbon particles, and a miscellaneous assortment of products that have been released from the material involved. Most visible smoke is a suspension of small particles that can be in solid or liquid form. The solid particles provide a location for the condensation of the gaseous products of combustion. However, some of the combustion products remain as droplets and do not condense on the solid particles. (**NOTE:** The following section on Toxic Gases discusses specific gases.)

Toxic particles can enter the body in three ways: by inhalation, by absorption through the skin, and by ingestion into the digestive tract. Recall the defense mechanisms of the body that were discussed in the previous chapter. Remember that gases and very small particles have a good chance of reaching the alveoli. With prolonged exposure, the body's defense mechanisms are overpowered by the particles and droplets. When enough contaminants reach the alveoli, the gas exchange process shuts down. In addition to the inhalation and absorption of smaller smoke particles, larger smoke particles can be ingested (swallowed), allowing contaminants to enter the blood from the digestive process. At the very least, swallowing smoke particulates causes nausea, vomiting, and diarrhea.

Tar particles or oil droplets are especially dangerous. Upon entering the alveoli, they may cause intense inflammation. Special cells in the alveoli attempt to remove these particles, but this defense mechanism can soon be overwhelmed. The condition that develops from this inflammation is known as lipid pneumonia.

Oil droplets can also cause the alveoli to dilate and rupture, thus decreasing the total surface available to exchange oxygen and carbon dioxide. It is recommended that firefighters who have been exposed to heavy, choking smoke for even a few seconds be examined by a physician, even if they feel well. There can be a delay of from one to six hours before symptoms develop.

TOXIC GASES

Toxic gases produced by the fire will be mixed with smoke. Some gases are colorless and odorless; others are quite irritating.

Exposure to one gas is bad enough, but most toxic gases are present in groups and in varying concentrations. When these toxins enter the body, some can cause a synergistic effect. A synergistic effect occurs when the combined effect of two or more substances is more toxic or irritating than the total effect would be if each were inhaled separately.

Toxic gases can enter the body through the respiratory system in the same manner as smoke particles, or these gases can be absorbed through the skin (Figure 2.3). Therefore, full protective clothing is necessary.

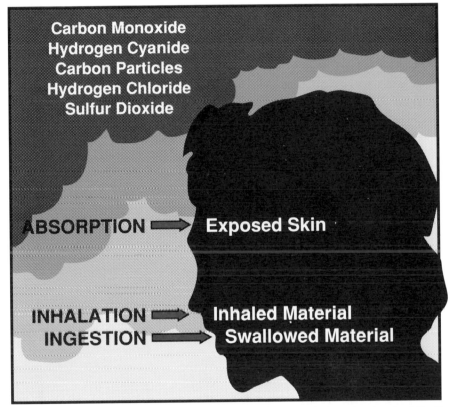

WARNING
Inhaling toxic gases can cause serious injury or death.

Carbon Monoxide
Hydrogen Cyanide
Carbon Particles
Hydrogen Chloride
Sulfur Dioxide

ABSORPTION ➡ Exposed Skin

INHALATION ➡ Inhaled Material
INGESTION ➡ Swallowed Material

Figure 2.3 Although SCBA cannot protect against substances that can be absorbed, it will protect the firefighter from substances that can be inhaled or ingested.

The type and amount of toxic gases given off at a fire vary according to four factors:

- Nature of the combustible source
- Rate of heating
- Temperature of the evolved gases
- Oxygen (O_2) concentration

When discussing amounts of gases in the air, a measurement is given in parts per million (ppm):

$$\frac{\text{level of contaminant}}{1,000,000 \text{ parts air}}$$

Parts per million (ppm) is actually a very small number. The following analogy will help illustrate how small ppm is: 1 ppm could be compared to 1 cent in $10,000.

Exposure to toxic gases and chemicals is not a new problem. People who work in chemical plants, refineries, or pesticide manufacturing plants have been exposed to toxic chemicals and gases for years. How much exposure is acceptable? There are guidelines established for human exposure to many chemicals.

Fires produce large concentrations of toxic gases; these concentrations almost always exceed maximum allowable exposure limits and require the use of protective equipment. Table 2.2 shows a listing of exposure limits for common fire gases. Two levels are shown: the Short-Term Exposure Limit (STEL) and the Immediately Dangerous to Life and Health (IDLH). The IDLH concentration represents a maximum level from which one could escape within 30 minutes without suffering any escape-impairing symptoms or irreversible health effects. STEL is defined as a 15-minute time-weighted average that should not be exceeded at any time during a workday. (**NOTE:** See Table 2.2 for additional definitions of the terms and abbreviations used in the table.) Exposures at the STEL should not be longer than 15 minutes and should not be repeated more than four times per day with at least 60 minutes between exposures.

Fire fighting operations usually expose firefighters to very high levels of toxic gases. In many cases, the concentrations of these gases are so high that even a brief exposure of only a few minutes can cause injury. The IDLH concentrations listed reflect the maximum concentration level of exposure. It should be noted that exposure includes skin and eyes as well as the respiratory system.

Obviously, firefighters without SCBA should never enter an atmosphere containing toxic gases at the IDLH level. Atmospheres containing concentrations up to the STEL level may be tolerated only very briefly. Most fire gases will reach or exceed IDLH levels.

The vapor density (VD) of a gas tells whether it is heavier or lighter than air. Air has a value of 1. Gases with a vapor density greater than 1 will be found low, near the floor. Gases with a vapor density less than 1 are lighter than air and will be found near the ceiling.

Many fire gases are not only toxic but also explosive (Figure 2.4). Table 2.2 also gives explosive limits for common fire gases. The explosive limits (upper and lower) indicate the percentage of gas that must mix with air in order to cause an explosion; these limits are boundaries of the explosive range. Gases with wide explosive ranges are the most dangerous.

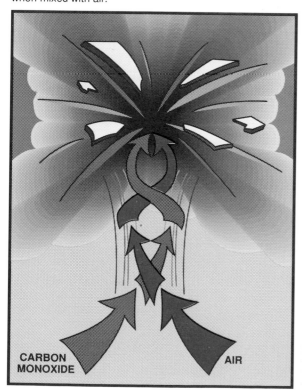

Figure 2.4 Some fire gases, such as carbon monoxide, can cause an explosion when mixed with air.

CARBON MONOXIDE

AIR

TABLE 2.2
CHART OF COMMON FIRE GASES

Chemical	TLV and/or PEL (ppm)	STEL (ppm)	IDLH (ppm)	Chemical Properties		Target Organs
				(VD, SG)	(LEL, UEL)	
Carbon Monoxide (CO)	50	400	1,500	VD: 1.0 SG: GAS	LEL: 12.5% UEL: 74%	Blood, Lungs, Cardio-vascular System, Central Nervous System
Carbon Dioxide (CO$_2$)	5,000	30,000	50,000	VD: 1.5 SG: GAS	Nonflammable	Lungs, Cardiovascular System
Hydrogen Chloride (HCl)	5	--	100	VD: 1.3 SG: GAS	Nonflammable	Respiratory System, Skin, Eyes
Hydrogen Cyanide (HCN)	10	--	50	VD: 0.9 SG: 0.7	LEL: 5.6% UEL: 40%	Liver, Kidney, Central Nervous System, Cardio-vascular System
Nitrogen Dioxide (NO$_2$)	1	5	50	VD: 1.6 SG: 1.4	Nonflammable	Respiratory System, Cardiovascular System
Ammonia (NH$_3$)	25	35	500	VD: 0.6 SG: --	LEL: 16% UEL: 25%	Respiratory System, Eyes
Phosgene (COCL$_2$)	0.1	--	2	VD: 3.4 SG: GAS	Nonflammable	Respiratory System, Skin, Eyes
Acrolein (CH$_2$CHCHO)	0.1	0.3	5	VD: 1.9 SG: 0.8	LEL: 2.8% UEL: 31%	Heart, Eyes, Skin, Respiratory System
Formaldehyde (HCHO)	1	2	100	VD: -- SG: 1.1	LEL: 7% UEL: 73%	Respiratory System, Eyes, Skin
Hydrogen Sulfide (H$_2$S)	10	15	300	VD: 1.2 SG: GAS	LEL: 4.3% UEL: 46%	Respiratory System, Eyes
Benzene (C$_6$H$_6$)	1	--	2,000	VD: 2.7 SG: 0.9	LEL: 1.3% UEL: 7.1%	Blood, Skin, Bone Marrow, Eyes, Respiratory System, Cardiovascular System
Acetic Acid (CH$_3$COOH)	10	15	1,000	VD: 2.1 SG: 1.0	LEL: 5.4% UEL: 16%	Respiratory System, Skin, Eyes, Teeth
Acetaldehyde (CH$_3$CHO)	100	150	10,000	VD: 1.5 SG: 0.8	LEL: 4% UEL: 60%	Respiratory System, Skin, Kidneys
Formic Acid (HCOOH)	5	--	100	VD: 1.6 SG: 1.2	LEL: 18% UEL: 57%	Respiratory System, Skin, Kidney, Liver, Eyes

VD: Air = 1   SG: Water = 1

TLV (Threshold Limit Value) — A time-weighted average concentration under which most people can work consistently for 8 hours a day, day after day, with no harmful effects.

PEL (Permissible Exposure Limit) — The maximum time-weighted concentration at which 95 percent of exposed, healthy adults suffer no adverse effects over a 40-hour week — an 8-hour time-weighted average concentration, unless otherwise noted.

ppm (parts per million) — A ratio of the volume of contaminants (parts) compared to the volume of air (million parts).

STEL (Short-Term Exposure Limit) — A 15-minute time-weighted average that should not be exceeded at any time during a workday. Exposures at the STEL should not be longer than 15 minutes and should not be repeated more than four times per day with at least 60 minutes between exposures.

IDLH (Immediately Dangerous to Life and Health) — Any atmosphere that poses an immediate hazard to life or produces immediate irreversible, debilitating effects on health.

VD (Vapor Density) — The weight of a given volume of pure vapor or gas compared to the weight of an equal volume of dry air at the same temperature and pressure. A figure less than 1 indicates a vapor lighter than air; a figure greater than 1 indicates a vapor heavier than air.

SG (Specific Gravity) — The weight of a substance compared to the weight of an equal volume of water. If the specific gravity is less than 1, the material is lighter than water and will float; if it is greater than 1, the material is heavier than water and will sink.

LEL (Lower Explosive Limit) — Below the flammability range or lower explosive limit, a gas or vapor is too lean to burn (too little fuel and too much oxygen).

UEL (Upper Explosive Limit) — Above the flammability range or upper explosive limit, a gas or vapor is too rich to burn (too much fuel and too little oxygen).

Gas concentrations above or below the explosive range are too lean or too rich to burn. Flammable fire gases provide fuel for flashover and backdraft conditions.

The term *target organ* refers to the organ or system the gas will affect. Note that quite a number of these gases affect the eyes and skin. Wearing SCBA protects the eyes as well as the respiratory system. Since many of these gases are directly absorbed into the skin without the firefighter's knowledge, full protective clothing should always be worn. In addition to SCBA, gloves and hoods give some protection to the skin against these toxic gases during fire fighting operations.

Determining the concentration of toxic gases in an atmosphere requires specialized equipment and a thoroughly trained, knowledgeable operator. Generally, this equipment cannot be used during fire fighting operations; therefore, firefighters should be aware of symptoms that result from overexposure to toxic gases. Recognizing these symptoms will alert firefighters to the need for obtaining proper medical attention.

Symptoms can be classified as acute (immediate) and chronic (long-term). Acute symptoms may be an immediate reaction from overexposure to a toxic substance, or they may occur several hours after exposure. Firefighters should be able to recognize abnormal reactions in themselves as well as other firefighters. The following section contains a description of some toxic gases found in most fire situations and symptoms that may occur with overexposure. Chronic symptoms may not be readily detectable without medical testing. Therefore, it is recommended that firefighters receive regular medical examinations by a qualified physician. Such examinations are required for firefighters acting as hazardous material response teams.

The list of toxic gases presented in Table 2.2 is by no means complete. Further information can be obtained by consulting an industrial hygienist. Nonetheless, it should be clear that even an ordinary house contains many products that will produce toxic gases during a fire (Figure 2.5). Because of the injuries these gases can cause, firefighters should *never* enter a hazardous atmosphere without wearing SCBA.

Carbon Monoxide (CO)

More fire deaths occur from carbon monoxide (CO) poisoning than from any other toxic product of combustion. This colorless, odorless, and tasteless gas is present at all fires. The poorer the ventilation and the more inefficient the burning, the greater the quantity of carbon monoxide formed. A rule of thumb, although subject to much variation, is that the darker the smoke the higher the carbon monoxide levels. Black smoke is high in particulate carbon and carbon monoxide because of incomplete combustion.

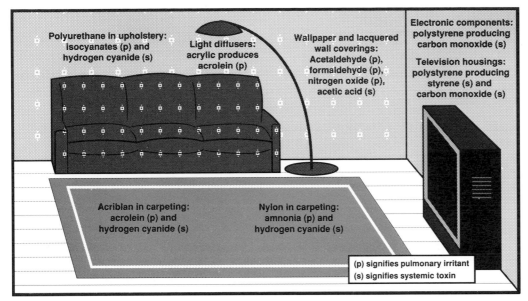

Figure 2.5 Common products in today's households will produce many toxic gases during a fire.

Carbon monoxide combines with the blood's hemoglobin much more readily than does oxygen. The blood's hemoglobin combines with and carries oxygen in a loose chemical combination called oxyhemoglobin. The most significant characteristic of carbon monoxide is that it combines with the blood's hemoglobin so readily that the available oxygen is excluded. The loose combination of oxyhemoglobin becomes a stronger combination called carboxyhemoglobin (COHb). In fact, carbon monoxide combines with hemoglobin about 200 times more readily than does oxygen.

Carbon monoxide does not act on the body directly; rather, it crowds oxygen from the blood and leads to eventual hypoxia of the brain and tissues, followed by death if the process is not reversed.

Exposure to a 5 percent carbon monoxide atmosphere can cause a 50 percent carbon monoxide level in the blood within 30 to 90 seconds. A room air concentration of 1 percent carbon monoxide will cause a 50 percent carbon monoxide blood level in 2½ to 7 minutes. Table 2.3 shows the effects of carboxyhemoglobin, a compound formed in the blood when carbon monoxide occupies the positions normally taken by oxygen.

Carbon monoxide exposure is not cumulative; however, because it takes the body some

TABLE 2.3
EFFECTS OF CARBOXYHEMOGLOBIN

Carboxyhemoglobin (COHb) in Bloodstream (Percent)	Symptoms
0-10	No symptoms
10-20	Shortness of breath during physical exertion; tightness across the forehead
20-30	Headache, shortness of breath
30-50	Confusion, severe headache, dizziness fatigue, collapse from exertion
50-70	Unconsciousness, respiratory failure, and death if exposure continued

time to rid itself of carbon monoxide, exposure to two or three fires a few hours apart would have the same effect as one exposure to a large fire. Table 2.4 shows the toxic effects of carbon monoxide. The characteristic cherry red or mottled skin color is not always a reliable indicator of exposure, particularly in cases of long exposures to low concentrations. Other symptoms of exposure include shortness of breath, mild to throbbing headache, irritability, emotional instability, rapid fatigue, weakness, nausea, dizziness, confusion, and collapse. Heavy exposure can permanently damage the cardiovascular system and/or lead to respiratory arrest.

WARNING
Do not remove SCBA during the overhaul stage of fire fighting. Carbon monoxide levels are extremely high during this stage due to incomplete combustion.

TABLE 2.4
TOXIC EFFECTS OF CARBON MONOXIDE

Carbon Monoxide (CO) (ppm)	Carbon Monoxide (CO) in Air (Percent)	Symptoms
100	0.01	No symptoms — no damage
200	0.02	Mild headache; few other symptoms
400	0.04	Headache after 1 to 2 hours
800	0.08	Headache after 45 minutes; nausea, collapse, and unconsciousness after 2 hours
1,000	0.10	Dangerous — unconsciousness after 1 hour
1,600	0.16	Headache, dizziness, nausea after 20 minutes
3,200	0.32	Headache, dizziness, nausea after 5 to 10 minutes; unconsciousness after 30 minutes
6,400	0.64	Headache, dizziness, nausea after 1 to 2 minutes; unconsciousness after 10 to 15 minutes
12,800	1.26	Immediate unconsciousness, danger of death in 1 to 3 minutes

ppm - parts per million

Treatment for exposure to carbon monoxide should include 100 percent oxygen given by mask at high flow rates. The firefighter should also be evaluated further by a physician.

Hydrogen Chloride (HCl)

Hydrogen chloride (HCl) is produced as a byproduct of the combustion of plastics, most commonly polyvinyl chloride (PVC). Polyvinyl chloride is used in many household furnishings such as wall coverings, upholstery materials, electrical insulation, and furniture laminates. In addition to the usual presence in the home, firefighters can expect to encounter plastics containing polyvinyl chloride in drug, toy, and general merchandise stores. The overhaul stage of fire fighting is especially dangerous because breathing apparatus is often removed, and toxic fumes may linger in a room. For example, heated concrete can remain hot enough to decompose the plastic in telephone or electrical cables, thus releasing more hydrogen chloride.

Hydrogen chloride is colorless but can be detected by its pungent odor. It causes irritation of the eyes and respiratory tract. When hydrogen chloride gas is inhaled, it mixes with the moisture in the respiratory tract to form hydrochloric acid. Hydrochloric acid can cause severe burns to the respiratory tract and lungs. These burns can lead to pulmonary edema, shock, and even death.

When the burning vapors are first inhaled, the body attempts to protect itself by closing off the airway. This protective reaction is known as a laryngospasm, a spasm of the laryngeal muscles. Because this spasm reduces the oxygen that can enter the respiratory system, the firefighter will also suffer the effects of oxygen deficiency.

With an increase in the use of plastics today, hydrogen chloride is present at practically every fire. Early signs of hydrogen chloride exposure are burning, irritated eyes, nose, and throat. Treatment for hydrogen chloride exposure should include high-flow, high-concentrate oxygen and irrigation of the eyes.

Hydrogen Cyanide (HCN)

Hydrogen cyanide (HCN) is produced by the combustion of nitrogen-bearing substances. These substances include synthetic fibers such as nylon, some plastics (particularly those in aircraft), and natural fibers such as wool. Hydrogen cyanide can also be produced by polyurethane foam, rubber, and paper. Hydrogen cyanide is a colorless gas but has a faint odor similar to bitter almonds.

Hydrogen cyanide interferes with respiration at the cellular and tissue levels. It deactivates certain enzymes, thereby preventing the use of oxygen by the cells. At lower concentrations, hydrogen cyanide can cause an increase in pulse rate, gasping respirations, headache, and confusion. Exposure to higher levels of hydrogen cyanide can lead to respiratory failure and death; however, exposure to even small quantities can be fatal.

Hydrogen cyanide has an IDLH level of 50 ppm. A person who has been exposed should receive immediate treatment and transport to a hospital. Immediate treatment requires administering artificial respiration to nonbreathing victims or oxygen to victims who are having difficulty breathing.

Carbon Dioxide (CO_2)

Although it is not a toxic gas, carbon dioxide (CO_2) must be considered because it is an end product of complete combustion (CO is incomplete) and can be dangerous at high levels. Carbon dioxide is a necessary part of respiration, but at high exposure levels it possesses a dangerous synergistic effect. Carbon dioxide is nonflammable, colorless, and odorless. Free-burning fires generally produce more carbon dioxide than do smoldering fires.

The chief danger of carbon dioxide exposure is that it causes increased respiratory rates. Recall that the carbon dioxide level in the blood stimulates the breathing center in the brain. When increased carbon dioxide levels are present (20,000 ppm), respirations can be increased by as much as 50 percent. This increased respiratory rate helps increase the amount of smoke and other toxic gases entering the body. Table 2.5 shows the effects of carbon dioxide. Because it is an asphyxiant, carbon dioxide in excessive amounts can also create an oxygen-deficient atmosphere that will not support life. Firefighters should anticipate high carbon diox-

TABLE 2.5
EFFECTS OF CARBON DIOXIDE

Carbon Dioxide (CO_2) (ppm)	Carbon Dioxide (CO_2) in Air (Percent)	Symptoms
5,000	0.5	No symptoms
20,000	2.0	Breathing rate increased by 50 percent
30,000	3.0	Breathing rate increased by 100 percent
50,000	5.0	Vomiting, dizziness, disorientation after 30 minutes
80,000	8.0	Headache, vomiting, dizziness, breathing difficulties after short exposure
100,000	10.0	Death in a few minutes

ppm - parts per million

ide levels when a carbon dioxide total-flooding system has been activated. These systems are designed to exclude oxygen from the fire and will also, in the process, exclude oxygen from the firefighters.

Signs of carbon dioxide poisoning include dizziness and difficulty breathing. Because exposure can cause suffocation, victims should be moved to fresh air and given artificial respiration if not breathing or oxygen if breathing is difficult.

Phosgene ($COCl_2$)

Phosgene ($COCl_2$), also known as carbonyl chloride, is produced when refrigerants such as freon, plastics containing polyvinyl chloride (PVC), or electrical wiring insulation contact flames. Phosgene's chief effect is in the lungs: When inhaled, phosgene converts to hydrogen chloride in the alveolar spaces and then into hydrochloric acid and carbon monoxide when it contacts the lungs. The hydrochloric acid produced when phosgene combines with moisture causes pulmonary edema, which prevents the exchange of oxygen in the lungs. The carbon monoxide produced prevents the red blood cells from accepting oxygen and causes cyanosis. Phosgene can also be absorbed through the skin, particularly at high concentrations.

Phosgene is a colorless, tasteless gas with a musty hay odor. This odor is perceptible at 6 ppm. Note from Table 2.2 that the IDLH level of phosgene is 2 ppm. By the time the body can tell its presence, the gas is already above the IDLH level.

Exposure to a relatively high concentration (10 to 12 ppm) is likely to produce prompt vomiting, followed by a dry throat, pain in the chest, coughing, and shortness of breath. Exposure at the IDLH level will produce the cough and irritation after a short exposure but will not cause serious discomfort in the time required to absorb a dangerous or lethal dose; in other words, a lethal dose can be absorbed before the body has time to react. Additional symptoms include severe eye and skin irritation, inability to breathe properly, and cyanosis (skin discoloration from oxygen deficiency in the blood). Although inhalation exposure damages the respiratory tract, the effects may be delayed from 2 to 24 hours or longer, depending on the length and level of exposure. The victim should be kept under observation during this time.

Treatment of phosgene poisoning requires moving the victim to fresh air and administering artificial respiration to nonbreathing victims or oxygen to those having difficulty breathing. The eyes and any skin contacted should be flushed thoroughly with running water.

Oxides Of Nitrogen (NO_2, NO)

There are two oxides of nitrogen (NO_2, NO) that are dangerous: nitrogen dioxide (NO_2) and nitric oxide (NO). Nitrogen dioxide is the more significant of the two because nitric oxide readily converts to nitrogen dioxide in the presence of oxygen and moisture. Nitrogen dioxide can mix with moisture in the air and in the respiratory tract and form nitric and nitrous acids. These acids can then burn the lungs and cause pulmonary edema, which can lead to death.

Nitrogen dioxide gas has a characteristic reddish brown color and an odor similar to that of household bleach. Nitrogen dioxide is commonly referred to as "silo gas." It forms under nonfire situations in grain bins and silos. It is most commonly associated with corn but forms during the storage of other crops as well. It is most concentrated within one to three days after the crop has been placed in the silo, although it may be present for as long as three weeks after storage.

In addition to causing pulmonary edema, nitric and nitrous acids may enter the bloodstream. The body will attempt to neutralize these acids and in doing so will cause formation of nitrites and nitrates. These substances chemically attach to the blood and can induce nausea, abdominal pains, vomiting, and cyanosis, which can lead to collapse and coma. Nitrates and nitrites can also cause arterial dilation, variation in blood pressure, headaches, and dizziness.

Nitrogen dioxide is especially dangerous because its irritating effects in the nose and throat can be tolerated even though a lethal dose is being inhaled. Therefore, the hazardous effects from its pulmonary irritation action or chemical reaction may not become apparent for several hours. The IDLH level for nitrogen dioxide is 50 ppm.

Treatment of nitrogen dioxide poisoning requires moving the victim to fresh air and administering artificial respiration to nonbreathing victims or oxygen to those having difficulty breathing. Because effects may not be apparent for several hours, the victim should be transported to a hospital and kept under observation.

Acrolein (CH_2CHCHO)

Acrolein (CH_2CHCHO) is produced when wood, paper, cotton, plastic materials, and oils and fats burn. Acrolein is a colorless, highly irritating gas with a piercing, disagreeable odor.

Inhaling acrolein can cause nose and throat irritation, nausea, shortness of breath, lung damage, pulmonary edema, and can eventually lead to death. The IDLH level for acrolein is very low (5 ppm). A mild cough may be the only symptom at the time of exposure.

Treatment of acrolein poisoning requires moving the victim to fresh air and administering artificial respiration to nonbreathing victims or oxygen to those having difficulty breathing. The eyes and any skin contacted should be flushed with running water for 15 minutes. The victim should be transported to a hospital and kept under observation as symptoms of edema may be delayed from 5 to 72 hours, depending on the level of exposure.

Formaldehyde (HCHO)

Formaldehyde (HCHO) is produced when wood, cotton, and newspaper burn. Formaldehyde is a colorless gas that has a characteristic pungent odor. It is an irritant to the eyes, nose, and throat. At higher concentrations (near 100 ppm), nausea and vomiting can result. Prolonged exposure can result in loss of consciousness. Formaldehyde does not have an IDLH level, but inhalation of formaldehyde in a 10-20 ppm concentration causes severe difficulty in breathing, intense lacrimation (tearing of the eyes), and severe cough. Formaldehyde can also be absorbed through the skin and is a known carcinogen.

Emergency treatment requires moving the victim to fresh air and thoroughly flushing the eyes with running water.

Hydrogen Sulfide (H$_2$S)

Hydrogen sulfide (H$_2$S) is produced when rubber insulation, tires, and woolen materials burn. It is also commonly produced by the decomposition of sulfur-bearing organic material and is often found in sewers, sewage disposal plants, and oil drilling operations. Hydrogen sulfide gas is colorless and has a strong rotten egg odor. It is dangerous because it quickly deactivates the sense of smell, as a result, the firefighter can be exposed to high concentrations without realizing it. The IDLH level for hydrogen sulfide is 300 ppm.

Inhalation of a high concentration of hydrogen sulfide will produce sudden asphyxiation—the firefighter falls, apparently unconscious immediately, and may die without moving again. There is a complete arrest of respiration, which can often be overcome by prompt application of artificial respiration. In less sudden poisoning, the signs may be nausea, profuse salivation, diarrhea, belching, cough, headache, dizziness, conjunctivitis of the eyes, and blistering of the lips. Emergency treatment at this level requires moving the victim to fresh air, giving oxygen to victims having difficulty breathing, flushing the eyes with running water, and transporting the victim to a hospital for observation.

Sulfur Dioxide (SO$_2$)

Sulfur dioxide (SO$_2$) is produced when sulfur-containing materials burn. Sulfur dioxide is a colorless gas with a highly irritating odor that makes it detectable below its lethal dosage. The IDLH level for sulfur dioxide is 100 ppm.

Inhaled sulfur dioxide acts mainly to irritate the eyes, skin, and mucous membranes. At the time of exposure, a mild cough may be the only symptom. Later symptoms may include rapid respirations, severe cough, and pulmonary edema. When combined with the moisture in the respiratory tract, sulfur dioxide acts as a corrosive, causing edema of the respiratory tract and lungs and producing respiratory paralysis.

Emergency treatment includes moving the victim to fresh air and administering artificial respiration to nonbreathing victims or oxygen to victims having difficulty breathing. The eyes should be thoroughly flushed with running water.

Benzene (C_6H_6)

Benzene (C_6H_6) is produced when PVC plastics and gasoline burn. It is a colorless gas with a fairly pleasant aromatic odor. Benzene can be inhaled or absorbed through the skin.

A single, heavy exposure may produce a serious acute effect, similar to an anesthetic, with special affinity for the central nervous system. The first sign is usually exhilaration, followed by sleepiness, dizziness, vomiting, tremors, hallucinations, seizures, and unconsciousness. Inhaling high levels of benzene gas can cause unconsciousness and death from respiratory paralysis and cardiovascular collapse. Lesser exposure levels cause irritation to the eyes, nose, and respiratory system, as well as headache, nausea, dizziness, weakness, and trembling.

Although it does not have an IDLH level, benzene is particularly dangerous because it is a known carcinogen. The National Institute for Occupational Safety and Health (NIOSH) has identified benzene as an agent that causes leukemia.

The main emergency treatments in acute poisoning are removal of the victim to fresh air, administration of oxygen, and maintenance of body warmth.

Asbestos

Although asbestos is not a fire gas, firefighters can be exposed to asbestos fibers during overhaul operations. Asbestos can be found in older buildings where it was used for insulation. Asbestos is classified as a carcinogen. When asbestos fibers are inhaled, they travel to the lungs, causing scarring that reduces lung capacity. The effects of asbestos exposure may not show up for many years.

RESPIRATORY HAZARDS NOT ASSOCIATED WITH FIRE
Oxygen-Deficient Atmospheres

Occasionally, a firefighter may have to enter an oxygen-deficient atmosphere that is not part of a fire fighting operation. This type of entry is usually made for rescue purposes. Entering caves, sewers, and confined spaces requires the use of SCBA. A confined space is any space having little or no natural ventilation and that can produce dangerous atmospheres. It is almost impossible to measure oxygen levels in a confined space without a meter, so SCBA must be worn for protection. *Just having to rescue a person who has lost consciousness in a particular space should be warning enough that the atmosphere of that space will not support life.* Table 2.6 lists concentrations of oxygen in the atmosphere and their various definitions or effects.

TABLE 2.6
CONCENTRATIONS OF OXYGEN AND THEIR EFFECTS

Concentration of Oxygen (Percent)	Effect
21	Usual content in air
19.5	OSHA recommended minimum oxygen content for entry
18	ANSI Z117.1-1977 definition of oxygen-deficient atmosphere
17	Medical problems begin

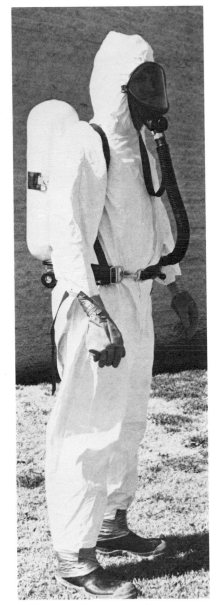

Figure 2.6 Wearing SCBA is mandatory (from both safety and legal standpoints) when working a hazardous materials incident.

Hazardous Materials Incidents

The U.S. Department of Transportation (DOT) defines a hazardous material as "any substance or material in any form which may pose an unreasonable risk to health and safety or property when transported in commerce." Because hazardous materials are routinely transported by rail, water, air, and road, every area is a potential site of a hazardous materials incident. Such fixed locations as industrial sites are also likely to present firefighters with a variety of hazardous materials situations.

Hazardous materials can range from chemicals in liquid or gas form to radioactive materials to etiologic (disease-causing) agents. When these materials burn, they can pose an even greater danger. Wearing SCBA is *mandatory* when dealing with hazardous materials incidents—both from a safety standpoint and because its use is required by law (Figure 2.6). Current hazardous materials regulations require extensive training and equipment for *anyone* responding to a hazardous materials incident.

When firefighters see a placard on a vehicle involved in an accident, it should serve as a warning that the atmosphere may be toxic and that SCBA should be worn. In industrial facilities, placards may also be placed on containers warning of the dangerous materials inside (Figures 2.7 a and b). Buildings may also be placarded with NFPA 704 diamonds. This placard informs responders about the substance's fire, life, and reactivity potential as well as special hazards (Figure 2.8). For more information on hazardous materials incidents, see the IFSTA validated **Hazardous Materials for First Responders**.

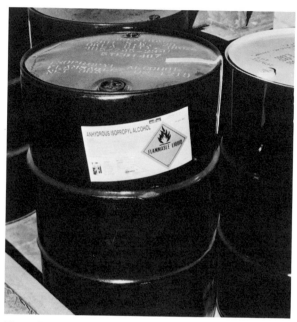

Figure 2.7a Drums containing dangerous chemicals must be marked with appropriate labels.

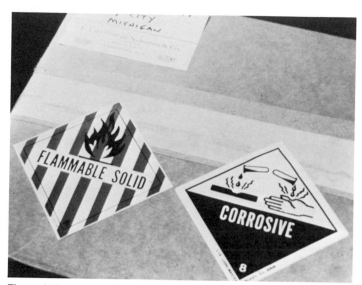

Figure 2.7b Labels indicating dangerous hazards (explosive, poisonous, combustible, and so on) are placed on shipping containers.

Figure 2.8 The NFPA 704 system gives vital information about chemicals stored in fixed facilities. *Reprinted with permission from NFPA 704-1985, Standard System for the Identification of Fire Hazards of Materials, Copyright 1985, National Fire Protection Association, Batterymarch Park, MA 02269. This warning system is intended to be interpreted and applied only by properly trained individuals to identify fire, health and reactivity hazards of chemicals. The user is referred to a certain limited number of chemicals with recommended classifications in NFPA 49 and NFPA 325.*

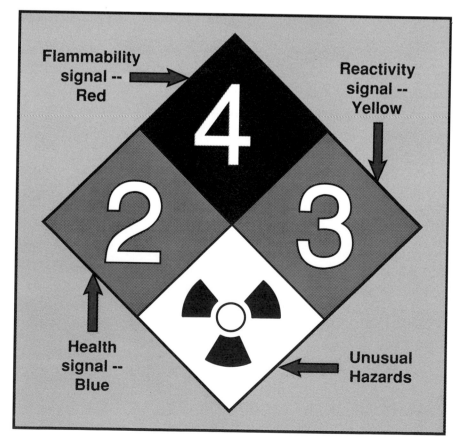

Do not limit the use of SCBA to hazardous materials incidents. Common calls, such as gas leaks or carbon monoxide poisonings, may also require the use of SCBA. Attempting rescues without proper protection will rapidly make the rescuers part of the problem, rather than part of the solution.

> # WHEN IN DOUBT, WEAR SCBA.

SUMMARY

Firefighters can encounter respiratory hazards almost anywhere because of the widespread manufacture, use, and transportation of hazardous materials. These hazards may arise from fire or nonfire incidents. Respiratory hazards from fires are categorized into oxygen-deficient atmospheres, elevated temperatures, flashover, backdraft, smoke, and toxic atmospheres. Respiratory hazards not associated with fire include oxygen-deficient atmospheres and hazardous materials incidents. Firefighters should not assume an atmosphere is safe whenever there is *any* possibility of respiratory hazards being present. SCBA must be worn in any atmosphere that may contain respiratory hazards.

Chapter 2 Review

Answers on page 347

TRUE-FALSE: Mark each statement true or false. If false, explain why.

1. Flashover and "rollover" are names for the same thing.

   ☐ T ☐ F _____

   _____

2. More fire deaths occur from carbon monoxide poisoning than from any other toxic product of combustion.

   ☐ T ☐ F _____

   _____

3. Carbon monoxide levels have already fallen and are relatively low during the overhaul stage of fire fighting.

   ☐ T ☐ F _____

   _____

4. Hydrogen chloride is colorless; however, it can be detected by its odor.

   ☐ T ☐ F _____

   _____

5. At high exposure levels carbon dioxide possesses a dangerous synergistic effect.

   ☐ T ☐ F _____

   _____

6. The effects of asbestos exposure are usually apparent within hours of exposure.

   ☐ T ☐ F _____

   _____

MULTIPLE CHOICE: Circle the correct answer.

7. Which of the following toxic gases can be produced when freon or polyvinyl chloride (PVC) plastics contact flames?

   A. Formaldehyde

   B. Phosgene

   C. Hydrogen sulfide

   D. Hydrogen chloride

8. Which of the following toxic substances can form acids that burn lung tissue, can enter the bloodstream and cause cyanosis, and has a reddish-brown color?

    A. Hydrogen sulfide

    B. Formaldehyde

    C. Acrolein

    D. Nitrogen dioxide

9. The combustion of paper, wood, or cotton can produce any of the following toxic substances **except** _____.

    A. formaldehyde

    B. acrolein

    C. hydrogen sulfide

    D. carbon dioxide

LISTING

10. List the conditions that indicate the possibility of a backdraft.

    A. _____

    B. _____

    C. _____

    D. _____

    E. _____

11. List the three ways in which toxic particles can enter the body.

    A. _____

    B. _____

    C. _____

12. What are the four factors that determine the type and amounts of toxic gases given off during a fire?

    A. _____

    B. _____

    C. _____

    D. _____

FILL IN THE BLANK: Fill in the blanks with the correct response.

13. Gases with vapor densities of less than 1 are _____ than air; those with vapor densities greater than 1 are _____ than air.

14. Inhaled hydrogen chloride mixes with moisture in the respiratory tract to form _____.

15. Hydrogen cyanide is produced by the combustion of _____ substances, including synthetic fibers such as _____ and natural fibers such as _____.

16. _____ is produced when PVC plastics and gasoline burn.

SHORT ANSWER: Answer each item briefly.

17. In what ways can inhaling heated air injure a firefighter?

_____

_____

_____

_____

18. When several different toxins enter the body, some can cause a synergistic effect. Explain synergistic effect.

_____

_____

_____

_____

19. What is the chief danger of exposure to excessive levels of carbon dioxide?

_____

_____

_____

_____

20. What is a "hazardous material" as defined by the U.S. Department of Transportation?

_____

_____

_____

_____

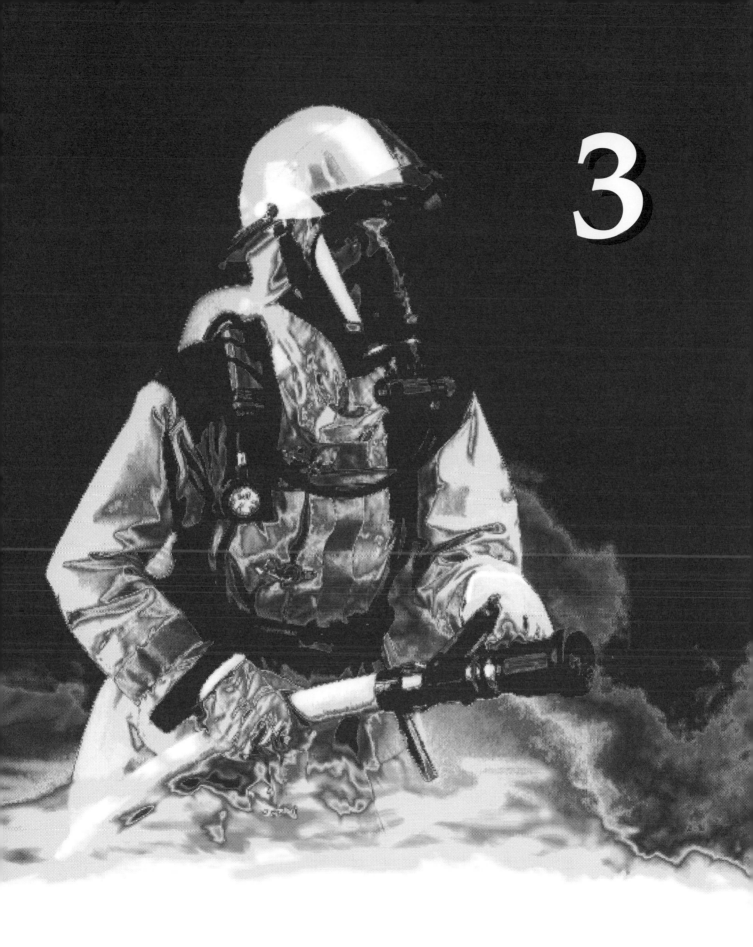

3

Types Of SCBA

This chapter provides information that addresses the following standards:

NFPA STANDARD 1001
Fire Fighter Professional Qualifications
1987 Edition

Chapter 3—Fire Fighter I

3-6.2

3-6.3

Chapter 5—Fire Fighter III

5-6.1

NFPA STANDARD 1404
Fire Department Self-Contained Breathing Apparatus Program
1989 Edition

Chapter 2—Provisions of SCBA

2-1.4

2-1.5

2-2.1

2-4.1

2-4.2

Chapter 3—Emergency Scene Use

3-1.4

Chapter 4—SCBA Training

4-2.3

4-2.4

4-2.5

4-6

4-9

4-10

4-12.1

NFPA STANDARD 1500
Fire Department Occupational Safety and Health Program
1987 Edition

Chapter 5—Protective Clothing and Protective Equipment

5-3.2

NFPA STANDARD 1981
Open-Circuit Self-Contained Breathing
Apparatus for Fire Fighters
1987 Edition

Chapter 2—General Requirements
2-3.1

2-3.2

2-3.3

2-3.4

ANSI STANDARD Z88.5-1981
Practices for Respiratory Protection for the Fire Service

Section 3—SCBA Program
3.1.6

Section 4—Selection of SCBA

Section 6—Maintenance of SCBA
6.7

Section 9—Special Problems
9.6

ANSI STANDARD Z88.2-1980
Practices for Respiratory Protection

Section 3—Respirator Program Requirements
3.5.4

3.5.5

Section 6—Selection of Respirators
6.1

6.2

6.9

6.14

Code of Federal Regulations
Title 29, Part 1910

Section 156—Fire Brigades

Chapter 3
Types of SCBA

INTRODUCTION

The many types of incidents to which a fire department responds will dictate the type of respiratory protection required. Fire departments routinely respond to fires, but they also respond to hazardous materials incidents and perform rescues. These latter types of incidents often demand respiratory protection with duration longer than standard 30- or 60-minute self-contained breathing apparatus. For these situations, either closed-circuit SCBA or airline systems attached to large air supplies are necessary.

There are two types of self-contained breathing apparatus used in the fire service: open-circuit and closed-circuit. Open-circuit SCBA is used much more frequently than closed-circuit SCBA. Open-circuit SCBA uses compressed air; closed-circuit SCBA uses compressed or liquid oxygen. Closed-circuit SCBA is also known as "rebreather" apparatus because the user's exhaled air stays within the system for reuse. Regardless of the type of SCBA used, training in its use is essential.

Until July 1, 1983, two types of open-circuit SCBA were used by the fire service: demand and positive pressure. Since that date, demand units have not been in compliance with Occupational Safety and Health Administration (OSHA) requirements and should not be in use. NFPA and ANSI standards also require that only positive-pressure breathing apparatus be used in the fire service. (**NOTE:** Any departments still using demand apparatus should be aware that these units can and should be converted to positive-pressure units as rapidly as possible.)

The main reason for the change to positive pressure is the greater protection factor afforded by the positive-pressure units. Positive-pressure SCBA maintains a slightly increased pressure (above atmospheric) in the user's facepiece. This positive pressure helps prevent contaminants from entering the facepiece if a leak develops.

Various factors need to be considered when selecting the type and/or make of SCBA for a fire department. This chapter describes the uses, components, and various accessories of open-circuit SCBA, airline equipment, and closed-circuit SCBA. Some important considerations for selecting or upgrading SCBA are also described.

DURATION OF AIR SUPPLY

Knowing the amount of air supplied by a particular type of breathing apparatus is critically important to the firefighter. Having an adequate air supply may literally make the difference between life and death. Closed-circuit SCBA and airline equipment are capable of providing the longest air supplies; standard open-circuit SCBA worn on the back, the least.

It can be difficult to determine just how much breathing air is available, even if a cylinder is full. The rated air supply generally does not correspond to the actual duration of the air available. Air duration varies with individual breathing rates and with the amount of physical activity performed. For example, a 30-minute-rated unit may supply only 15 minutes of air, and a 60-minute-rated unit may supply only 45 minutes of air. The National Institute for Occupational Safety and Health (NIOSH) and the Mine Safety and Health Administration (MSHA) even require a manufacturer's statement to this effect:

"The user should not expect to obtain exactly 30-minute service life from this apparatus for each use. The work being performed may be more or less strenuous than that used in the MSHA-NIOSH test. Where work is more strenuous, the duration may be shorter, possibly as short as 15 minutes."

The rating on an open-circuit unit is the *maximum* level of protection that can be expected. As a rule of thumb, expect no more than one minute per 100 psi (700 kPa) registered on the cylinder pressure gauge. On the other hand, a one-hour closed-circuit unit is designed to provide a *minimum* of 60 minutes of protection, regardless of the level of exertion.

Firefighters should have an understanding of the variables that affect air supply duration. With proper training, firefighters can estimate how long their air supply will last under different situations. Among the factors that influence actual working time when wearing SCBA are the following:

- Physical condition of the user
- Degree of physical exertion
- Emotional stability of the user

- Condition of the apparatus
- Cylinder pressure before use
- Amount of training and experience with SCBA

Fire fighting is physical work and is very strenuous. Because extra work requires extra oxygen, physical conditioning and training are two ways firefighters can improve their air supply duration (Figure 3.1). A firefighter who is not physically fit will deplete his or her air supply more rapidly than a firefighter who is physically fit. The ability to maintain composure and avoid panic will also help the firefighter achieve greater duration of air supply. Training enables the firefighter to remain calm.

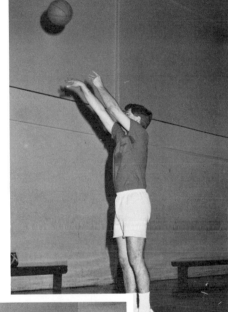

Figure 3.1 A firefighter following an aerobic conditioning program will be able to improve his or her air supply duration.

Condition Of SCBA

SCBA must be properly maintained to ensure safety and to avoid wasting the air supply. Improperly maintained apparatus may develop leaks that waste air and pose a potential hazard to the user. A faulty diaphragm or exhalation valve, or other mechanical failure, may also allow leaks. More dangerous is a cylinder filled with contaminated air. For example, if excessive carbon dioxide were present in the compressed air, the body would be triggered to breathe faster, thus wasting air.

Cylinder Pressure

Some departments allow a slightly used cylinder to stay in service until the pressure falls below a stated refill level, considering that to be a reasonable compromise between duration and convenience. Although many incidents require use of SCBA for only a short time, firefighters never know when they will need a full cylinder to provide maximum working time, so this procedure is not recommended. Table 3.1 shows the air volume theoretically possible when a 30-minute cylinder is at less-than-full pressure.

The time duration losses are based on manufacturers' information that low-pressure bottles lose approximately 1.5 minutes of use with each 100 psi (700 kPa) reduction. High-pressure bottles lose approximately 45 seconds with each 100 psi (700 kPa) reduction of pressure. Fire departments should recharge cylinders to full capacity after every use.

TABLE 3.1
AIR VOLUME OF 30-MINUTE CYLINDER
AT VARIOUS PRESSURES

Cylinder Pressure		Air Volume	
psi	kPa	ft³	L
2,200	15 180	45	1 275
1,500	10 350	32	905
1,000	690	23	650

OPEN-CIRCUIT BREATHING APPARATUS

Open-circuit SCBA are currently the most commonly used in the fire service. The air supply in open-circuit systems is compressed air. Exhaled air is vented to the outside atmosphere.

Several companies manufacture SCBA, each with different design features or mechanical construction. Certain parts, such as cylinders and backpacks, are interchangeable; however, such substitution voids NIOSH/MSHA certification and is not a recommended practice. Substituting different parts may also void warranties and leave the department or firefighter liable for any injuries incurred. Different makes of SCBA are discussed in Appendix E.

COMPONENTS

There are four basic SCBA component assemblies (Figures 3.2 a and b):

- *Backpack and harness assembly*
- *Air cylinder assembly*, including cylinder, valve, and pressure gauge
- *Regulator assembly*, including high-pressure hose and low-pressure alarm
- *Facepiece assembly*, including low-pressure hose (breathing tube) and exhalation valve (for SCBA with harness-mounted regulator) and head harness

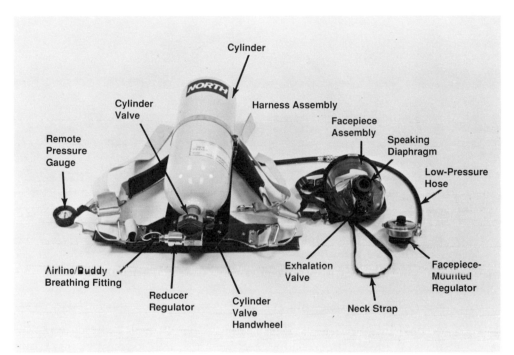

Figure 3.2a This open-circuit SCBA has the facepiece and regulator assemblies combined.

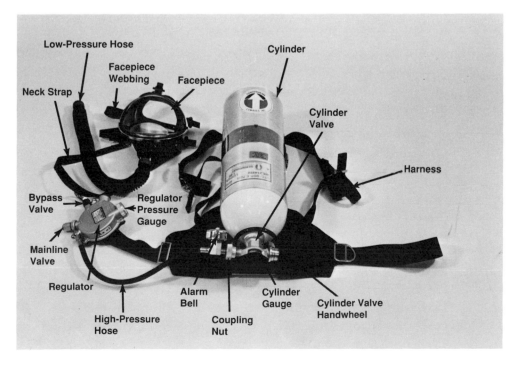

Figure 3.2b This open-circuit SCBA has distinct facepiece, regulator, and air cylinder assemblies.

Backpack And Harness Assembly

The backpack assembly is designed to hold the air cylinder on the firefighter's back as comfortably and securely as possible. Adjustable harness straps provide a secure fit for whatever size the individual requires. The waist straps are designed to help properly distribute the weight of the cylinder or pack (Figure 3.3). One problem is that waist straps are often not used or are removed. Remember that NIOSH and MSHA certify the entire SCBA unit, and removal of waist straps could void warranties.

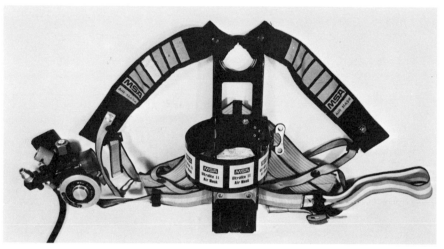

Figure 3.3 The backpack assembly uses adjustable harness and waist straps to provide security and proper weight distribution.

Air Cylinder Assembly

Air cylinders come in different sizes and with a variety of high-pressure hose connections. Because the cylinder must be strong enough to safely contain the high pressure of the compressed air, it constitutes the main weight of the breathing apparatus. A 2,216 psi (15 290 kPa), 30-minute cylinder when full may range from as little as 9.6 pounds (4.3 kg) for an MSA™ composite cylinder to 23.8 pounds (10.7 kg) for a steel Survivair® cylinder. Most composite cylinders weigh about 16 pounds (7.2 kg), while steel and aluminum cylinders weigh about 20 pounds (9 kg).

Fully charged, the typical 30-minute-rated cylinder contains 45 cubic feet (1 275 L) of breathing air at 2,216 psi (15 290 kPa). Cylinders rated for 60 minutes contain 88 cubic feet (2 490 L) of breathing air at 4,500 psi (31 000 kPa).

Lightweight aluminum and combination fiberglass-wrapped aluminum cylinders are the most common cylinder types and are 10 percent stronger than steel. A typical cylinder is rated at either 2,216 or 4,500 psi (15 290 kPa or 31 000 kPa), and the cubic foot rating depends upon the physical size of the cylinder. Manufacturers offer cylinders of various sizes, air volumes, and features to correspond to their varied uses in fire and rescue responses (Figures 3.4 and 3.5).

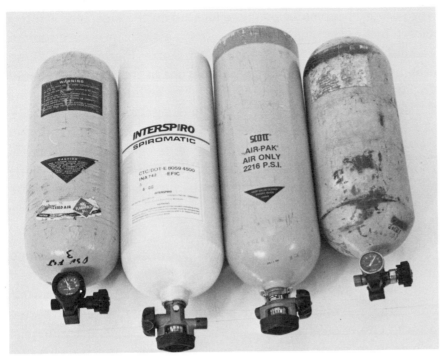

Figure 3.4 Air cylinders are available in various sizes, volumes, and compositions.

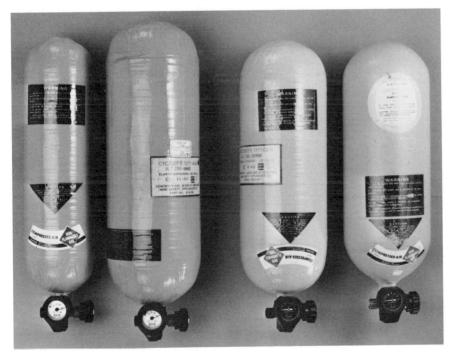

Figure 3.5 Composite air cylinders of various sizes and volumes are shown. *Photo courtesy of MSA.*

Regulator Assembly

The regulator reduces the pressure of the cylinder air to slightly above atmospheric pressure and controls the flow of air to meet the respiratory requirements of the wearer. Air from the cylinder travels through the high-pressure hose to the regulator. When the firefighter inhales, pressure is reduced in the facepiece and the regulator supplies more air to compensate for the pressure drop. The exhalation valve located on the facepiece is forced closed by spring tension, which causes a slight pressure buildup inside the facepiece, hence positive pressure (Figure 3.6). Exhalation by the firefighter increases pressure in the facepiece enough to overcome the spring tension in the exhalation valve. This causes the valve to open and allow waste gases to be expelled. As soon as pressure within the facepiece is less than the force applied by the exhalation valve spring, the valve closes, preventing the outside atmosphere from entering the facepiece. Some SCBA units have regulators that fit into the facepiece. On other units, the regulator is on the firefighter's chest or waist strap (Figures 3.7 and 3.8).

On many models, two external knobs, differing in color, shape, and location, control operating and emergency functions. These are the mainline valve and the bypass valve. During normal operation, the mainline valve is fully open and locked, if there is a lock. The bypass valve is closed. On some SCBA, the bypass valve controls a direct airline from the cylinder in the event that

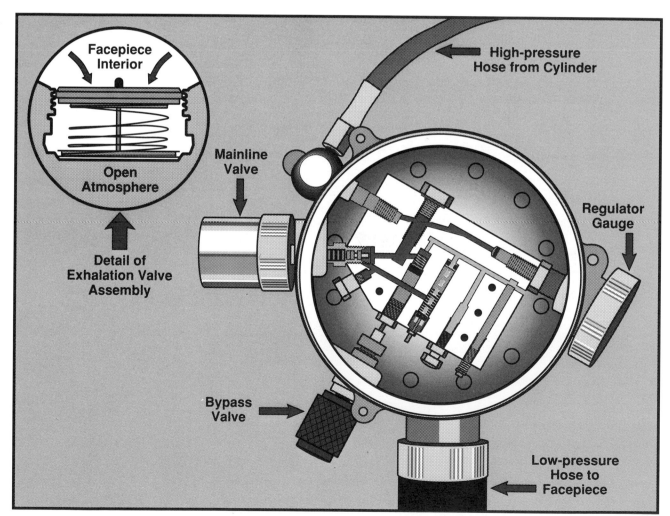

Figure 3.6 A cutaway drawing of an open-circuit regulator with the air pathway highlighted. A facepiece exhalation valve is shown in greater detail.

the regulator fails. Once the valves are set in their normal operating position, they should not be changed unless the emergency bypass is needed (Figure 3.9).

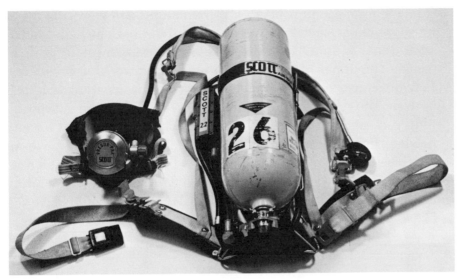

Figure 3.7 This SCBA has a mask-mounted regulator.

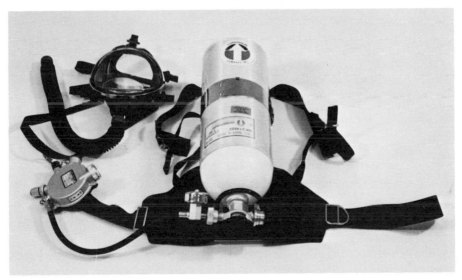

Figure 3.8 This SCBA has the regulator mounted on the waist strap.

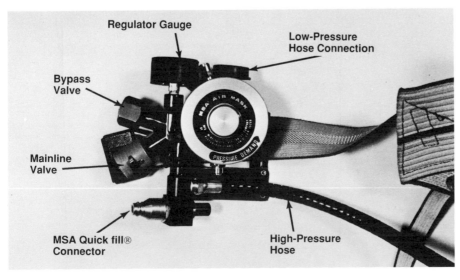

Regulator Gauge

Low-Pressure
Hose Connection

Bypass
Valve

Mainline
Valve

MSA Quick fill®
Connector

High-Pressure
Hose

Figure 3.9 An SCBA regulator with its mainline valve and bypass valve is shown. These knobs may be in different colors, shapes, and locations, depending on the SCBA model.

A pressure gauge is usually mounted on or near the regulator or on the high-pressure hose and shows the air pressure remaining in the cylinder (Figures 3.10 and 3.11). The regulator pressure gauge should read within 100 psi (700 kPa) of the cylinder gauge if increments are in psi (kPa). If increments are shown in other measurements, such as percents or fractions, both measurements should be the same. These pressure readings are most accurate at or near the upper range of the gauge's rated working pressures. Low pressures in the cylinder may cause inconsistent readings between the cylinder and regulator gauges. If they are not consistent, rely on the lower reading and check the equipment for any needed repair before using it again. All modern units have an audible alarm that sounds when the cylinder pressure decreases to a preset level: 450 to 550 psi (3 100 kPa to 3 795 kPa), depending on the manufacturer (Figure 3.12). SCBA teams should leave the fire area *immediately* after the first firefighter's alarm sounds.

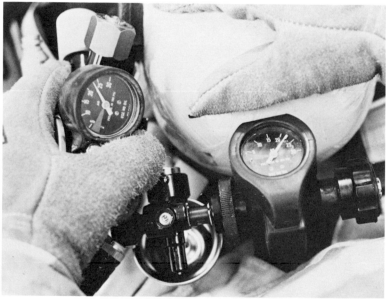

Figure 3.10 The SCBA pressure gauge shows the air pressure at the regulator. Pressure measurements may be in psi, percents, or fractions.

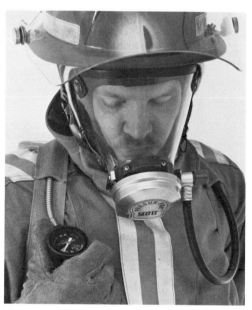

Figure 3.11 The pressure gauge can be mounted on the regulator or on the shoulder strap, as shown here, for quick access by the firefighter.

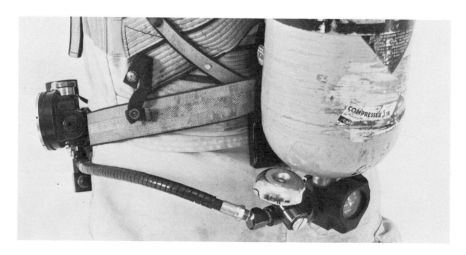

Figure 3.12 The low-pressure alarm will sound when the cylinder pressure reaches a certain level, usually about 25 percent of total capacity.

Facepiece Assembly

The facepiece assembly consists of the facepiece lens, an exhalation valve, and, if the regulator is separate, a low-pressure hose to carry the air from the regulator to the facepiece. The facepiece lens is made of clear safety plastic and is connected to a flexible rubber mask. The facepiece is held snugly against the face by a head harness with adjustable straps, net, or some other arrangement. The lens should be protected from scratches during use and storage. Some facepieces, such as the one shown in Figure 3.13, have a speech diaphragm to make communication easier.

The low-pressure hose brings air from the regulator into the facepiece; therefore, it must be kept free of kinks and away from contact with abrasive surfaces. The hose is usually corrugated to prevent collapse when a person is working in close quarters,

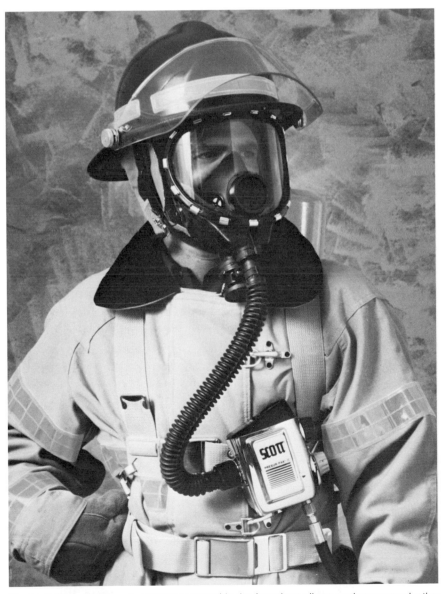

Figure 3.13 A speaking diaphragm mounted in the facepiece allows easier communication among firefighters. *Courtesy of Scott Aviation.*

breathing deeply, or leaning against a hard surface. Like the facepiece, this hose is oil-resistant rubber, neoprene, silicone, or plastic resin, all of which are referred to generically as elastomer.

The exhalation valve at the chin of the facepiece is a simple, one-way valve that releases an exhaled breath without admitting any of the contaminated outside atmosphere. Dirt or foreign materials can cause the valve to become partially opened, which will permit the contaminated outside atmosphere to enter the facepiece. Therefore, it is important that the valve be kept clean and free of foreign material. It is also important that the exhalation valve be tested by the firefighter during facepiece-fit tests prior to entering a hazardous atmosphere. See Chapter 4, Safety and Training, for a more detailed description of exhalation valve testing.

Facepieces provide some protection from facial burns and hold in the cool breathing air. Protective hoods complete the protective envelope for the head and neck area, along with the helmet and ear flaps.

An improperly sealed facepiece or a fogged lens can cause problems for the wearer. The different temperatures inside and outside the facepiece, where the exhaled air or outside air is moist, can cause the facepiece lens to fog, which hampers vision. Internal fogging occurs when the lens is cool, causing the highly humid exhaled breath to condense. As the cooler dry air from the cylinder passes over the facepiece lens, it often removes the condensation. External fogging occurs when condensation collects on the relatively cool lens during interior fire fighting operations. External fogging can be removed by wiping the lens.

Three methods are used to prevent or control internal fogging of a lens: releasing cylinder air, using a nosecup, and applying an antifogging chemical. Quickly opening and closing the bypass valve to release a brief flow of cylinder air removes internal fogging; however, *this technique uses valuable air and its use should be restricted.* Facepieces can be equipped with a nosecup that deflects exhalations away from the lens. If the nosecup does not fit well, however, it will permit exhaled air to leak into the facepiece and condense on the lens. Last, special antifogging chemicals recommended by the manufacturer can be applied to the lens of the facepiece. Some SCBA facepieces are permanently impregnated with an antifogging chemical.

The most dangerous problem with facepieces involves the seal between the facepiece and the contours of the user's face. It is unreasonable to expect one facepiece size to fit all faces during the kinds of activity required of a firefighter. Even when one facepiece size seems adequate, it should be remembered that all facepieces are subtly different even though they may come from the same manufacturer working with the same specifications. ANSI recommends that firefighters have their own properly fitted facepieces. For more information on facepiece fitting, see Chapter 4, Safety and Training.

ACCESSORIES

Most SCBA manufacturers sell accessories and products for improving communication, reducing facepiece fogging, and aiding vision. *Before installing or using any of these devices, be aware that altering the SCBA in any way may void the SCBA certification and the manufacturer's warranty.* The SCBA should have been approved with the accessory installed before the accessory is adopted for department use. The manufacturer's instructions should be strictly followed when installing such accessories.

Improving Communication

The facepieces of some SCBA have speaking diaphragms that let firefighters communicate over short distances with little voice distortion. Some manufacturers also sell electronic devices that can either amplify or transmit the voice. One transistorized, battery-operated unit has an electrical cord that plugs into the facepiece and connects to a clip-on voice amplifier (Figure 3.14). Still another device is a battery-powered transceiver that transmits voice signals through an ear plug. One combination unit amplifies the voice and has a connection for a portable radio that can be attached to transmit and receive messages (Figure 3.15). Also available are microphones that firefighters can wear on their throats. All battery-powered communication devices must be certified as intrinsically safe.

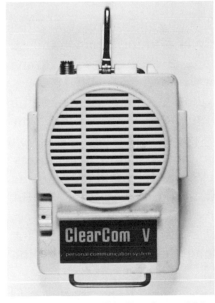

Figure 3.14 The MSA ClearCom™ Voice Amplification Unit can be used alone for amplified voice communications among close-by workers or combined with the ClearCom™ RI radio system.

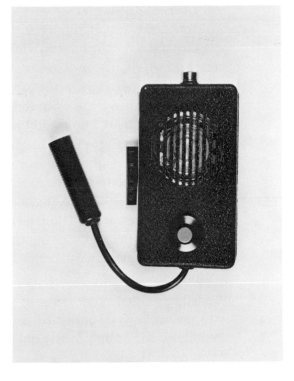

Figure 3.15 The radio interface unit attaches to a hand-held walkie-talkie for clear radio communications.

Hand-held communicators such as walkie-talkies can also be used to help improve communications. ANSI advises that such devices can best be used to transmit by pressing the microphone directly against the facepiece lens, instead of against the exhalation valve. If the transmitter comes in a leather case, the firefighter can improve transmission by cutting out the perforated leather over the microphone and cementing a thin strip of foam rubber around the outside edge of the hole.

Reducing Facepiece Fogging

Many firms sell antifogging compounds that firefighters can use to coat the inside of the facepiece lens. However, ANSI warns that some compounds can damage facepiece lenses and that personnel using them should follow the manufacturer's instructions carefully.

Many antifogging compounds do little good at temperatures below 32°F (0°C). At these temperatures, firefighters use nosecups, which direct exhalation away from the lens and out the exhalation valve. Nosecups can usually be installed without tools.

Aiding Vision

Firefighters cannot wear ordinary eyeglasses with SCBA because standard eyeglass frames prevent a proper facepiece seal. Special lens mounts for glasses can be obtained from almost all manufacturers of SCBA. See Chapter 4, Safety and Training, for a detailed discussion of eyeglass and contact lens regulations for wearers of SCBA.

AIRLINE EQUIPMENT

Incidents involving hazardous materials or rescues often require a longer air supply than can be obtained from standard open-circuit SCBA. In these situations, an airline attached to one or several air cylinders can be connected to an open-circuit facepiece, regulator, and egress cylinder. Airline equipment enables the firefighter to travel up to 300 feet (90 m) from the *regulated* air supply source (Figure 3.16). This type of respiratory protection enables the firefighter to work for several hours if necessary without the encumbrance of a backpack. If greater mobility is needed, however, the firefighter can also wear a standard SCBA with an airline option. Then, he or she can temporarily disconnect from the airline supply, using the SCBA to provide breathing air, and perform necessary tasks beyond the range of the airline equipment.

The number and sizes of air cylinders used with airline equipment vary from several small bottles to large, cascade-type cylinders. Air supply is available as long as there are spare full cylinders. All airline units should be capable of using more than

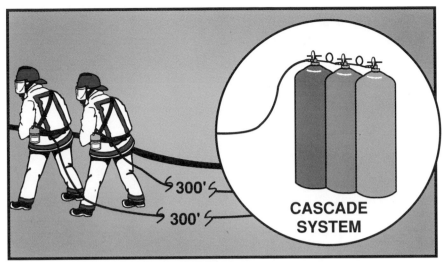

Figure 3.16 During incidents requiring a longer air supply than allowed by a standard SCBA, airline equipment is used. A firefighter can work for several hours up to 300 feet from an air source.

one cylinder in order to provide a continuous air source to the wearer. A small 45 cubic-foot (1 275 L) cylinder at 2,216 psi (15 290 kPa) is rated for 30 minutes. A large 240 cubic foot (6 792 L) cylinder at 2,400 psi (16 560 kPa) is rated for approximately 2½ hours. The smallest cylinders are rated for 5 minutes and are to be used only for escape purposes. (**NOTE:** A small cylinder here refers to a 45 cubic-foot (1 275 L) cylinder, not the 5-minute escape cylinder of some airline units that is worn on the hip.)

Small SCBA cylinders are easily and readily transported, but have a limited capacity and require frequent changing. The larger cylinders are difficult to maneuver in small spaces and may not be readily available, but they permit extended operations without cylinder changes. Any airline respirator that is used in an IDLH atmosphere must provide enough breathing air for the wearer to escape the atmosphere in the event the airline is severed. This requirement is usually accomplished by attaching the very small breathing cylinders, rated for 5 minutes, to the airline unit. Almost all airline units used in rescue situations will require the 5-minute escape cylinder. The 5-minute escape cylinders cannot be disconnected from the air supply line for untethered work — they are for escape only! To perform untethered work, a 30- or 60-minute SCBA that can be augmented by an airline should be used.

CLOSED-CIRCUIT BREATHING APPARATUS

Closed-circuit breathing apparatus are not used in the fire service as commonly as open-circuit breathing apparatus. However, they are becoming more popular for hazardous materials incidents because of their longer air supply duration. Closed-circuit SCBA are available with durations of 30 minutes to 4 hours. Closed-circuit units also generally weigh less than open-circuit units of similarly rated service time. They weigh less because a smaller cylinder containing pure oxygen is used (Figure 3.17).

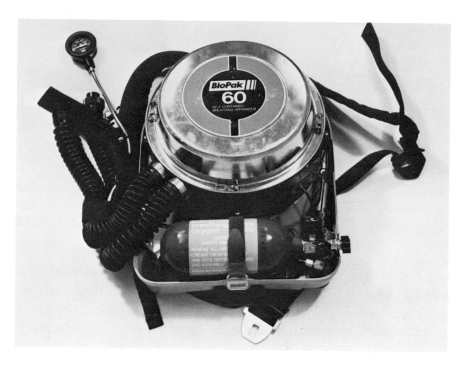

Figure 3.17 Closed-circuit SCBA use a small cylinder of pure oxygen.

Operation

Closed-circuit SCBA operate differently than open-circuit apparatus. In closed-circuit SCBA, the oxygen leaves its container and passes through a pressure regulator that supplies the desired amount of oxygen through the inhalation valve. Exhaled gas flows back through the valve and into a carbon dioxide absorption pack (Figure 3.18). The carbon dioxide is removed, and unused oxygen

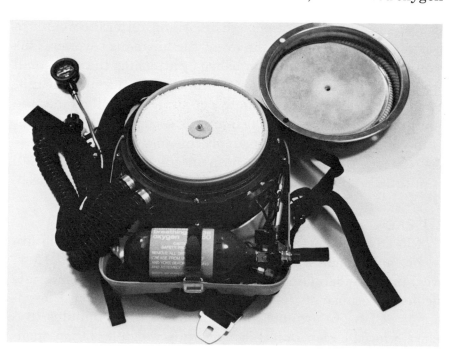

Figure 3.18 A Biomarine™ closed-circuit SCBA with cover removed is pictured. After carbon dioxide is removed by the absorption pack, fresh oxygen is added. The renewed air passes back through the inhalation valve ready to repeat the cycle.

flows into a "rebreather" bag, where fresh oxygen is added. The "renewed" breathing air passes back through the inhalation valve, and the cycle is repeated.

None of the oxygen or exhaled waste gas used in the closed-circuit system is released into the outside atmosphere, except for that released when excessive pressure is vented through the relief valve. For all practical purposes, all gases in the system stay in the system, traveling in a closed circuit. The oxygen within the system comes from a cylinder of compressed oxygen. Reuse of the exhaled air results in longer duration of air supply and allows lower unit weight.

Positive Pressure

Positive pressure in closed-circuit units serves the same purpose as positive pressure in open-circuit units. The compressed oxygen in the system is supplied at a rate greater than that needed solely for breathing. The extra breathing air increases the pressure in the facepiece during inhalation and exhalation. This slight positive pressure is maintained mechanically in the breathing chamber by a device that exerts a force on the breathing diaphragm.

Maintenance

Oxygen-cylinder closed-circuit SCBA was designed to let the firefighter carry a relatively small supply of breathable oxygen, yet make it last longer per operation. This is accomplished by removing the carbon dioxide from the exhaled breath with a chemical scrubber so that the air can be rebreathed (Figure 3.19). The exhaled air is still relatively high in oxygen and can be

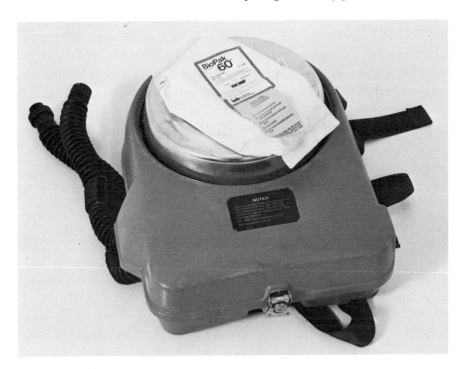

Figure 3.19 A chemical scrubber in the Biomarine™ closed-circuit SCBA removes the carbon dioxide from the exhaled air so it can be used again.

supplemented with a small quantity of the oxygen stored in a compressed-oxygen cylinder. Rebreathing a quantity of the exhaled air is possible because carbon dioxide and moisture are removed. Therefore, the firefighter needs less oxygen directly from the cylinder for breathing. To maintain this system, the carbon dioxide scrubber must be changed and the oxygen cylinder recharged or replaced after each use.

Advantages And Disadvantages

There are advantages and disadvantages to using closed-circuit SCBA. Closed-circuit SCBA provides longer air supply duration and is lighter in weight than open-circuit SCBA. On the negative side, closed-circuit SCBA is generally more expensive to purchase and maintain and requires more training and maintenance than open-circuit SCBA.

SELECTION OF SCBA

Many factors enter into the process of selecting the appropriate and most effective SCBA unit for a particular fire department:

- Geographical area and climate
- Response hazards typically encountered
- Economic factors
- Operational considerations
- Desired features and accessories
- Manufacturer's reliability

Geographical Area And Climate

Basic considerations regarding geographical area (i.e., city, rural, industrial, mining, wildland, mountain, or coastal regions) and climate must be weighed. Departments in cold northern regions have different requirements than those in hot southern regions. Those in the thin air of high altitudes face different problems than those departments located in the humid, salt air of a southern coast. Those in smoggy, heavily polluted industrial areas have different requirements than those departments in open rural areas or sandy desert areas. Ask how various atmospheres and temperatures affect the operation and maintenance of the SCBA being considered. Look for SCBA with features and accessories compatible with the geographical area and climate.

Response Hazards Typically Encountered

Does the department fight mostly brush and forest fires? Fires in large multistory inner city structures? Residential fires? Is the department called to hazardous materials incidents? Does it respond to fires in confined spaces such as mines and grain storage facilities? The typical response hazards encountered dictate, to a degree, the type of SCBA used and the length of time SCBA use will be required in any fire fighting situation. For example, a firefighter would need a longer-duration air supply to allow escape from a large warehouse than from a smaller residential structure. Closed-circuit SCBA may be more suitable for responses to hazardous materials incidents or confined space situations.

Economic Factors

Economic factors are, of course, prime considerations. Must the department purchase all new SCBA or supplement already existing equipment? Are some of the equipment parts (such as facepieces, tools, and cylinders) compatible with newer models? Can any parts be sold or used as trade-in on new equipment? Are conversion packages available, and are they more economically feasible than complete replacement? What will be the cost of training service personnel on new equipment?

Operational Considerations

Along with economic considerations, operational factors should be considered. What type of equipment is used in surrounding areas? Would there be problems or confusion for firefighters working in mutual aid situations at a fire scene if everyone had different equipment? Incremental replacement of units within a department could cause the same type of problems as well. Surveying the actual users of particular equipment will provide answers to questions about ease of operation, advantages, disadvantages, and personal experiences with the equipment.

Desired Features And Accessories

The particular SCBA itself should be studied to learn about its capabilities, safety features, and limitations. The model chosen should contain features and accessories tailored to the department's needs. Does the SCBA meet NFPA standards? Is it certified by NIOSH/MSHA?

Manufacturer's Reliability

The manufacturer's history, reliability, and repair capabilities should be researched carefully. Facts about the manufacturer are important. What is their history of reliability, speed of maintenance/repairs, and availability of parts? Do they provide good user support and help with training? Are they responsive to the firefighter's needs as technology and lifestyle change?

Meeting Standards

If a department carefully analyzes its requirements and looks closely at the above selection factors, it will be able to provide firefighters with SCBA equipment that will serve them and their area in the safest, most appropriate, and most economical manner.

SUMMARY

The two types of SCBA used in the fire service are open-circuit and closed-circuit, with open-circuit being the most commonly used. Both open-circuit and closed-circuit breathing apparatus used in the fire service must be positive pressure.

The basic components of SCBA are the backpack assembly, air cylinder, regulator, and facepiece. Because types of SCBA will differ, parts must not be interchanged. Firefighters should always follow manufacturers' instructions and recommendations when working with SCBA.

Open-circuit and closed-circuit SCBA differ in their design and method of operation. Open-circuit SCBA uses compressed air, while closed-circuit apparatus uses compressed oxygen. Closed-circuit units are generally more expensive and require more maintenance.

Various accessories are available for SCBA to improve communication, reduce facepiece fogging, and aid vision. Accessories must be approved by NIOSH; otherwise, there is risk of voiding certification and warranty of the apparatus.

Many factors should be considered in selecting the most effective SCBA unit for a department. Among factors to consider are climate and geographical location, response hazards typically encountered, and economic and operational considerations. The physical characteristics of the SCBA and the performance history of the manufacturer regarding reliability and user support must also be considered. Surveying neighboring departments and firefighters themselves will provide answers to many questions on SCBA selection.

Chapter 3 Review

Answers on page 348

TRUE-FALSE: Mark each statement true or false. If false, explain why.

1. Closed-circuit is the most commonly used type of self-contained breathing apparatus.

   ☐ T ☐ F _____

   _____

2. Altering SCBA in any way may void SCBA certification and the manufacturer's warranty.

   ☐ T ☐ F _____

   _____

3. The rated air supply of an SCBA air cylinder generally does not correspond to the actual available air supply of the cylinder when fully charged.

   ☐ T ☐ F _____

   _____

4. When wearing SCBA, the firefighter must periodically adjust the mainline valve and the bypass valve.

   ☐ T ☐ F _____

   _____

LISTING

5. What are the four basic components of an SCBA?

   A. _____

   B. _____

   C. _____

   D. _____

6. List the two main functions of an SCBA regulator.

   A. _____

   _____

   B. _____

   _____

7. What are the three methods used to prevent or control internal fogging of a facepiece lens?

   A. _____

   B. _____

   C. _____

8. What are the factors that affect air supply duration when wearing SCBA?

   A. _____

   B. _____

   C. _____

   D. _____

   E. _____

   F. _____

SELECT: Circle the correct response.

9. The rating on an open-circuit unit is the (minimum, maximum) level of protection that can be expected.

10. A 1-hour closed-circuit unit is designed to provide a (minimum, maximum) of 60 minutes of protection, regardless of the level of exertion.

11. Closed-circuit SCBA generally weigh (less, more) than open-circuit units of similarly rated service time.

FILL IN THE BLANK: Fill in the blanks with the correct response.

12. The air supply for closed-circuit SCBA is either_____ or _____ oxygen; the air supply for open-circuit SCBA is _____ _____.

13. Fully charged, the typical 30-minute-rated cylinder contains _____ cubic feet (_____ L) of breathing air at 2,216 psig (15 290 kPa), and fully-charged cylinders rated for 60 minutes contain _____ cubic feet (_____ L) of breathing air at 4,500 psig (31 000 kPa).

14. The regulator gauge should read within _____ psi (_____ kPa) of the cylinder gauge if gauge increments are in psi.

15. The facepieces of some SCBA have _____ _____ that let firefighters communicate over short distances without much voice distortion.

16. In a closed-circuit system, the carbon dioxide is removed from the exhaled air with a(n) _____.

SHORT ANSWER: Answer each item briefly.

17. What is the advantage of using positive pressure open-circuit breathing apparatus over using demand units?

_____

_____

_____

_____

18. Self-contained breathing apparatus are manufactured by several companies. Similar parts available from different manufactures are interchangeable. Is it advisable to interchange such parts? Why or why not?

_____

_____

_____

_____

19. What are some advantages of using airline equipment?

_____

_____

_____

_____

20. Why is a closed-circuit SCBA sometimes called a "rebreather" apparatus?

_____

_____

_____

_____

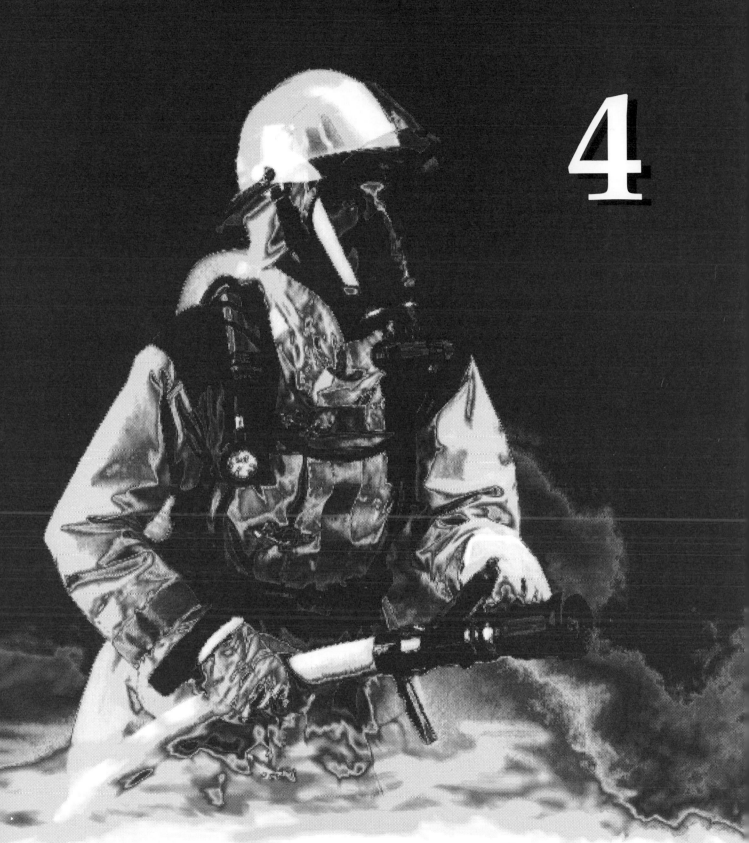

4

Safety And Training

This chapter provides information that addresses the following standards:

NFPA STANDARD 1001
Fire Fighter Professional Qualifications
1987 Edition

Chapter 3—Fire Fighter I
3-6.2
3-6.5
3-6.6

NFPA STANDARD 1404
Fire Department Self-Contained Breathing Apparatus Program
1989 Edition

Chapter 1—Introduction
1-4.4
1-4.5
1-4.6
1-4.6.1

Chapter 2—Provisions of SCBA
2-3.2
2-4.1
2-4.2

Chapter 4—SCBA Training

4-1.1	4-4.2
4-1.2	4-4.3
4-1.3	4-5
4-2.3	4-6
4-2.4	4-7
4-2.6	4-9
4-2.7	4-10
4-2.8	4-12.1
4-3.1	4-12.2
4-3.2	4-12.3
4-3.3	4-13
4-3.4	4-14
4-4.1	

Chapter 8—Program Evaluation
8-1.1
8-1.2
8-1.3
8-1.4

NFPA STANDARD 1500
Fire Department Occupational Safety and Health Program
1987 Edition

Chapter 3—Training and Education
3-1.1
3-1.2

3-1.3
3-1.4
3-1.5
3-4.2
3-4.3
3-4.4
3-4.5

Chapter 5—Protective Clothing and Protective Equipment
5-1.3
5-2.5
5-3.9
5-3.10
5-4.1

Chapter 6—Emergency Operations
6-3.1

ANSI STANDARD Z88.5-1981
Practices for Respiratory Protection for the Fire Service

Section 3—SCBA Program
3.1.1	3.2.1
3.1.2	3.2.2
3.1.3	3.2.3
3.1.4	3.2.4
3.1.5	

Section 6—Maintenance of SCBA
6.1.1
6.1.2
6.3.1

Section 7—Fitting of SCBA Facepieces
7.1
7.2
7.2.1
7.2.2
7.3
7.4
7.5
7.5.1
7.5.2

Section 8—Training and Education in Proper Use of SCBA
8.1
8.1.1
8.1.2
8.1.3
8.1.4
8.2
8.3

Section 9—Special Problems

9.1

9.2

9.3

9.4

9.5

9.6

9.7

Section 10—Program Evaluation

10.2

10.4

10.5

ANSI STANDARD Z88.2-1980
Practices for Respiratory Protection

Section 3—Respirator Program Requirements

3.3.1	3.5.1
3.3.2	3.5.6
3.3.3	3.5.7
3.4.1	3.5.8
3.4.2	3.5.10
3.4.3	3.5.14

Section 6—Selection of Respirators

6.11

6.12

Section 7—Use of Respirators

7.1	7.3.4
7.2	7.3.5
7.2.3	7.3.6
7.2.3.1	7.3.7
7.3	7.3.8
7.3.1	7.4
7.3.2	7.6
7.3.3	

Section 9—Special Problems

9.1

9.2

9.3

9.5

9.6

Section 10—Evaluation of Respirator Program Effectiveness

10.1

10.3

Code of Federal Regulations
Title 29, Part 1910

Section 120—Hazardous Waste Operations and Emergency Response

Section 134—Respiratory Protection

Chapter 4
Safety and Training

INTRODUCTION

SCBA safety and training are so closely interrelated that one cannot be discussed without discussing the other. Firefighters need to be trained in correct procedures for using SCBA and must be confident of their abilities in order for SCBA to be both safe and effective. Proper training and skill mastery help firefighters avoid or reduce injuries and survive life-threatening situations. On the other hand, lack of training — or failing to wear SCBA in hazardous atmospheres — can result in serious injury or even death.

Even with the best possible SCBA, firefighters can be seriously or fatally injured if they have not been properly trained or do not follow safety procedures. NFPA 1404, *Standard for a Fire Department Self-Contained Breathing Apparatus Program*, states the minimum requirements for a fire service respiratory protection program. (**NOTE:** An example of a fire department SCBA program is given in Appendix C.) This standard should be referenced for all SCBA training programs. In addition, every fire department should have a policy for mandatory SCBA use. This policy should be introduced and enforced in training.

The Phoenix (Arizona) Fire Department discovered the significance of SCBA use within five years of starting its mandatory SCBA program. Before starting the program in 1974, the department averaged 34 respiratory injuries a year, many of them requiring hospitalization and lost time. But during the five years following the institution of mandatory SCBA use, **not one firefighter** lost time from smoke inhalation or contact with toxic materials.

Recruit firefighters begin learning about SCBA the day they enter the fire service, sometimes from overheard station house comments. But for firefighters to adequately learn about SCBA requires formal training. Formal training should go beyond knowing basic fire fighting skills and learning how to don and doff the apparatus. Firefighters must be certain of their fire fighting skills, but they must also be aware of their capabilities and limitations and know when to avoid overextending themselves. They should have the same awareness of their psychological abilities and limitations. Firefighters who receive comprehensive SCBA training built on a foundation of pre-incident planning and basic fire fighting skills have confidence in their abilities. This confidence helps them use SCBA safely.

SCBA training should do more than make firefighters proficient with their equipment. Training should take into consideration the psychology of SCBA use — the anxieties produced when the human body is reliant on a mechanical source of breathing air. Training should make firefighters aware of how their bodies work when they breathe and how contaminants can damage the respiratory and circulatory systems. Training should teach firefighters how to breathe properly while wearing SCBA. In short, training that covers the mental as well as the mechanical aspects of SCBA use gives firefighters a psychological edge: confidence in their equipment and the ability to concentrate on the task at hand without the nagging fear that they or their equipment will fail.

A planned program is required that teaches firefighters to use SCBA step by step, focuses on safety, builds confidence, and reduces apprehension. This chapter will focus on how these training and safety goals can be met by both the firefighter and the department. Firefighters who have gradually become accustomed to the circumstances in which they will work show fewer signs of stress and act calmly, confidently, and safely in emergency situations.

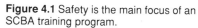

Figure 4.1 Safety is the main focus of an SCBA training program.

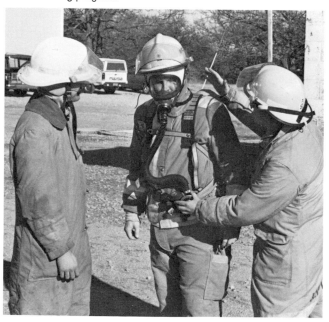

GENERAL SAFETY

All aspects of an SCBA training program should focus on safety (Figure 4.1). Safety procedures should be drilled and practiced until they become second nature to each firefighter. Trainees should be taught that using SCBA safely includes donning and wearing the apparatus properly, following established safety procedures while at the incident, and maintaining the apparatus in proper working order.

Facial And Long Hair

In order to seal properly, the facepiece must fit against the bare skin. Long sideburns, mustaches, beards, or hair over the forehead that comes in contact with the seal prevents the facepiece from sealing properly. There is evidence that even a one-day growth of beard can cause an ill-fitting facepiece (Figure 4.2). Most departments have written policies regarding hair length and facial hair. OSHA, NIOSH, NFPA, and ANSI all require or recommend that firefighters wear short hair and be clean shaven.

Protective Clothing

Today, more departments than before issue protective hoods for use by firefighters. A hood protects the neck and ears from burns. In order for the hood to be effective, the facepiece should be donned first, with the protective hood donned over it. The helmet should fit snugly but comfortably over the hood and facepiece straps (Figure 4.3). Nothing should interfere with the head straps or the seal of the facepiece.

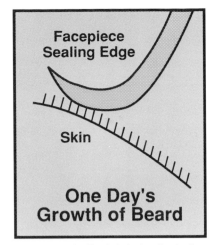

Figure 4.2 Facial hair, including sideburns, mustaches, beards, hair over the forehead, and even a one-day growth of beard can prevent a facepiece from sealing properly. *Courtesy of the International Association of Fire Fighters.*

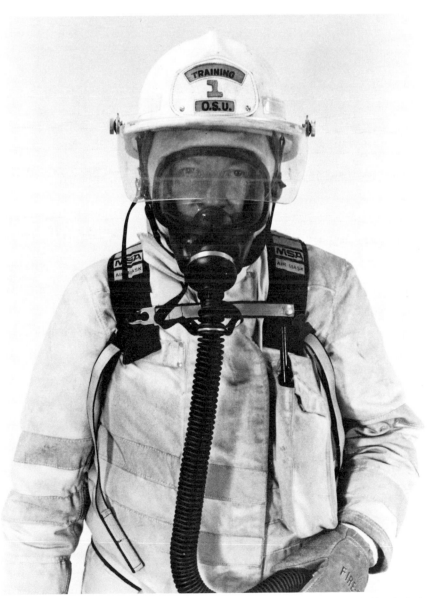

Figure 4.3 Along with a proper fitting facepiece, the firefighter's protective clothing includes hood and helmet. The hood and helmet are donned after the facepiece for maximum effectiveness.

Donning

SCBA must always be donned and airflow started in fresh air. The practice of firefighters rigging up in fresh air but not putting on their facepieces and starting their regulators until they reach the smoky or other hazardous atmosphere is extremely dangerous and should be prohibited.

Eyeglasses And Contact Lenses

Presently OSHA and ANSI standards prohibit firefighters from wearing contact lenses while using a respirator. This regulation has been repeatedly challenged by users, however. In 1985, OSHA reevaluated their position after funding a study conducted by Robert A. da Roza and Catherine Weaver of the Lawrence Livermore National Laboratory, Livermore, California.

Weaver and da Roza surveyed 9,100 firefighters in the United States and Canada regarding their use of contact lenses with SCBA. Of the 403 respondents who wore contacts despite the regulation, 6 reported that contact lens-related problems had caused them to remove the facepiece in an environment in which the facepiece would normally have been worn. However, 30 respondents reported safety-related problems regarding mask-mounted eyeglasses (which are legal) in SCBA. The researchers concluded that the prohibition against wearing contacts while using SCBA should be discontinued.

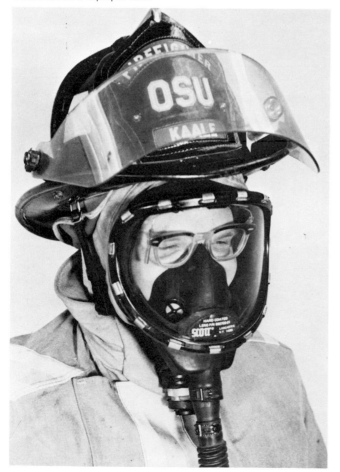

Figure 4.4 Firefighters wearing eyeglasses use special holders mounted inside the facepiece; regular temple bars would not allow a proper seal.

Based on the results of the Livermore study and the review of other reports and studies, OSHA intends to modify the regulation (1910.134) to permit firefighters to use soft, extended-wear contact lenses with SCBA. The issue with nongas-permeable, hard contact lenses will also be resolved in the revision effort, which is presently underway. Until the revised regulation is printed, OSHA will follow an interim enforcement policy that states:

"Violations of the respirator standard involving the use of gas-permeable and soft contact lenses shall continue to be documented in the case file and recorded as *de minimis* [the smallest infraction]; citations shall not be issued."

For those firefighters needing corrected vision, special holders inside the facepiece are made for eyeglasses (Figure 4.4). Regular eyeglasses, of course, cannot be worn because the temple bars do not permit a proper seal.

Use In High Or Low Temperatures

Firefighters should have special training to make them aware of the complications that can result from using SCBA in high or low temperatures. For an additional discussion of SCBA use in high and low temperatures, see the section on temperature extremes in Chapter 8, Using SCBA.

Accidental Submersion

Firefighters should have special training to prepare them for survival should they fall into water while wearing SCBA. For a detailed discussion of correct procedures for accidental submersion, see Chapter 9, Emergency Conditions Breathing.

Communication

Wearing SCBA may decrease the firefighter's ability to communicate. This can cause problems because messages, orders, or warnings may not be heard or understood. While a portable radio held against the facepiece can keep a firefighter in radio contact, it ties up the firefighter's hands and can be inconvenient (Figure 4.5). State-of-the art technology now provides users of certain brands of SCBA with attachable or built-in radios (Figure 4.6). In addition, some manufacturers have built speaking diaphragms into the apparatus to improve communications. Electronic devices that amplify the voice are also available. Refer to Chapter 3, Types of SCBA, for details on SCBA accessories that improve communications.

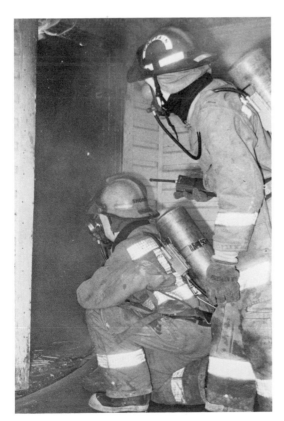

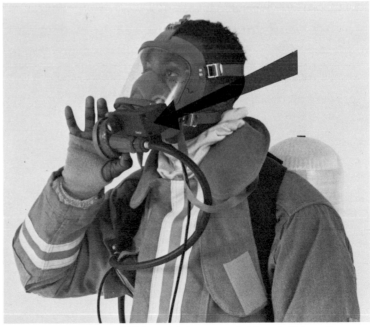

Figure 4.6 Some newer SCBA models have attachable or built-in radios.

Figure 4.5 A portable radio is one method of communication while wearing SCBA, but it can be inconvenient because it ties up the firefighter's hands.

In addition to these communications methods, a hand signaling system can be used. Specific hand signals should be written into the department policies and procedures so that the system is standardized. All firefighters should be taught to use and recognize the signals.

Working In Teams

Firefighters wearing SCBA should *always* operate in teams of two. Team members should *never* leave their partners. When one team member has to leave the area because of low air or problems with the apparatus, his or her partner must also leave. The team should also have a way to communicate with the outside. Contact can be made by face-to-face visual or verbal communications or by lifeline/guide line or radio.

Personal Alert Safety Systems (PASS)

Personal alert safety systems (PASS) sound an audible alarm when the firefighter remains motionless for a predetermined length of time. This loud alarm alerts other firefighters that a fellow firefighter is in trouble and may be injured. Many departments attach the PASS device to the harness of the SCBA rather than allowing the firefighter to carry the PASS in a pocket (Figure 4.7). Firefighters should be trained to activate the PASS device when they don an SCBA. NFPA 1982, *Standard on Personal Alert Safety Systems (PASS) for Fire Fighters*, specifies minimum performance standards for PASS devices.

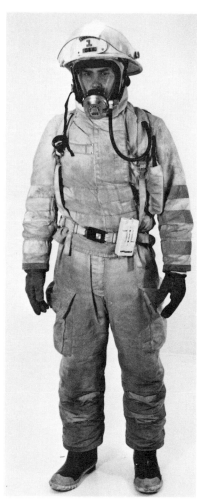

Figure 4.7 A personal alert safety system (PASS) device attached directly to the harness of the SCBA. Some firefighters carry them in a pocket.

Doffing

The firefighter should *not* take off the facepiece nor remove the SCBA as soon as the fire is out or knocked down. There are still toxic gases in the air, and there may not be enough oxygen for the firefighter to breathe. SCBA must always be worn inside buildings during overhaul. Firefighters should doff their SCBA only after buildings are well ventilated with fresh air and it has been established through monitoring or air sampling that toxic gases have been removed and the atmosphere is not oxygen deficient. This rule applies also to removing the facepiece in confined spaces, below ground level, or in *any* situation where the possibility of a contaminated atmosphere exists. The rule of thumb should be: *"When in doubt, wear SCBA."*

Physical Conditioning

Firefighters must be in top physical shape to meet the demands of fire fighting. The firefighter with healthy cardiovascular and respiratory systems has more stamina when wearing SCBA and is less likely to suffer respiratory distress or cardiovascular problems than the firefighter whose respiratory system is damaged by smoking or whose cardiovascular system is taxed by obesity. Proper diet, physical conditioning, and not smoking help make wearing SCBA safe (Figure 4.8).

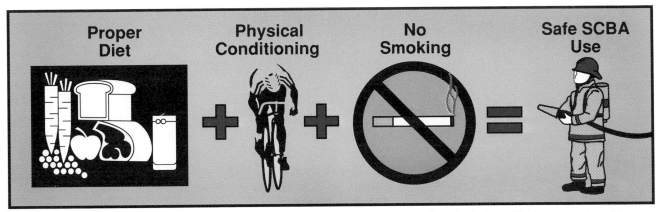

Figure 4.8 The keys to top physical fitness, which equals safe SCBA use, include proper diet, physical conditioning, and not smoking.

THE FIREFIGHTER'S SAFETY RESPONSIBILITIES

Safety is the responsibility of both the individual firefighter wearing SCBA in a hazardous atmosphere and of the fire department official monitoring or directing operations at the scene of an emergency. Both must know their responsibilities if firefighters are to perform their jobs safely and efficiently. The firefighter's SCBA safety responsibilities include the following:

- Using the provided SCBA in accordance with instructions and training
- Knowing SCBA protection limits and safety features
- Knowing air supply duration
- Calculating point of no return
- Ensuring facepiece fit
- Following basic safety guidelines
- Protecting the SCBA from damage as appropriate
- Reporting any malfunctions or damage
- Inspecting and maintaining the SCBA in accordance with department standard operating procedures (SOPs)

Knowing SCBA Protection Limits And Safety Features

The firefighter's first responsibility is to know what SCBA can and cannot do. Although SCBA protects firefighters from most hazardous atmospheres and from inhaling superheated air, it cannot protect them from certain toxic gases or chemicals, radioactive materials that can be absorbed through the skin, or contaminated air entering the respiratory tract through ruptured or punctured eardrums. For protection from these hazards, firefighters must wear proper protective equipment and use appropriate procedures. Additionally, the firefighter must be thoroughly familiar with warning devices required on SCBA.

Knowing Air Supply Duration

SCBA are rated by their air supply duration. Firefighters must know how much air is available in their breathing apparatus and must know their individual air consumption rates under various conditions *prior* to an actual emergency.

Air supply duration in SCBA generally ranges from 30 minutes to 1 hour. Longer-duration SCBA that can provide protection for up to 4 hours are also available. The type of apparatus — open-circuit or closed-circuit — also has an impact on air supply duration. Closed-circuit apparatus are capable of providing longer-duration air supply than open-circuit apparatus. Refer to Chapter 3 for a more in-depth discussion of SCBA air supply.

When using open-circuit breathing apparatus, firefighters should realize that the ratings seldom correspond to the time they can actually use the equipment. Hard work uses up the air supply much faster than the rating indicates. Controlled breathing techniques — consciously reducing air consumption by forcing exhalation from the mouth and allowing natural inhalation through the nose — stretch the air supply somewhat. However, the working air supply usually depends on the firefighter's training, physical condition, activity, and mental state under the stressful conditions of an emergency.

Calculating Point Of No Return

Firefighters in hazardous atmospheres must always be aware of how much air they have remaining for use. Cylinders should always be fully charged before the firefighter enters the danger area. As the firefighter enters the hazardous atmosphere, readings on the air cylinder and regulator pressure gauges should correspond with each other. Once in the hazardous atmosphere, the firefighter must listen for signals from the low-pressure alarm that the unit is low on air. Then the firefighter must know how much time is left to get out of the area when the alarm sounds. The low-pressure alarm sounds a warning when approximately 20 to 25 percent of the air supply is left.

However, *the low-pressure alarm should not be depended on to warn the firefighter in time for a safe exit.* In most residential fires, the low-pressure warning bell is adequate to signal the point of no return because the firefighter should be able to exit a house-sized structure easily after the alarm sounds. However, in large structures — shopping malls, warehouses, high-rise buildings — the firefighter may need more time to exit than would be allowed if the firefighter relied solely on the low-pressure alarm. This situation is compounded for hazardous materials teams working in encapsulated suits requiring decontamination. OSHA 1910.120 *Standard for Hazardous Waste Operations and Emergency Response* (HAZWOPER) requires that a designated person monitor responding hazardous materials team members and calculate their remaining air supply in order to determine at which point they should be recalled. NFPA 1404 also requires that a designated person monitor fire fighting teams inside a structure and calculate their remaining air supply. See "Monitoring Systems in the United States and Canada" in this chapter for more details on monitoring SCBA teams at the incident scene.

Despite a required monitoring system, however, each firefighter is responsible for determining his or her individual point of no return. A simple method for determining the point of no return is for the firefighter to check the pressure gauge before entering the contaminated atmosphere and again on arrival at the objective (Figure 4.9). The amount of air the firefighter used to get to the objective is the *least* amount needed to get back to a nonhazardous atmosphere. However, a calculated consumption rate is more accurate and is recommended over the simpler method because it takes more variables into consideration.

Generally, firefighters learn to calculate their own consumption rates in SCBA training courses. This is accomplished by

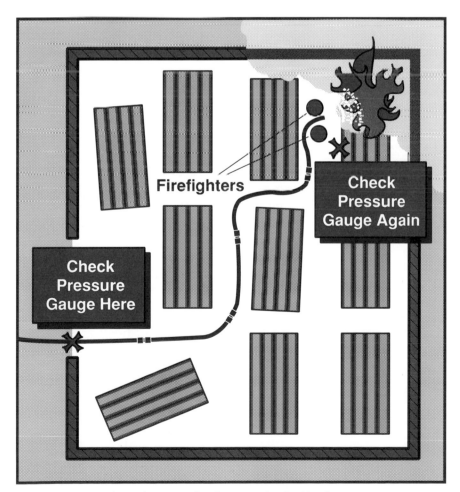

Figure 4.9 Always determine your point of no return by checking the pressure gauge as you enter and again when you arrive at the interior objective. At minimum, allow at *least* as much air for escape as has been used to reach the objective.

having the firefighter use several cylinders of air while working vigorously — the work punctuated with appropriate rest breaks. The idea is to simulate the body stresses of a working fire so that the firefighter can find the *average* time it takes him or her to consume a cylinder of air. For example, if Firefighter Tom Waters consumes six full cylinders of air, and the average time each cylinder lasts is 18 minutes, then Tom's individual consumption rate is 2,250 psi (15 525 kPa) divided by 18 minutes, or 125 psi/min (863 kPa/min).

When a firefighter's individual air consumption rate is known, the firefighter can then predict how many minutes of air he or she has available at any given time and can determine the point of no return. Knowing individual air consumption rates also allows firefighters to watch the regulator pressure gauge and pace themselves accordingly. Firefighters must know their individual consumption rates and know how to calculate their point of no return *before* participating in any live fire training or responding to an actual emergency.

Ensuring Facepiece Fit

Firefighters are also responsible for making sure that their facepieces fit well enough to keep out hazardous atmospheres. It is recommended that firefighters test their facepiece fit each time before entering a hazardous atmosphere or anytime they have a change in their facial characteristics. Testing for facepiece fit and for positive pressure are covered in Chapter 5, Donning and Doffing.

Figure 4.10 Firefighters following basic safety guidelines always work in groups of at least two people.

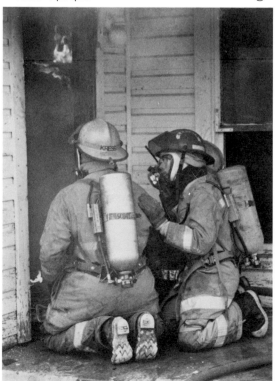

Following Basic Safety Guidelines

Firefighters are responsible for knowing and applying the following basic safety rules when wearing SCBA:

- Before entering a hazardous atmosphere, don the apparatus, start the airflow, and *make sure that the equipment is operating properly*.
- Always *work in pairs* (Figure 4.10).
- *Stay in contact* with a wall, hoseline, lifeline/ guide line, or SCBA team member.
- *Work to control breathing* and conserve air.
- *Be extremely cautious* if forced to breathe through the bypass valve, and exit immediately.
- *Do not take off the facepiece* while still in a hazardous atmosphere.
- *Report any malfunctions or apparent damage*, and immediately take the unit out of service.

THE DEPARTMENT'S RESPONSIBILITIES AT THE STATION

The department is responsible for creating a written SCBA/respiratory protection program that meets the standards set out in NFPA 1404 and OSHA 1910.134(b). In addition, it should have and should enforce written standard operating procedures (SOPs) for training, use, and testing of SCBA and related equipment. Department SOPs should stress mandatory SCBA use. All personnel who use SCBA should be made familiar with the department's SOPs and be required to follow them. An example of an SCBA SOP is shown in Appendix D.

The department's responsibilities at the station include the following:

- Creating a written SCBA/respiratory protection program

- Enforcing written SOPs

- Qualitatively or quantitatively testing facepiece fit at least once a year

- Keeping fit test records

- Keeping facepiece records

- Keeping inspection, maintenance, and repair records

- Following general safety guidelines in the training of personnel, the purchase of SCBA, the maintenance of records, and the maintenance, upgrading, transportation, and storage of SCBA

Testing Facepiece Fit

The department is responsible for conducting annual facepiece fit testing as required by NFPA 1404 and 1500. Department fit tests may be qualitative or quantitative, although OSHA 1910.134 recommends that only quantitative fit testing provides adequate wearer protection. In addition, while ANSI Z88.2 (6.11)-1980 does not require any fit testing for positive-pressure respirators, NFPA requires at least one qualitative facepiece fit test annually.

QUALITATIVE FACEPIECE FIT TESTS

Qualitative fit tests involve a test subject's response (either voluntary or involuntary) to a chemical outside the respirator facepiece. These tests are fast, easy to perform, and use inexpensive equipment. However, because they are based on the respirator wearer's subjective response to the test substance, accuracy may vary. Three of the most popular qualitative facepiece fit test methods are the irritant smoke test, the odorous vapor test, and the taste test.

Irritant Smoke Test. This qualitative fume test is a subjective test used for yearly or periodic tests of facepiece-to-face seal. The test is conducted in a well-ventilated room, and the smoke for the test usually comes from a stannic or titanium tetrachloride smoke tube. The following procedure is used:

Step 1: Ensure that the firefighter to be tested dons the SCBA in fresh air and starts the flow of breathing air.

Step 2: Enter the well-ventilated room chosen for testing. Instruct the wearer to close his or her eyes and to keep them closed for the duration of the test. (The wearer's eyes must be kept closed because the smoke is an eye irritant.)

Step 3: Activate the smoke tube.

Step 4: Pass the smoke tube over the firefighter's facepiece from about 2 feet (0.6 m) away.

Step 5: Gradually move the tube closer while making sure that the wearer is not feeling any discomfort. (If the smoke penetrates the seal, the wearer will usually react involuntarily by coughing or sneezing.)

Step 6: If the wearer does not react to the smoke fumes when the smoke tube is 6 inches (150 mm) from the facepiece, move the tube close to areas around the facepiece that are likely to leak: under the chin and near the cheeks, temples, and forehead.

Step 7: Direct the wearer to breathe deeply, turn or nod the head, or talk to make sure that the facepiece does not leak.

Step 8: If the smoke penetrates the seal, have the wearer redon or adjust the facepiece in fresh air and perform the test a second time.

Step 9: If smoke still penetrates the seal, the facepiece fit is unsatisfactory.

Odorous Vapor Test. The odor test is another simple check used yearly or periodically for proper facepiece seal. However, the odor test is less foolproof and may be more stressful than the smoke test. Isoamyl acetate (banana oil) is most commonly used. Some people become sick with the smell of banana oil. In addition, although most people can smell a banana oil concentration as low as 0.1 percent, some firefighters may not be able to smell the banana odor as well as others. The following procedure is used:

Step 1: Check the firefighter's ability to detect the odor agent several hours before the fit test.

Step 2: Ensure that the firefighter to be tested dons the SCBA in fresh air and starts the flow of breathing air.

Step 3: Enter the well-ventilated room where testing is to take place.

Step 4: Dampen a cloth or sponge with isoamyl acetate and pass the cloth or sponge near areas of potential leaks in the facepiece.

Step 5: Direct the wearer to breathe deeply, turn or nod the head, or talk to make sure that the facepiece does not leak.

Step 6: If the banana oil odor can be detected by the wearer, have the wearer redon or adjust the facepiece in fresh air and perform the test a second time.

Step 7: If the odor still penetrates the seal, the facepiece fit is unsatisfactory.

Taste Test. The taste test is another simple qualitative test. This test relies on the respirator wearer detecting the taste of a chemical substance — usually sodium saccharin — inside the respirator. The taste test is the least reliable of the qualitative tests because there is no involuntary response, and individual taste thresholds vary widely. The following procedure is used:

Step 1: Instruct the firefighter being tested not to smoke, eat, drink, or chew gum or tobacco for 15 minutes before the test.

Step 2: Fill an atomizer (a clean plant mister may be used) with the sodium saccharin solution.

Step 3: Ensure that the firefighter to be tested dons the SCBA in fresh air and starts the flow of breathing air.

Step 4: Enclose the respirator wearer's head and shoulders in a hood (a large plastic bag works well).

Step 5: Spray the saccharin solution into the enclosed space under the hood.

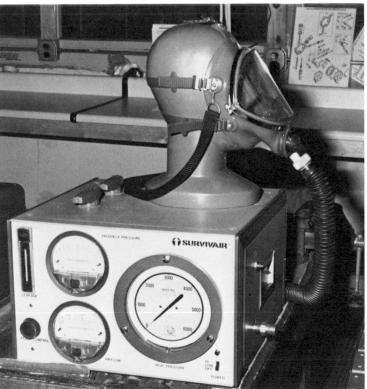

Figure 4.11 A portable test machine used for quantitative tests of facepiece seal.

Step 6: If the saccharin taste is detected by the wearer, have the wearer redon or adjust the facepiece in fresh air and perform the test a second time.

Step 7: If the taste can still be detected, the facepiece fit is unsatisfactory.

QUANTITATIVE FACEPIECE FIT TESTS

Because all qualitative fit testing is subjective, quantitative fit tests are better — although much more expensive and complex — methods of testing facepiece seal. In quantitative tests, the respirator is equipped with a sampling probe, which is connected with flexible tubing to a portable (Figure 4.11) or nonportable test instrument. While wearing the probe-equipped respirator in a controlled test atmosphere (a test chamber containing a required concentration of test agent), the wearer performs a series of required exercises. The test instrument records test agent facepiece penetration values in parts per million (ppm). These values are then converted to a protection factor that indicates how well the facepiece is sealed.

Because quantitative fit testing is highly technical and requires specific testing agents, test atmospheres, test booth designs, and exacting mathematical computations, it is recommended that fire departments have the testing done by personnel trained by the test machine manufacturer. For a general quantitative test procedure, refer to ANSI Z88.2-1980.

Firefighters must not be sent into a hazardous atmosphere with SCBA unless they have been fit-tested annually, either qualitatively or quantitatively. If a facepiece-to-face seal cannot be obtained, the cause must be determined and the problem remedied. The most common causes of seal failure are facial hair, a change in the facial contour, or improper facepiece size. After the cause of the failure has been remedied, the fit test should be conducted again.

Record Keeping
FIT TEST RECORDS

It is important to keep records of all fit tests. Information should include the firefighter's name, the type of test used, the makes, models, and facepiece sizes of SCBA used, and the results of the tests. A fit test assures that an individual is capable of getting a seal with a particular facepiece, brand, or model. All fit test records should be retained for an extended period of time, the same as are medical records of the employee.

FACEPIECE RECORDS

Department officers are responsible for keeping accurate and complete records for each SCBA facepiece. These records should include inventory or serial numbers, date of purchase, location, maintenance and repairs, replacement parts, upgrading, and test performance.

INSPECTION, MAINTENANCE, AND REPAIR RECORDS

The department is responsible for establishing an SCBA maintenance program in accordance with NFPA 1404 and ANSI Z88.5. This program should be reflected in the department's SOPs and should include the following record-keeping responsibilities:

- Maintaining an inventory of SCBA adequate to provide one SCBA to each department member who may be exposed to respiratory hazards.

- Maintaining individual records of each SCBA cylinder, regulator and harness assembly, and facepiece.

- Establishing a replacement and upgrading program in compliance with NFPA 1981, *Standard on Open-Circuit Self-Contained Breathing Apparatus for Fire Fighters.*

- Maintaining records for each air compressor, fill station, cascade cylinder, purification system, and related equipment used to produce or store breathing air. The record should contain the date of purchase, location, inspection, maintenance, and testing of the device.

See Chapter 6, Inspection, Care, and Testing of SCBA, for a more detailed discussion of a preventive maintenance program.

Following General Safety Guidelines

Overall, the department is responsible for purchasing SCBA; training personnel; maintaining records; and maintaining, upgrading, transporting, and providing safe storage for all department SCBA and related equipment. The following general guidelines should be followed:

CLEANING AND SANITIZING
- Train firefighters in the department's SOPs for cleaning and sanitizing.

- Ensure that facepiece cleaning and sanitizing is performed after each use.

- Provide firefighters with cleansers recommended by the manufacturer to clean and sanitize facepieces.

- Maintain inventory so that extra facepieces and breathing hoses are available to replace those being cleaned.

INSPECTION AND TESTING FOR DEFECTS
- Train firefighters in the department's SOPs for inspection.

- Inspect all new SCBA and related equipment for defects before placing them in service.

- Ensure that routine, after use, monthly, and annual inspections are performed by trained personnel.

- Have breathing air quality tested every three months by a qualified laboratory.

- Keep accurate records of air quality tests.

- Remove any defective SCBA from service.

REPAIR AND RECONDITIONING
- Carry out replacement or repairs in strict accordance with the manufacturer's instructions.

- Allow repairs only by personnel certified by the SCBA manufacturer.

- Use exact replacement parts purchased from the manufacturer.

- Use a person trained or certified by the manufacturer to recondition or rebuild an SCBA.

STORAGE

- Train firefighters in the department's SOPs for storage.
- Rigidly follow the manufacturer's instructions for storing individual units after each use.
- Ensure that straps are in good condition *and fully extended* before storing.
- Thoroughly train personnel handling storage cylinders.
- Store air cylinders securely above ground in dry, cool, well-ventilated, and fire-resistant places (Figure 4.12).
- Place the storage rack or locate the storage area out of the way so that the cylinders cannot be accidentally hit, cut, punctured, or dented.
- Locate and store the breathing-air compressor in an area free from contamination.
- Be sure that cylinders do not touch electrical sources.

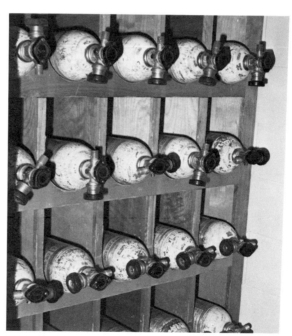

Figure 4.12 Air cylinders properly stored at a fire station.

RECHARGING

- Train personnel according to the department's SOPs for recharging.
- Avoid dropping or abusing the air cylinder in any way.
- Before recharging individual SCBA, be sure that the storage cylinders are secured.
- Never bang on sticky valve wheels with hammers. Instead, check with the manufacturer for the proper procedure for opening the valve.

- Be sure that connections are tight (without forcing them) and that the hoses are in good condition.

- Close the cylinder valve and release air pressure in the regulator before removing it from the cylinder.

See Chapter 7, Air Cylinder Recharging Systems, for more safety precautions to take while recharging individual air cylinders.

THE DEPARTMENT'S SAFETY RESPONSIBILITIES AT THE EMERGENCY SCENE

The department is responsible for monitoring the activities of firefighters using SCBA at the incident scene. Officers must know where SCBA wearers are at all times and are responsible for providing relief personnel when necessary.

At incidents having hazardous atmospheres, all departments should assign an officer to keep track of those firefighters using SCBA, as required by OSHA 1910. A monitoring system should be designed so that a designated officer knows at all times which firefighter has entered the hazardous area, when the firefighter entered the hazardous area, where the firefighter is going, how long the air supply should last, and when the firefighter should be ready for relief. Such a system reduces losses from smoke inhalation, protects firefighters from injury, and facilitates search and rescue for a downed firefighter if it becomes necessary.

Entry Control

A model monitoring system is used throughout the United Kingdom (U.K.), and similar systems are used in Australia and New Zealand. In all three systems, each SCBA comes equipped with an information tally that the wearer fills in and hands to an entry control officer as the firefighter enters a hazardous area (Figure 4.13). The officer slides the tally into a slot on a control board, writes down the time the firefighter went in, and calculates — by using a table on the control board (see Figure 4.14 on next page) — the approximate time the firefighter's low-pressure alarm should sound. Firefighters leaving the danger area take back their tallies so that the control officer knows who is safely outside and

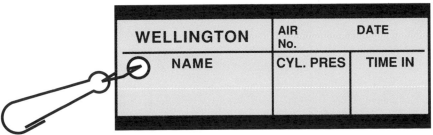

Figure 4.13 An SCBA information tally for entry control. Completed by New Zealand firefighter and given to breathing apparatus control officer before the firefighter enters the building. *Courtesy of New Zealand Fire College.*

who is still in the danger area. Relief crews are sent in before the time estimated for the low-pressure alarm to sound.

At a major fire covering a large building or area or when more than one entry point is used, several control boards may be set up

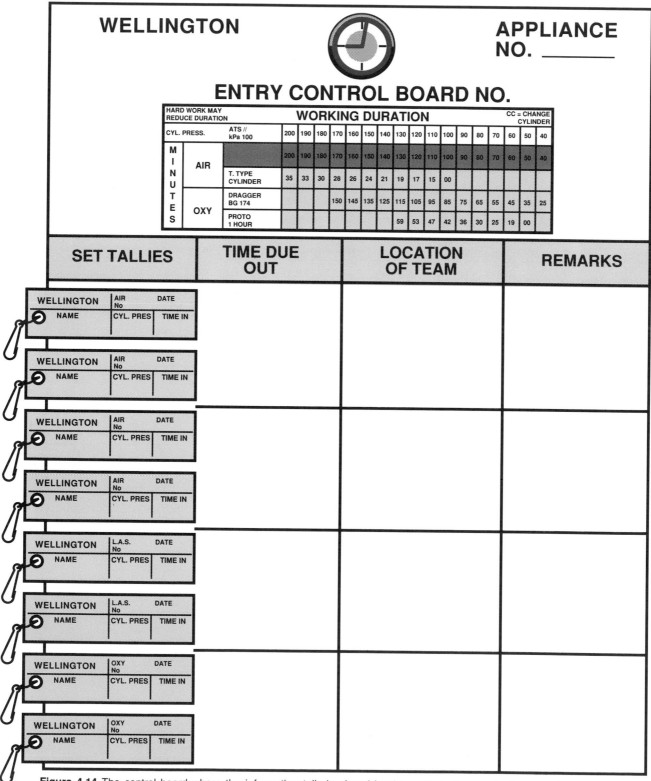

Figure 4.14 The control board where the information tally is placed by the control officer; entry times and point-of-no-return calculations are recorded for each firefighter. *Courtesy of New Zealand Fire College.*

and used by control officers wearing color-coded armbands printed with contrasting identifying initials (i.e., E.C.O. for Entry Control Officer; B.A. for Breathing Apparatus). Another officer stationed at a main control board coordinates efforts if necessary (Figure 4.15). This officer keeps in touch with the assistant control officers and makes sure that relief crews are on hand when needed. For instance, the Australian Control Officer is responsible for having at least two other firefighters rigged in SCBA and standing by for emergency purposes.

Guide Line System

In addition to the entry control system, United Kingdom, Australian, and New Zealand departments use an SCBA guide line system. In this system, firefighters use a series of guide ropes

NEW ZEALAND FIRE SERVICE BREATHING APPARATUS CONTROL BOARD						
OFFICER IN CHARGE OF INCIDENT _____ LOCATION _____ COMMUNICATION _____						
ENTRY CONTROL POINT	COMM	LOCATION	NO OF SETS IN USE AIR OXY AIRLINE	RELIEFS REQUIRED SENT NO TYPE TIME NO TYPE TIME	NOTES	
1 ECO						
2 ECO						
3 ECO						
4 ECO						
5 ECO						

EMERGENCY STAND-BY CREWS				BA OPERATORS			
NO OF OPERATORS	SETS AIR OXY	STAND-BY LOCATION	NOTES		AIR	OXY	AIRLINE
				WORKING			
				AT INCIDENT			
				RELIEFS AVAIL			
				RESERVES REQ			

BREATHING APPARATUS AVAILABILITY							FIRE GROUND
TYPE	TOTAL BRIGADE AREA	AT INCIDENT IN USE BRIG AREA	RESERVES BRIG AREA	RECHARGING LOCATION NO EST RETURN HOW SENT			
CABA	SETS CYL				hrs		
OXY 1 HR	SETS CYL				hrs		
OXY 2 HR	SETS CYL				hrs		
INSPECTION SETS	SETS CYL				hrs		
	SETS CYL				hrs		
AIRLINES				REMARKS			
CHEMICAL SUITS							
AMMONIA SUITS							

Figure 4.15 The master control board used at large incidents when several entry points and control boards are needed. The officer at this board coordinates relief crews. *Courtesy of New Zealand Fire College.*

and personal ropes to stay together, make searches more methodical and thorough, and provide escape and rescue routes. The guide line is a special rope that may be used either as a main guide line to indicate a route between the entry control point and the scene of operations or as a branch line (personal line) when it is necessary to traverse or search deeply off the main guide line. Guide lines are unnecessary when an SCBA team lays a hoseline or while in single-unit residential and other small premises.

Using the guide line system, the first SCBA team leader to enter the danger area carries a rope coiled in a container on his or her back. The line is attached to an immovable object outside the emergency area and reels out as the team leader advances. The second team member secures the rope at different intervals at a convenient height from the ground. The tie-off points are spaced at sufficient intervals to keep the line off the ground.

Firefighters mark the guide rope at its source with lettered disks (Figure 4.16). Inside, the team leader can tie the 200-foot (60-m) guide rope to an object so that other teams can follow it to the area of operations. Other firefighters, when they see the guide rope, know the route to follow to the initial team and know that the area is being searched or has already been searched.

Individual firefighters have 20-foot (6-m) personal ropes that they can snap to the guide rope. If they have to move farther than 20 feet (6 m) from the guide rope, they can call for secondary guide ropes (branch lines) to follow through other parts of the emergency area. Branch guide lines are identified with cards or disks punched with different numbers of holes so that firefighters can feel them in dark, smoky atmospheres (Figure 4.17). Each guide rope is spliced every 8 feet (2.4 m) with two cords that dangle down a few inches (millimeters) apart. One cord is longer than the other; the shorter cord indicates the direction of safety (Figure 4.18).

Monitoring Systems In The United States And Canada

Unlike the U.K., the United States and Canada do not have specific, standardized SCBA monitoring systems. Each fire department is responsible for developing its own comprehensive

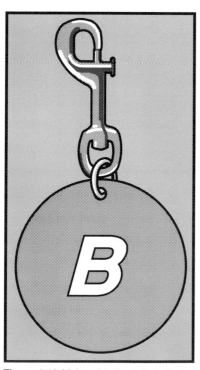

Figure 4.16 Main guide line tally indicator used in the guide line system.

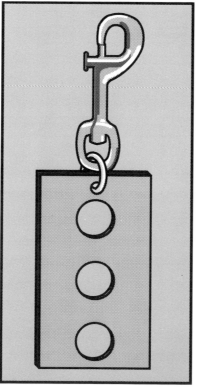

Figure 4.17 Branch line tally punched with holes for firefighters to feel in the dark.

SCBA incident scene monitoring system and SOPs to meet OSHA 1910 and NFPA 1404, which require the monitoring of personnel wearing SCBA.

NFPA 1404 designates that "at least one person must remain outside the area where respiratory protection is being used." This person — variously known as the Breathing Apparatus Officer or the Breathing Apparatus Monitor — is responsible for knowing the number and identity of all personnel using SCBA, their location and function in the fire building, and their entry time. Some departments have each firefighter report his or her assignment and individual consumption rate to the Breathing Apparatus Officer before entering the structure. Other departments provide the Breathing Apparatus Officer with the individual air consumption rates of all personnel who may be involved in the response. In the latter case, before entering the structure, firefighters need only identify themselves and their assignment to the Breathing Apparatus Officer, who already has their consumption statistics.

The Breathing Apparatus Officer is responsible for monitoring the length of time each firefighter spends in the structure and predicting each firefighter's maximum safe operating time. This officer is also responsible for referring to the entry time and air consumption statistics and calculating, at intervals, the remaining air available for each firefighter. If the Breathing Apparatus Officer notes that a firefighter inside the structure is low on air, the officer is responsible for recalling the team and replacing it with a new team. NFPA 1404 also stipulates that additional personnel must be available for rescue, if necessary. In addition to monitoring for air consumption, the Breathing Apparatus Officer should monitor SCBA personnel for indications of fatigue and other factors that could lead to unsafe conditions (Figure 4.19).

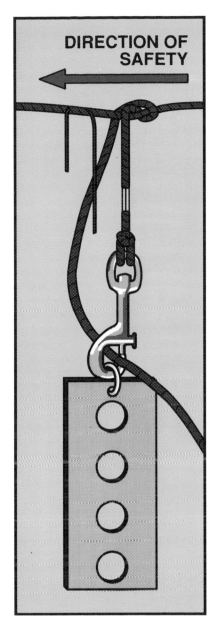

Figure 4.18 An arrangement of guide and personal lines with different length cords to indicate the direction of safety.

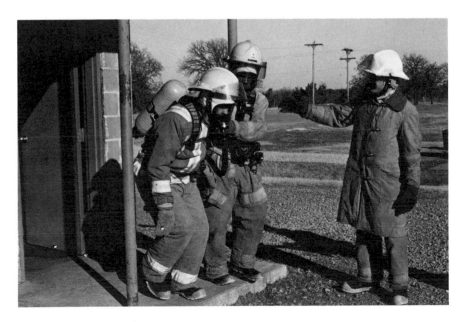

Figure 4.19 The Breathing Apparatus Officer monitors users of SCBA for fatigue or other unsafe conditions and removes them from duty when necessary.

The essential NFPA requirement is that departments assign at least one member to remain outside the fire building or emergency scene to maintain accountability and to direct help, if needed (Figure 4.20). NFPA stipulates that during the initial stages of emergency scene operations, this person may assume additional responsibilities, such as operating pumps, preparing equipment, or commanding operations. However, as operations progress, these responsibilities should be assigned to specific personnel according to the department's SOPs. Members assigned to rescue can also be assigned other duties at the incident scene, as long as they are properly suited up and available for reassignment. The requirement for additional personnel to be available for rescue can also be satisfied by additional companies or members who are responding to the scene and will arrive within the safe operating time of initial entry teams.

Each fire department is responsible for developing a workable system for monitoring and safeguarding their personnel wearing SCBA. More information about the systems described above can be obtained in NFPA 1404 and by writing to the addresses in Appendix B.

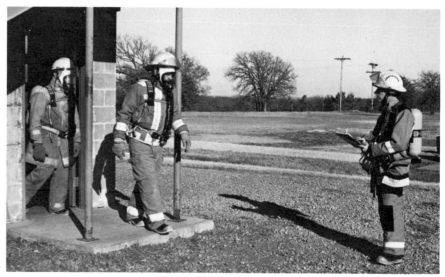

Figure 4.20 At least one SCBA monitor remains outside as SCBA teams work in the fire building.

SCBA TRAINING

During preliminary training, training officers should remember that individuals react differently to wearing and working with SCBA. This is the time to build confidence, not a time to use scare tactics. The training officer should prepare trainees by calming fears, answering questions, telling trainees what is expected, explaining what is going to happen, and praising trainees on tasks done well (Figure 4.21). Words of encouragement and positive reinforcement go a long way toward building confidence.

Most new firefighters experience at least some physical or mental discomfort, and training officers should learn to recognize

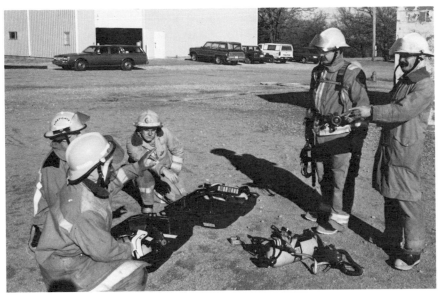

Figure 4.21 SCBA training officers preparing trainees during preliminary training by answering questions, explaining what is going to happen, and giving encouragement about working with SCBA.

signs of anxiety so that they can prevent potentially dangerous reactions later in the training session. The most obvious discomfort signals are apprehensive looks, excessive breathing rates, repeated yawning, or even vomiting when trainees face a smoke room (Figure 4.22). Other trainees may seem calm, but may indicate their nervousness by constantly readjusting their harness straps, facepieces, or other equipment. The training officer should also watch for those who often repeat questions about procedures.

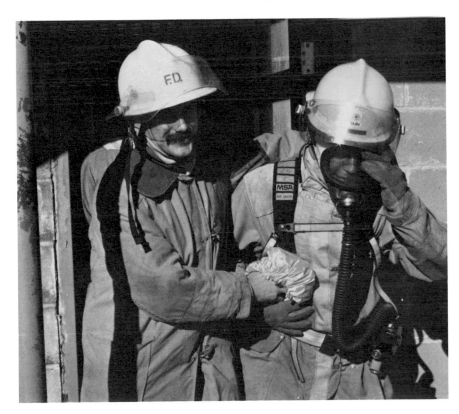

Figure 4.22 During training, a new firefighter may show signs of anxiety; the training officer should be alert to these signs.

The training officer must also overcome some of the fears firefighters may have about the SCBA itself. Trainees should be allowed to examine and try several different SCBA — donning, doffing, and using the apparatus until they are thoroughly familiar and comfortable with it. However, they should train with the equipment for which they have been fit-tested, which is the same equipment they have used, or will use, in their actual fire service responses.

In addition to learning about different types and styles of SCBA, trainees should be made aware of the hazards of breathing smoke and toxic gases. The training officer should stress that wearing SCBA can prevent injury and even death; and, when used properly, SCBA can be a significant factor in keeping the firefighter alive under the worst conditions. Training officers may want to stress the saying: "SCBA is protective equipment, and the life it protects is *yours*."

Training Sequence

SCBA training should be sequential to build endurance and to dispel the psychological fears that can lead to adverse reactions or panic. Firefighters may believe that they have inadequacies, they may lack confidence in themselves or in their equipment, or they may fear the hostile environment they must enter — flames, high heat, toxic gases, or the possibility of structural failure.

Before being exposed to smoke or live fire training, firefighters must have a thorough working knowledge of SCBA and should be able to calculate their individual point of no return. Training should progress in increments so that firefighters can make a gradual educational, physical, and mental adjustment to unfamiliar equipment and new procedures. Crash courses can be recipes for disaster. Trainees may feel claustrophobic just being strapped into an SCBA facepiece. Adding darkness and smoke too soon could further heighten trainees' feelings of anxiety. The classroom training and practices that follow are listed in the sequential order recommended to introduce trainees gradually to SCBA use.

- Introduction to the history, development, and use of SCBA (This is a nice-to-know but not a critical competency.)

- Introduction to different SCBA systems and parts (Demonstrate and allow trainees to examine different systems.)

- Instruction in proper safety precautions

- Practice in cleaning the apparatus after use

- Practice of controlled breathing techniques

- Practice wearing the facepiece with the breathing tube disconnected from the regulator (Make sure that the trainee does not allow the hose to drag on the ground [Figure 4.23].)

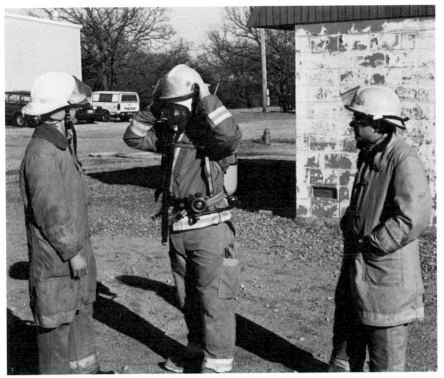

Figure 4.23 An SCBA trainee practicing wearing the facepiece with the breathing tube disconnected from the regulator—a way to gradually introduce SCBA use.

- Practice in wearing the facepiece with the lens covered and the low-pressure hose disconnected from the regulator

- Practice in wearing the facepiece attached to the regulator

- Practice in wearing the facepiece with the lens covered and the low-pressure hose attached to the regulator

- Practice in donning the entire SCBA over protective clothing within a set time limit

- Practice in wearing all protective equipment and breathing from an air cylinder while the facepiece is covered (This is a good time to incorporate an obstacle course.)

- Exercises to allow the firefighter to adjust to working in total darkness, "see" by feel, gain self-confidence, and practice controlled breathing

- Performance of fire fighting tasks in full protective equipment under smoky (machine-made smoke), but controlled, conditions

- Calculation of individual points of no return

- Instruction and practice in maintaining SCBA

When firefighters are comfortable and familiar with the weight and proper breathing style used with the SCBA, they can take part in more strenuous activity. For instance, individual firefighters with covered facepieces can be drilled in obstacle courses. They can follow hoselines through furnished rooms, their facepieces temporarily blocked with photographic diffusion paper (available at photo supply stores) to simulate smoky conditions. Some training organizations use shower caps or bags with a drawstring to cover the lenses, and others have used masking tape or dark green or black plastic bags (Figure 4.24). While training officers watch, advise, correct, assist, and evaluate the trainees' techniques, trainees crawl through the room, traveling around obstacles. They learn to move as rapidly as possible, without acting too hastily, using their hands as their eyes.

As the training advances, exertion levels are increased. The trainees climb ladders, handle hoselines, or work in heated training rooms while wearing breathing apparatus (Figure 4.25). They soon learn that to use SCBA efficiently in all fire fighting and rescue situations, good physical conditioning and controlled breathing techniques are necessary.

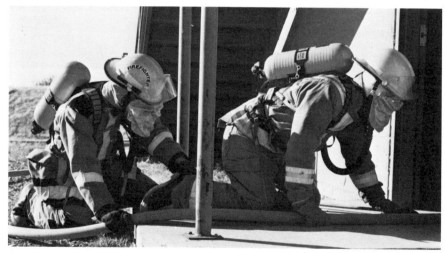

Figure 4.24 One way to simulate smoky conditions during training is to cover the facepiece with a shower cap.

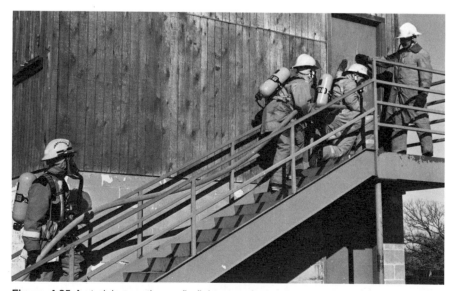

Figure 4.25 As training continues, firefighters perform more and more strenuous activities while wearing their SCBA.

Facilities

SCBA training facilities can range from elaborate structures costing hundreds of thousands of dollars to buildings that are about to be torn down for community improvement projects. All buildings used for SCBA training should be inspected and a safe condition ensured. NFPA 1403, *Standard on Live Fire Training Evolutions in Structures* and NFPA 1404 should be referenced when applicable. NFPA 1500, *Standard on Fire Department Occupational Safety and Health Program*, must also be used to determine the safety of individuals when using breathing apparatus in training situations and real emergencies. Fire departments around the country have effectively used all kinds of arrangements to train their firefighters to use SCBA. Fixed and mobile training equipment is as varied as the number of agencies using breathing apparatus.

No matter how elaborate or basic the training facility, firefighters should receive training on the proper uses of SCBA on an ongoing basis and have a performance evaluation quarterly or at least once a year.

PERMANENT TRAINING CENTERS

Departments that are financially capable can construct ideal permanent training centers that can be used to train firefighters in all types of fire fighting. Many centers, for example, have an academic building for classroom work and a fire building and training tower for more practical exercises. In the fire building are layouts using practically every feature a firefighter might find in a building — a variety of roofs, steps, ramps, fire escapes, and balconies. There are simulated store basements or utility vaults, rooms and hallways like those found in high-rise apartments, residential attics with attic ladders and scuttle holes, garden apartments, and elevator doors and shafts. Such a multilevel tower may also be used for stairwell and high-rise building evolutions. Many training centers include smoke rooms and mazes for special SCBA training.

MOBILE TRAINING LABORATORIES

Although some firefighters may travel to train at a permanent regional facility, training officers in a variety of states and provinces take their facilities to the firefighters. The permanent facility may be supplemented with mobile training laboratories complete with mazes and smoke rooms.

Mobile maze training units are often used to help train firefighters to use SCBA. A typical mobile maze may be a 45-foot (14-m) trailer, containing a three-level maze that can be arranged in numerous ways (see Figure 4.26 on next page). State and province fire schools use these mobile mazes to provide practical breathing apparatus training on location.

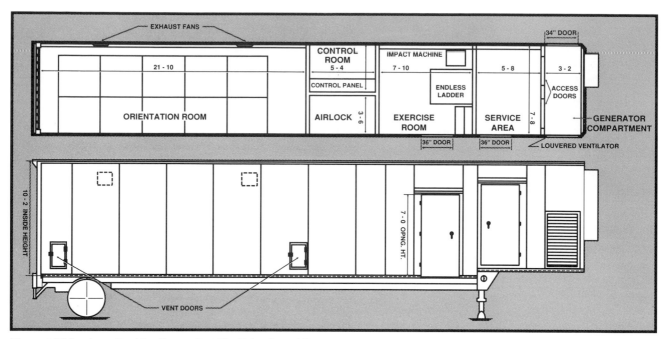

Figure 4.26 A schematic of the Connecticut Fire School's mobile maze training trailer. *Courtesy of Connecticut State Fire School.*

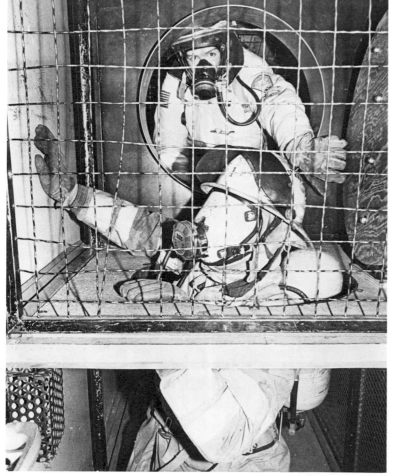

Figure 4.27 Firefighter in a mobile maze encountering a fence barrier as the instructor watches.

Firefighters encounter many obstacles in a mobile maze. The maze will have crawl spaces, hatchways, tunnels, various openings, and dead ends. Barriers in the maze may be made of fences or movable partitions (Figure 4.27). Firefighters must decide which way to go when they come to a barrier. The maze may also have a series of radiant heaters in the walls to simulate the high temperatures encountered in live fire conditions (Figure 4.28). Different noises may also be added to the maze, and closed-circuit television may allow observation of the firefighters from a control booth at the front of the trailer.

Firefighters navigate the maze in pairs, wearing full protective fire gear. The amount of air that firefighters use when going through the maze can be measured, thus giving trainees an idea of just how fast they can use their air supply when under exertion.

The Hanford Fire Department in Washington State has developed a state-of-the-art mobile breathing apparatus training unit as an integral

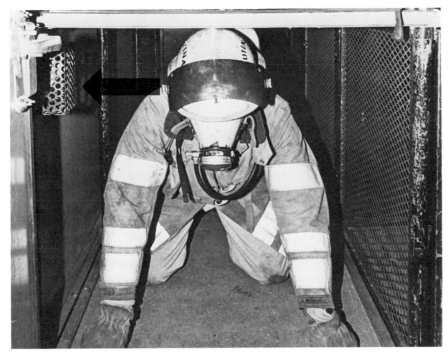

Figure 4.28 A mobile maze with a radiant heater on the wall to simulate the high temperatures of a live fire.

part of their firefighter safety and training program (Figure 4.29). This department is one of a growing number of departments that recognize the importance of ongoing, state-of-the-art SCBA training and firefighter conditioning.

Hanford's two-part mobile training facility consists of a control room, called the command module, and a training area. The command module allows the training officer to create and control the environment the trainees experience. The trailer's unique construction features movable panels that can be placed in seemingly unlimited positions to create mazes, tunnels, confined spaces, dead ends, and stairs or climbing obstructions.

Before trainees are allowed to enter the mobile training facility, they must first exercise to raise their heart rate to 60

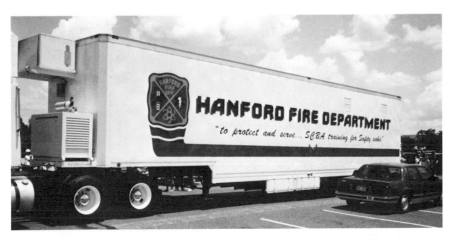

Figure 4.29 The Hanford (Washington) Fire Department state-of-the-art mobile unit.

percent of maximum aerobic state. A heart monitoring machine has been incorporated into a ladder climb exercise and is monitored from the command module. The trainees then negotiate these obstacles while their senses are besieged by heat, actual fireground sounds, and simulated radio traffic.

Firefighters using the mobile training facility are constantly monitored by the training officer from the command module via closed circuit television monitors and infrared cameras. Additionally, a safety officer is in constant attendance inside the training area when the unit is in use.

MAZES

Facilities — permanent and mobile — commonly have mazes to train firefighters to use SCBA. Mazes can be operated with or without machine-produced smoke to give firefighters experience in overcoming some of the obstacles they commonly find at fires. Smokeless mazes generally use darkened facilities that have black walls. All facilities need to allow maximum instructor/ trainee contact to enhance the training.

Trainees without hand lights have to feel their way through these mazes, generally monitored by two instructors posted inside in case a trainee encounters difficulties. In one mobile facility, trainees enter the two-level, 100-foot (30-m) maze and pass through a tunnel that decreases in height as they move forward. After climbing through a window, they ascend a flight of stairs to a second level and a simulated attic. There they crawl through tunnels, climb down a drop, and then crawl up an incline to more small tunnels on the second level. Trainees leave the maze after more drops and tunnels.

SMOKE ROOMS

Smoke rooms are smoke-filled training rooms or areas intended to simulate emergency conditions. Because NFPA 1500 prohibits hazardous or live fire smoke in SCBA training sessions, smoke-generating devices fill the rooms with nonhazardous smoke. Usually, trainees are grouped into teams of three or four members each and sent into the dark, smoky rooms to perform individual assignments such as search and rescue or gas shutoff. A standpipe connection, a gas meter with a shutoff valve, and several electrical boxes may be built into the rooms. Equipment in the smoke room is duplicated on the outside of the smoke room for briefing and practice before entering. Teams are expected to systematically search for victims or equipment and finish their assignments after reaching their objective. Furniture and room partitions provide an added touch of realism.

MAKESHIFT FACILITIES

Departments without the money for expensive, permanent training facilities have often found ingenious ways to use the equipment and facilities at hand to provide realistic SCBA training for their firefighters (Figure 4.30). For instance, an emptied apparatus bay provides a large, open area that can be laid out to depict a typical one-floor ranch-style residence. Walls, furniture,

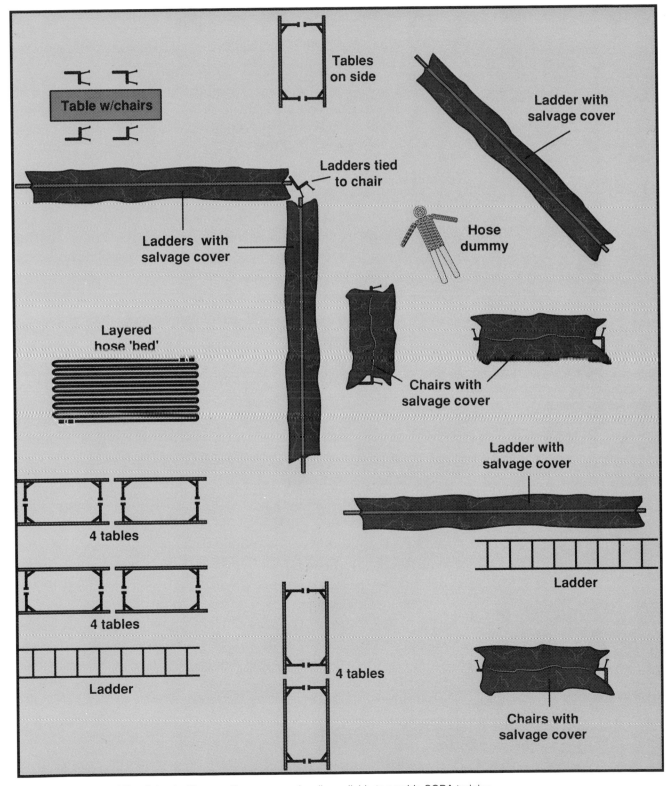

Figure 4.30 A makeshift training facility uses the resources locally available to provide SCBA training.

entrances, and confined spaces can be constructed with ordinary fire department equipment. The following are some suggested constructions:

- Ladders may be turned on the beam and covered with salvage covers to simulate a long wall.

- Tables may be turned on their sides to simulate short walls. When using tables for walls, sandwich the legs in the center of two tables to prevent injury to the trainee.

- Tables, chairs, and sofas from the fire department day room or lounge area may be used to "furnish" the rooms created, or salvage covers may be placed over chairs or SCBA boxes to represent furniture.

- Empty SCBA boxes may be strategically placed in the course as end tables or other obstacles.

- "Victims" can be created by coiling a length of hose and wrapping it in duct tape, rope, or hose straps. When creating such a victim, care should be taken to cover all hose couplings to prevent injury.

- Hoses may be laid through the rooms created and the trainee required to follow the hoseline through the structure or room.

- By placing a ladder on two chairs, a small entrance to an attic, basement, or some other confined space can be represented. The firefighter would be required to pass under the ladder and between the chairs. The chairs should be sturdy and the ladder secured with ropes to prevent it from falling on a trainee.

- Tables can be lined up, draped with salvage covers, and walled with ladders placed along both sides to represent a confined space such as an attic or crawlspace.

In addition to these methods of using the fire department equipment and rooms, resourceful training officers have developed other exercises with common structures locally available. For example, departments have used motels to conduct search-and-rescue training. Training officers simply waited until registrations were down or a wing of the motel was closed for remodeling. The machine-produced, nonhazardous smoke caused no damage to rooms and furnishings. One department put its firefighters into full protective gear and SCBA and sent them into a high-rise dormitory for search-and-rescue training. University students posed as victims.

Imagination is the key to creating a makeshift training facility. With creativity, it is possible to develop an innovative drill from the resources common to the fire department or community.

Advanced Training (Smoke Diver School)

The most common advanced training program available to firefighters is called Smoke Diver School (Figure 4.31). Many smoke diver schools are run by state fire service training institutions. However, some manufacturers have mobile training centers that tour the country and can offer training close to home.

Smoke diver schools introduce firefighters gradually to increasingly difficult tasks while wearing SCBA. At these schools, trainees learn more about their abilities and limitations while using SCBA, and they have more time to perfect their skills with the apparatus. For instance, trainees intensely practice techniques such as controlled breathing — making repeated and conscious efforts to reduce air consumption by forcing exhalation from the mouth and allowing natural inhalation through the nose. They also learn how to calculate their own point of no return and how to use the SCBA in varied, realistic situations.

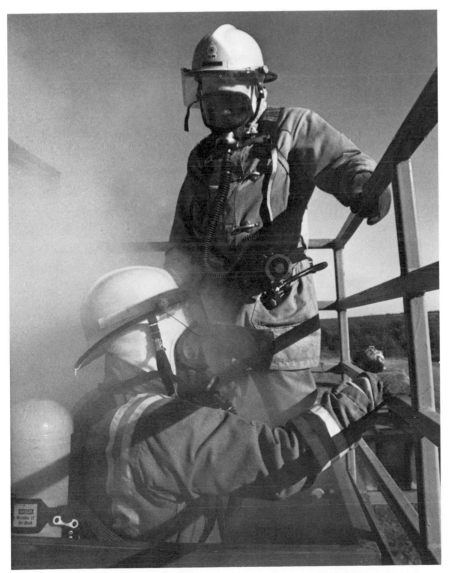

Figure 4.31 Smoke diver schools provide advanced SCBA training programs for firefighters.

In the Scandinavian countries, smoke diver trainees are chosen for their skill and stamina, and only those who finish smoke diver training are allowed to fight fires inside buildings with heavy smoke. Graduates are the elite of Scandinavian firefighters.

Typical U.S. smoke diver schools last between 30 and 45 hours, usually spread out over a week or several weekends. The first day's work can include the causes of firefighter collapse, the physical aspects of breathing and fatigue, and the fire environment — basically a review of what the firefighter should have learned in basic academy. Trainees then review and practice the basics of using SCBA and become proficient in donning and doffing the apparatus.

Routine training becomes increasingly more difficult as trainees progress in confidence and experience. First, trainees may review how to fit and test their facepieces and how to recharge their cylinders. Once they have reviewed the equipment, they are usually given a relatively simple task to perform while wearing the apparatus. As training progresses, trainees practice controlled breathing techniques and learn how to calculate their individual air consumption rates. For instance, trainees may be asked to don their breathing apparatus and spend two minutes chopping at a telephone pole with an axe. This exercise allows instructors to measure and evaluate how well the trainee can control breathing while wearing SCBA during heavy work. Instructors can get the same information by having trainees swing a sledgehammer at a tire section anchored to a heavy beam.

Another exercise to teach controlled breathing techniques involves having trainees in full SCBA walk several stories up and down a training tower. Their air consumption is then measured, and the exercise is repeated following controlled breathing training. Firefighters can learn to reduce their air consumption by as much as 50 percent.

At this point trainees may be shown how it feels to depend on their breathing apparatus while their vision is obscured. Instructors put cloth or translucent paper over the facepiece so that the trainee can see light but nothing else. Then the trainees are given another relatively simple task such as following a hoseline 100 feet (30 m) through an obstacle course. This exercise allows trainees to practice "seeing" with their hands. They learn to identify objects, obstacles, and — by feeling the couplings — to determine which direction they are traveling along the hose.

As trainees become more familiar with their equipment, they learn what to do if the equipment fails or if they run out of air. Theory is handled in a classroom lecture and supplemented with practice.

Trainees are generally given training and practice in team emergency conditions breathing procedures ("buddy breathing") after classroom instruction in emergency operations. At some schools this is done twice — once with machine-generated smoke and once without smoke. Other evolutions may include entering a tank through an opening too small for firefighters with cylinders strapped to their backs. Trainees remove their cylinders, crawl into the tank, and redon cylinders passed to them from outside. Trainees are also taught how to change cylinders in simulated hazardous atmospheres. See Chapter 5, Donning and Doffing, for a more detailed discussion of cylinder changing procedures.

At this point, trainees may be taught how to conduct search-and-rescue operations in full protective gear and breathing apparatus. Trainees first hear a classroom lecture on search patterns and rescue techniques. They then spend the rest of the day practicing. Some of the exercises may be performed in machine-made smoke with a clear facepiece; others may be performed with vision obscured.

The final day of smoke diver school may be all practice. Trainees usually perform combined evolutions. They may be shown how it feels to be lowered down a narrow shaft to perform a rescue while in breathing apparatus. They may be assigned to enter a smoky atmosphere, find firefighters who are "overcome" by smoke or toxic materials, and bring them out. They may be sent into a tunnel — such as a large culvert blocked at one end — to secure and remove a victim in a Stokes basket. In all exercises, trainees are forced to depend on their breathing apparatus in "hazardous" atmospheres. By the end of this intensive course, using SCBA in hazardous atmospheres and emergency situations becomes second nature to the trainee.

At the Greensburg Fire Department in Pennsylvania, the smoke divers concept was taken further by having even more advanced exercises for course graduates. To keep certified smoke divers proficient and interested in their training, the advanced work gave them practice in breaching walls, attacking fires, using small power tools, opening ceilings and walls, and rescuing victims from manholes, fire escapes, and stairways while using SCBA.

Keeping Training Records

As trainees progress through the stages of SCBA training, instructors should collect data on each trainee's breathing and air consumption. These air consumption records allow trainees to compare the amount of air they use at the beginning and end of the course. They learn how to decrease their air intake as they learn controlled breathing techniques, and they learn to use the air consumption statistics to calculate their point of no return. Not only do trainees learn to conserve air but they also gain more confidence in their equipment.

Regardless of the type of school the firefighter attends, an accurate training record should be kept by the fire department. Firefighters should also be allowed to review these records to check for accuracy. Record keeping can range from a simple handmade sheet kept by the training officer to computer records.

SUMMARY

Safety and training are very important and closely related areas of SCBA use. Both the training officer and the trainee must know and follow general safety guidelines, procedures, and standards. In addition, the firefighter is responsible for properly donning the apparatus; following basic safety guidelines; knowing the protection limits, safety features, and air supply duration of the apparatus; calculating individual point of no return; and ensuring facepiece seal before entering hazardous atmospheres.

The department is responsible for providing written SOPs and an SCBA/respiratory protection program that meet NFPA, ANSI, OSHA, and NIOSH standards regarding SCBA training, use, monitoring, and maintenance. In addition, the department is responsible for performing annual qualitative or quantitative facepiece fit tests to ensure facepiece seal and for keeping accurate and complete test records. At the incident scene, the department is responsible for monitoring and knowing the locations of all personnel wearing SCBA and for providing relief for SCBA personnel as necessary.

Safe and effective training requires a sequential approach in which the trainee is slowly introduced to equipment, theories, and practice and builds gradually from simple to more complex and strenuous tasks. Training facilities include permanent training centers, mobile training laboratories, mazes, smoke rooms, and carefully thought-out makeshift facilities. Advanced SCBA training is usually performed at smoke diver schools that provide intensive sequential training. All training should be ongoing and requires the training officer to keep accurate and complete records.

Chapter 4 Review

Answers on page 349SH

TRUE-FALSE: Mark each statement true or false. If false, explain why.

1. To conserve air, it is best to don the SCBA (except for the facepiece) in fresh air, and then don the facepiece after entering the fire area.

   ☐ T ☐ F _____

   _____

2. Regular eyeglasses cannot be worn with SCBA because the temple bars do not permit a proper facepiece seal.

   ☐ T ☐ F _____

   _____

3. A designated person should monitor firefighter teams inside the structure and calculate their remaining air supplies.

   ☐ T ☐ F _____

   _____

4. Each individual firefighter's point of no return should be determined by one specially designated person.

   ☐ T ☐ F _____

   _____

5. Quantitative fit testing is subjective, whereas qualitative fit testing, which requires using a special test instrument, is not.

   ☐ T ☐ F _____

   _____

MULTIPLE CHOICE: Circle the correct answer.

6. Firefighter A says that when the low-pressure alarm sounds, there is enough air remaining for the firefighter to safely exit the area. Firefighter B says that when the alarm sounds, there may not always be enough air for the firefighter to exit. Who is correct?

   A. Firefighter A

   B. Firefighter B

   C. Both A and B

   D. Neither A nor B

7. The best way for a firefighter to calculate his or her individual consumption rate is to _____.

    A. check the amount of air used 15 minutes after entering the fire area and divide this amount by 15 to determine amount of air used per minute

    B. check the average time cylinders last during several actual emergencies and divide the cylinder capacity (in psi) by this average time to determine amount of air used per minute

    C. check the average time cylinders last during vigorous activity (with appropriate rest breaks) and divide the cylinder capacity (in psi) by this average time to determine amount of air used per minute

    D. none of the above is correct

8. Firefighter A says that firefighters wearing SCBA should not be sent into a hazardous atmosphere unless they have had annual facepiece fit tests. Firefighter B says that fit testing may be either qualitative or quantitative. Who is correct?

    A. Firefighter A

    B. Firefighter B

    C. Both A and B

    D. Neither A nor B

9. Firefighter A says that SCBA protects firefighters from all toxic gases. Firefighter B says that SCBA does not protect firefighters from radioactive materials that can be absorbed through the skin. Who is correct?

    A. Firefighter A

    B. Firefighter B

    C. Both A and B

    D. Neither A nor B

LISTING

10. List four SCBA safety responsibilities of the firefighter.

    A. _____

    _____

    B. _____

    _____

    C. _____

    _____

    D. _____

    _____

11. SCBA duration ratings seldom correspond to the time a firefighter can actually use the equipment. The working air supply of the firefighter usually depends on what four factors?

A. _____

B. _____

C. _____

D. _____

12. List seven safety rules that firefighters should follow when wearing SCBA.

A. _____

_____

B. _____

_____

C. _____

_____

D. _____

_____

E. _____

_____

F. _____

_____

G. _____

_____

FILL IN THE BLANK: Fill in the blanks with the correct response.

13. The low-pressure alarm sounds a warning when _____ to _____ percent of the air supply is left.

14. The amount of air the firefighter used to get to the objective is the _____ amount needed to get back to a nonhazardous atmosphere.

15. The three most popular qualitative facepiece fit tests are the _____ _____ test, the _____ test, and the _____ test.

SHORT ANSWER: Answer each item briefly.

16. What is PASS?

_____

_____

_____

_____

_____

17. Should SCBA be worn during overhaul activities? Why or why not?

_____

_____

_____

_____

_____

18. Why is it important for a firefighter to know his or her air consumption rate?

_____

_____

_____

_____

_____

19. When not laying a hoseline, firefighters may use guide lines or ropes when working inside a structure. What is a guide line?

_____

_____

_____

_____

_____

_____

20. What are some of the principal duties of a Breathing Apparatus Officer?

_____

_____

_____

_____

_____

_____

_____

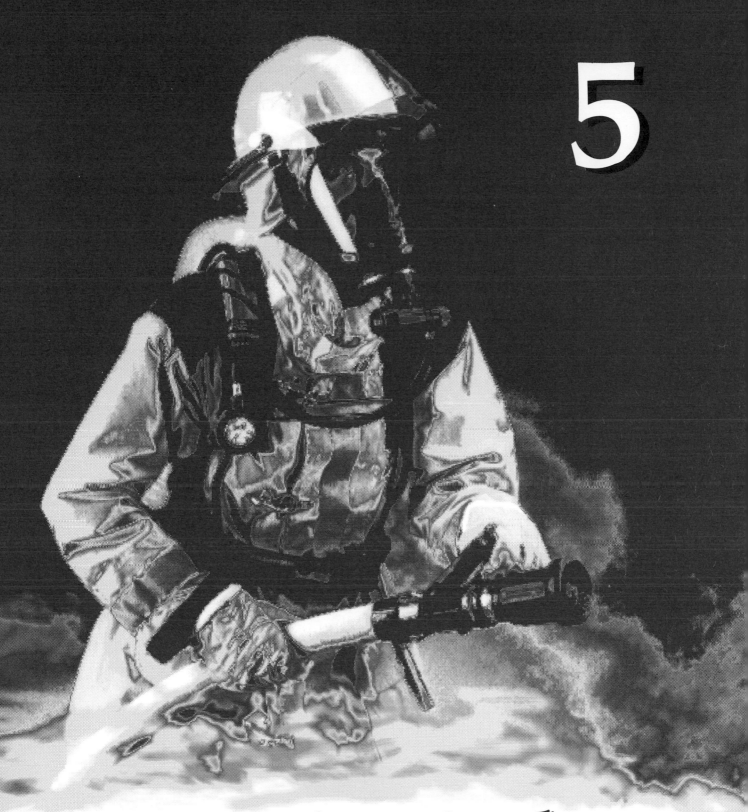

5

Donning And Doffing

This chapter provides information that addresses the following standards:

NFPA STANDARD 1001
Fire Fighter Professional Qualifications
1987 Edition

Chapter 3—Fire Fighter I
3-6.4

NFPA STANDARD 1404
Fire Department Self-Contained Breathing Apparatus Program
1989 Edition

Chapter 4—SCBA Training
4-1.3
4-11

ANSI STANDARD Z88.2-1980
Practices for Respiratory Protection

Section 7—Use of Respirators
7.2.3.1

Chapter 5

Donning and Doffing

INTRODUCTION

Firefighters must be able to don and doff self-contained breathing apparatus quickly and correctly. Several methods of donning the backpack can be used, depending upon how the SCBA is stored. These methods include the over-the-head method, coat method, and donning from a seat, side or rear mount, and compartment mount. The steps for donning differ with each method, but once the SCBA is on the body, the method of securing the unit will be the same. Methods for donning the facepiece differ, depending upon the manufacturer and whether the regulator is harness-mounted or facepiece-mounted.

The procedures in this chapter are intended to be general in nature; firefighters should be aware that there are different steps for donning different makes and models. Therefore, the instructions given in this chapter should be adapted to the specific type of SCBA used. Always follow the manufacturer's instructions when donning, doffing, and operating SCBA. For more information about donning procedures for some specific types of SCBA, see Appendix E.

DONNING THE OPEN-CIRCUIT SCBA

Because many firefighters prefer to don the SCBA backpack first, then the facepiece, procedures for donning the backpack are covered in this section. Methods for donning different types of facepieces are covered in the section that follows.

Donning The Backpack
OVER-THE-HEAD METHOD

SCBA must be stored ready to don. The backpack straps should be arranged so that they do not interfere with grasping the cylinder. The firefighter should put on his or her protective hood, pull it back, button the turnout coat, and turn the collar up so that the shoulder straps do not hold the collar down. The procedures for donning a backpack using the over-the-head method are as follows:

Step 1: Check the unit.

a. Crouch or kneel at the end opposite the cylinder valve, regardless of whether the unit is in its case or on the ground.

b. Check the cylinder gauge to make sure that the air cylinder is full. Open the cylinder valve *slowly* and listen for the audible alarm as the system pressurizes. Then, open the cylinder valve fully. If the audible alarm does not sound, or if it sounds but does not stop, place the unit out of service by tagging it and notifying an officer; use another unit.

c. Check the regulator gauge; both the cylinder and regulator gauges should register within 100 psi of each other — if increments are in psi — when the cylinder is pressurized to its rated capacity (Figure 5.1). If increments are in other measurements, such as fractions or minutes, they should correspond. If the unit has a donning switch (for units with facepiece-mounted regulators), leave the cylinder valve open and the unit in the donning mode. If the unit is positive pressure only, refer to the manufacturer's instructions concerning the cylinder valve.

NOTE: Positive-pressure SCBA that can supply air in a demand-type mode do not meet the requirements of NFPA 1981, 1987 edition.

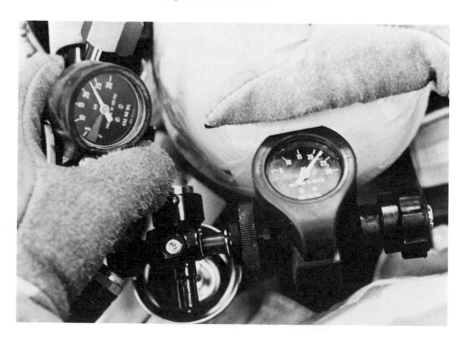

Figure 5.1 Pressure gauges on the regulator and cylinder should have corresponding readings when the cylinder is fully pressurized.

Step 2:   Spread the harness straps out to their respective sides.

Step 3:   Grasp the backplate or cylinder with both hands, one at each side (Figure 5.2). Make sure that the cylinder valve is pointed away from you. There should be no straps between your hands.

Step 4:   Lift up the cylinder, and let the regulator and harness hang freely (Figure 5.3).

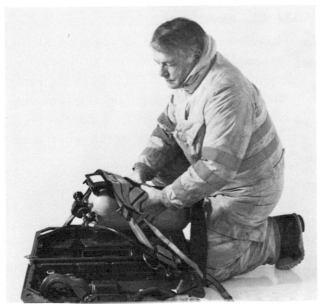

Figure 5.2 With straps spread, grasp the cylinder through the shoulder straps, and lift it from the case.

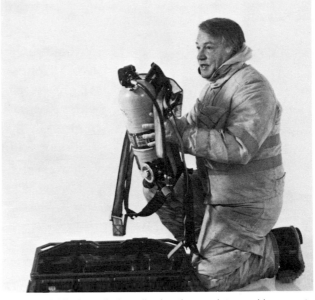

Figure 5.3 Lift the cylinder, allowing the regulator and harness to hang freely.

Step 5:   Raise the cylinder overhead, and let your elbows find their respective loosened harness shoulder strap loops (Figure 5.4). Keeping your elbows close to your body, tuck your chin and grasp the shoulder straps as the SCBA begins to slide down your back. Let the straps slide through your hands as the backpack lowers into place.

Step 6:   Lean forward to balance the cylinder on your back and partially tighten the shoulder straps by pulling them outward and downward (Figure 5.5). (**NOTE:** It is sometimes necessary to lean forward with a quick jumping motion to properly position the SCBA on the back while tightening the straps.)

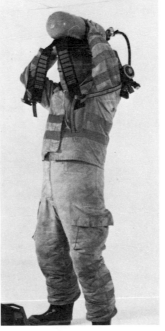

Figure 5.4 Stand and raise the cylinder overhead, allowing the shoulder straps to fall outside the arms.

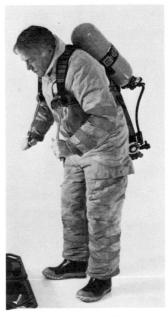

Figure 5.5 Lean forward for balance and partially tighten the shoulder straps by pulling outward and downward.

Step 7: Continue leaning forward, and then fasten the chest buckle if the unit has a chest strap (Figure 5.6). (**NOTE:** Depending upon the firefighter's physique, it may be more comfortable to fasten the chest buckle before tightening the shoulder straps.)

Step 8: Fasten and adjust the waist strap until the unit fits snugly (Figure 5.7).

Step 9: Don the facepiece. (**NOTE:** This procedure is covered in the next section.)

Some departments have removed waist straps from SCBA. Without a waist strap fastened, the SCBA wearer suffers undue stress from side-to-side shifting of the unit and from improper weight distribution of the unit. Even more important, removing waist straps permits the SCBA to be used in a nonapproved manner, which may violate NIOSH certification of the equipment and may void the manufacturer's warranty.

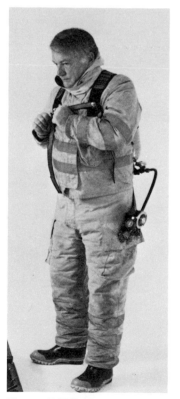

Figure 5.6 Connect the chest strap. The chest strap must be connected prior to fully tightening the shoulder straps.

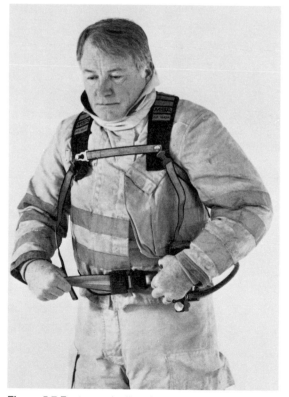

Figure 5.7 Fasten and adjust the waist strap. Readjust all other straps until the unit fits snugly.

CROSS-ARMED COAT METHOD

Self-contained breathing apparatus can be donned like a coat. The equipment should be arranged so that both shoulder straps can be grasped for lifting.

Step 1: Check the unit.

a. Crouch or kneel at the cylinder valve end of the unit, regardless of whether the unit is in its case or on the ground.

b. Check the cylinder gauge to make sure that the air cylinder is full (Figure 5.8). Open the cylinder valve *slowly* and listen for the audible alarm as the system pressurizes. Then, open the cylinder valve fully. If the audible alarm does not sound, or if it sounds but does not stop, place the unit out of service by tagging it and notifying an officer; use another unit.

c. Check the regulator gauge; both the cylinder and regulator gauges should register within 100 psi of each other — if increments are in psi — when the cylinder is pressurized to its rated capacity. If increments are in other measurements, such as fractions or minutes, they should correspond. If the unit has a donning switch, leave the cylinder valve open and the unit in the donning mode. If the unit is positive pressure only, refer to the manufacturer's instructions concerning the cylinder valve.

NOTE: Positive-pressure SCBA that can supply air in the demand-type mode do not meet the requirements of NFPA 1981, 1987 edition.

Step 2: Spread the harness straps out to their respective sides. Cross your arms, left over right. Grasp the shoulder straps at the top of the harness, left hand holding the left strap and right hand holding the right strap (Figure 5.9).

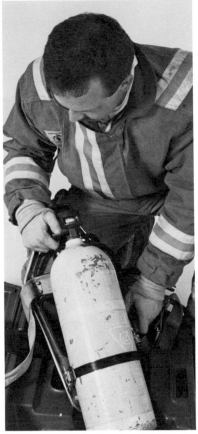

Figure 5.8 Always check the cylinder gauge prior to donning the SCBA. Open the valve fully before donning the unit.

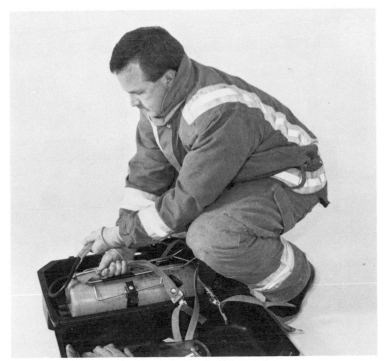

Figure 5.9 Kneel and grasp the shoulder straps with arms crossed, left over right.

Step 3: Lift the SCBA. Using both arms, swing the unit around your right shoulder, and raising your left arm, continue bringing the unit behind your head and onto your back. Both hands should still be grasping the shoulder straps high on the harness (Figures 5.10 a through d).

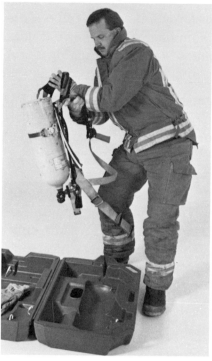

Figure 5.10a While rising to a standing position, lift SCBA, keeping wrists together.

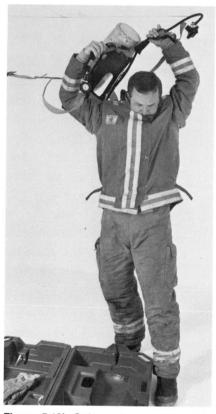

Figure 5.10b Swing unit around the right shoulder, allowing wrists to separate.

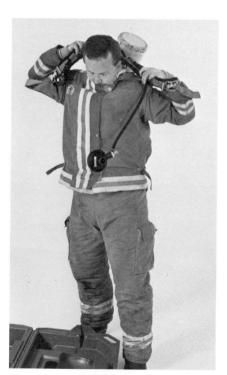

Figure 5.10c Guide unit onto back.

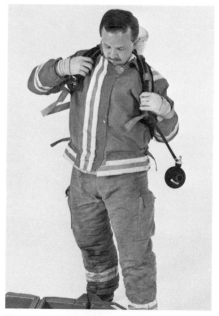

Figure 5.10d Let harness straps slide through hands until the SCBA is positioned on back.

Step 4:   Maintaining a firm grip on the straps, slide your hands down the straps to the shoulder strap buckles. Your elbows should be between the straps and the backpack (Figures 5.11 and 5.12).

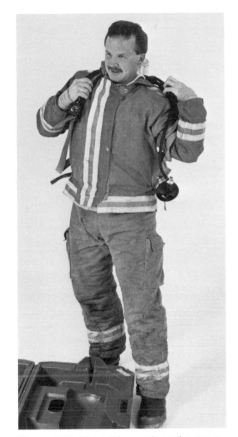

Figure 5.11 Maintaining a grip on the straps, straighten the straps as necessary.

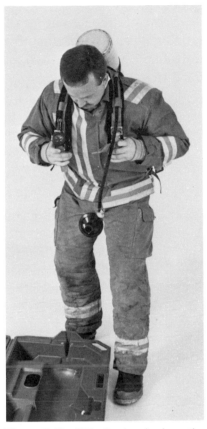

Figure 5.12 Slide the hands down the shoulder straps to the adjustment buckles.

Step 5:   Lean slightly forward to balance the cylinder on your back; tighten the shoulder straps by pulling them outward and downward (Figure 5.13). (**NOTE:** It is sometimes necessary to lean forward with a quick jumping motion to properly position the SCBA on the back while tightening the straps.)

Step 6:   Continue leaning forward, and fasten the chest buckle if the unit has a chest strap. (**NOTE:** It may be necessary to fasten the chest strap before completely tightening the shoulder straps.)

Step 7:   Fasten and adjust the waist strap until the unit fits snugly (Figure 5.14).

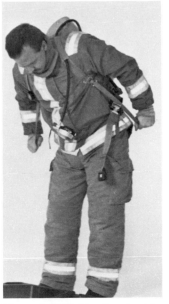

Figure 5.13 Tighten the shoulder straps by pulling them outward and downward.

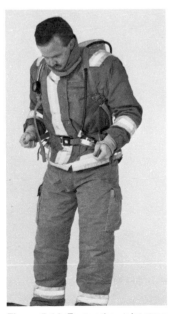

Figure 5.14 Fasten the waist strap and adjust until snug.

Step 8: Recheck all straps to see that they are correctly adjusted.

Step 9: Don the facepiece. (**NOTE:** This procedure is covered later in this chapter.)

REGULAR COAT METHOD

Self-contained breathing apparatus can be donned like a coat, putting one arm at a time through the shoulder strap loops. The unit should be arranged so that *either* shoulder strap can be grasped for lifting.

Step 1: Check the unit.

a. Crouch or kneel at the cylinder valve end of the unit, regardless of whether the unit is in its case or on the ground.

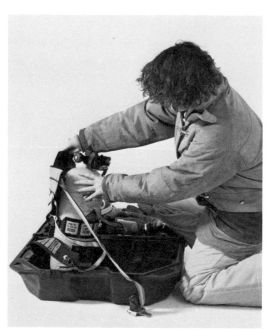

Figure 5.15 Check the cylinder gauge to verify the cylinder is full, and slowly open the cylinder valve to pressurize the system.

b. Check the cylinder gauge to make sure that the air cylinder is full (Figure 5.15). Open the cylinder valve *slowly* and listen for the audible alarm as the system pressurizes. Then, open the cylinder valve fully. If the audible alarm does not sound, or if it sounds but does not stop, place the unit out of service by tagging and notifying an officer; use another unit.

c. Check the regulator gauge; both the cylinder and regulator gauges should register within 100 psi of each other — if increments are in psi — when the cylinder is pressurized to its rated capacity. If increments are in other measurements, such as fractions or minutes, they should correspond. If the unit has a donning switch, leave the cylinder valve open and the unit in the donning mode. If the unit is positive pressure only, refer to the manufacturer's instructions concerning the cylinder valve.

NOTE: Positive-pressure SCBA that can supply air in a demand-type mode do not meet the requirements of NFPA 1981, 1987 edition.

Step 2: Spread the straps out to their respective sides, and position the upper portion of the straps over the top of the backplate (Figure 5.16). (**NOTE:** By doing this, the straps are less likely to fall, and the arms can go through the straps with less difficulty.)

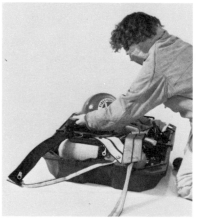

Figure 5.16 Spread the straps and position the upper part of the shoulder straps over the backplate.

NOTE: This procedure is written for those harnesses having the regulator attached to the left side of the harness. There are some SCBA that have the regulator mounted on the right. For these types, the right strap should be grasped with the right hand, and the backpack should be donned following the instructions in the next steps, but using directions opposite those indicated.

Step 3: At top of the harness, grasp the left strap with the left hand; grasp the lower portion of the same strap with the right hand (Figure 5.17). (**NOTE:** When kneeling at the cylinder valve end, the left harness strap will be to your right.)

Step 4: Lift the unit up; swing it around the left shoulder and onto the back. Both hands should still be grasping the shoulder strap (Figure 5.18).

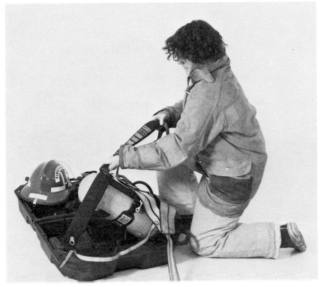

Figure 5.17 Grasp the top of the left shoulder strap with left hand. Grasp the lower part of the same strap with the right hand.

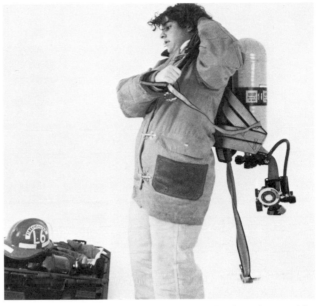

Figure 5.18 Lifting the SCBA by the straps, swing the unit around the left shoulder and onto the back while maintaining a firm grasp of the straps.

Step 5: Continue to hold the strap with your left hand, release your right hand, and insert your right arm between the right shoulder strap and the backpack frame.

Step 6: Lean slightly forward to balance the cylinder on your back (Figure 5.19); tighten the shoulder straps by pulling them outward and downward (Figure 5.20). (**NOTE:** It is sometimes necessary to lean forward with a quick jumping motion to properly position the SCBA on the back while tightening the straps.)

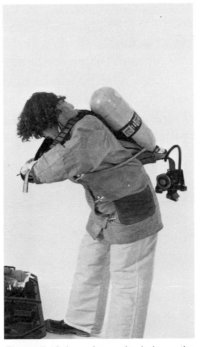

Figure 5.19 Lean forward to balance the unit while tightening the shoulder straps.

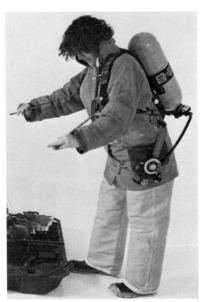

Figure 5.20 Tighten the shoulder straps by pulling them outward and downward.

Step 7: Continue leaning forward, and fasten the chest buckle if the unit has a chest strap (Figure 5.21). Tighten the shoulder straps further if necessary (Figure 5.22).

Step 8: Fasten and adjust the waist strap until the unit fits snugly (Figure 5.23).

Step 9: Recheck all straps to see that they are correctly adjusted.

Step 10: Don the facepiece. (**NOTE:** This procedure is covered in the next section.)

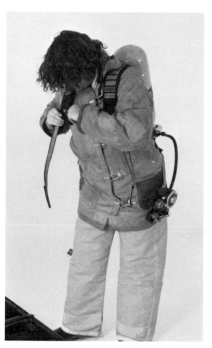

Figure 5.21 Connect the chest strap before the shoulder straps are completely tightened.

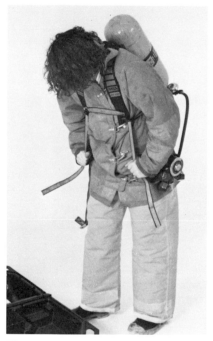

Figure 5.22 Continue tightening the shoulder straps, if necessary.

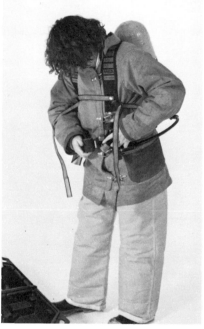

Figure 5.23 Fasten and adjust the waist strap until the unit fits snugly.

SEAT MOUNT

Valuable time can be saved if the SCBA is mounted on the back of the firefighter's seat in the vehicle (Figure 5.24). By having a seat mount, firefighters can don SCBA while en route to an incident. If the SCBA is not needed upon arrival, it can be removed quickly and remain mounted in its support.

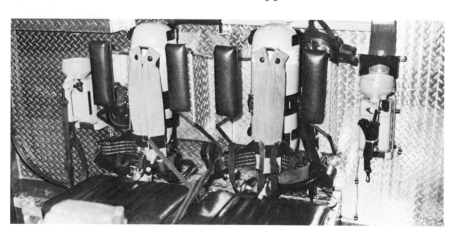

Figure 5.24 Seat-mounted SCBA are shown in the fire fighting vehicle.

Seat-mounting hardware comes in three main types: lever clamp, spring clamp, or flat hook. A drawstring or other quick-opening bag should enclose the facepiece to keep it clean and to protect it from dust and scratches. (**NOTE:** Do not keep the facepiece hooked to the regulator during storage. These parts must be separate to check for proper facepiece seal.)

Donning en route is done by inserting the arms through the straps while sitting with the seat belt on, then adjusting the straps for a snug fit (Figures 5.25 and 5.26).

WARNING

Never stand up to don SCBA while the vehicle is moving. Standing places both you and other firefighters in danger of serious injury in the event of a fall. NFPA 1500 requires firefighters to remain seated and belted at all times while the emergency vehicle is in motion.

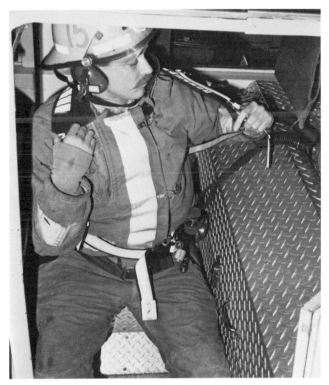

Figure 5.25 Donning en route, the firefighter inserts both arms through the straps and carefully connects the waist belt to avoid entanglement with the seat belt.

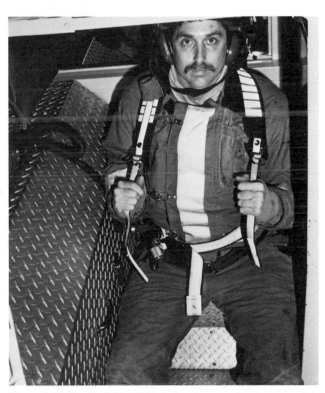

Figure 5.26 The firefighter adjusts the straps as snugly as possible while seated. Upon leaving the apparatus, straps may be adjusted again as necessary.

The cylinder's position should match the proper wearing position for the firefighter. The visible seat-mounted SCBA reminds and even encourages personnel to check the equipment more frequently. Because it is exposed, checks can be made more conveniently. When exiting the fire apparatus, be sure to adjust the straps for a snug and comfortable fit.

SIDE OR REAR MOUNT

Although it does not permit donning en route, the side- or rear-mounted SCBA may be desirable. Time is saved because the steps needed to remove the equipment case from the fire apparatus, place it on the ground, open the case, and pick up the unit are eliminated. However, because the unit is exposed to weather and physical damage, a canvas cover is desirable.

If the mounting height is right, firefighters can don SCBA with little effort. Having the mount near the running boards or near the tailboard allows the firefighter to don the equipment while sitting. The steps are essentially the same as those for seat-mounted SCBA.

COMPARTMENT OR BACKUP MOUNT

SCBA stored in a closed compartment can be ready for rapid donning by using any number of mounts (Figure 5.27). A mount on the inside of a compartment presents the same advantages as does side-mounted equipment. Some compartment doors, however, may not allow a firefighter to stand fully while donning SCBA. Other compartments may be too high for the firefighter to don the SCBA properly.

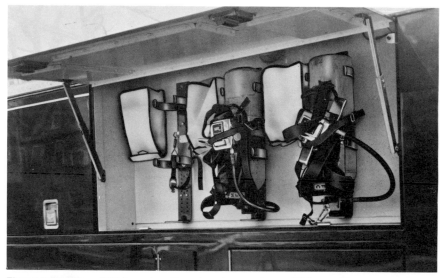

Figure 5.27 These SCBA are stored in a closed compartment. While providing good protection, this compartment may not be the correct height for proper donning. *Courtesy of Ziamatic Corporation.*

Other compartment mounts feature a telescoping frame that holds the equipment out of the way inside the compartment when it is not needed (Figure 5.28). One type of compartment mount telescopes outward, then upward or downward to proper height for quick donning.

The backup mount provides quick access to SCBA (some high-mounted SCBA must be removed from the vehicle and donned using the over-the-head or coat method). The procedure for donning SCBA using the backup method, with slight variation for

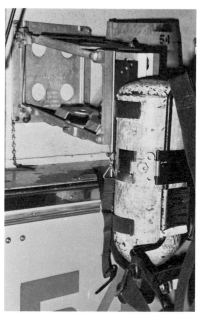

Figure 5.28 A compartment mount featuring a telescoping frame to hold the equipment inside the compartment provides the proper height for donning.

mounts from which the SCBA can be donned while seated, is as follows:

Step 1: Uncover the SCBA. Remove the facepiece and place it nearby.

Step 2: Check the unit.

  a. Open the cylinder valve *slowly* and listen for the audible alarm as the system pressurizes. Open the cylinder valve fully. If the audible alarm does not sound, or if it sounds but does not stop, place the unit out of service by tagging it and notifying an officer; use another unit.

  b. Check the regulator gauge; both the cylinder and regulator gauges should register within 100 psi of each other — if increments are in psi — when the cylinder is pressurized to its rated capacity. If increments are in other measurements, such as fractions or minutes, they should correspond. If the unit has a donning switch, leave the cylinder valve open and the unit in the donning mode. If the unit is positive pressure only, refer to the manufacturer's instructions concerning the cylinder valve.

  NOTE: Positive-pressure SCBA that supply air in the demand-type mode do not meet the requirements of NFPA 1981, 1987 edition.

Step 3: Back up against the cylinder backplate, and place your arms through the harness straps (Figure 5.29). As you lean slightly forward to balance the unit on your back, release the cylinder according to the kind of mounting device.

Step 4: Step forward to clear the unit from the mount while you fasten the chest buckle if the unit has a chest strap.

Step 5: Tighten the shoulder straps (see Figure 5.30 on next page).

Step 6: Fasten and adjust the waist strap until the unit fits snugly (see Figure 5.31 on next page).

Step 7: Don the facepiece. (**NOTE:** Donning the facepiece is covered in the next section.)

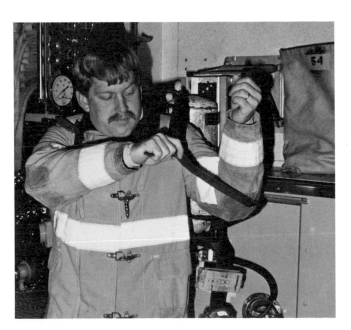

Figure 5.29 Back up against the cylinder backplate, and place arms through harness straps.

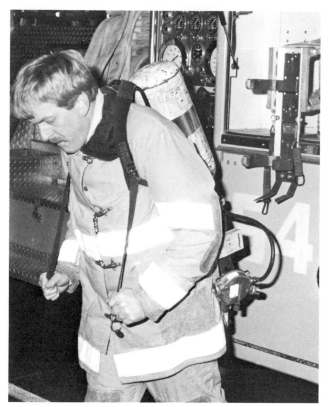

Figure 5.30 Tighten shoulder straps, and with a slight jerk, pull the SCBA away from the bracket.

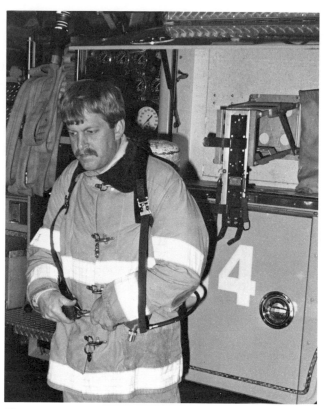

Figure 5.31 Fasten and adjust the waist strap until the unit fits snugly.

Donning The Facepiece

The facepieces for most SCBA are donned similarly. One important difference in facepieces is the number of straps used to tighten the head harness (Figure 5.32). Different models from the same manufacturer may have a different number of straps. Another important difference is the location of the regulator. The regulator may be attached to the facepiece or mounted on the waist belt. The shape and size of facepiece lenses may also differ. Despite these variations, the uses and donning procedures for facepieces are essentially the same.

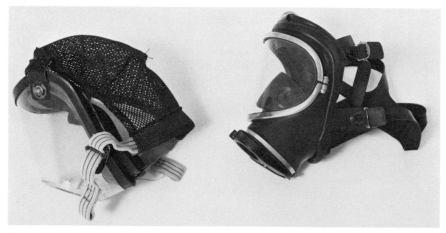

Figure 5.32 Two types of head harnesses are depicted — a nylon mesh or hairnet model and a traditional style with five straps, sometimes referred to as a web-type harness.

NOTE: Interchanging facepieces, or any other part of the SCBA, from one manufacturer's equipment to another makes any warranty and certification void.

An SCBA facepiece cannot be worn loosely or it will not seal against the face properly. An improper seal may permit toxic gases to enter the facepiece and be inhaled. Firefighters should not let long hair, sideburns, or beards interfere with the outer edges of the facepiece, thus preventing contact and a proper seal with the skin. Most fire departments simplify this policy by insisting that firefighters be clean shaven. Temple pieces of glasses and missing dentures can also affect facepiece fit.

A firefighter should not rely solely on tightening facepiece straps to ensure proper facepiece fit. A facepiece tightened too much will be uncomfortable or may cut off circulation to the face. Each firefighter must be fitted with a facepiece that conforms properly with the face shape and size. For this reason, many SCBA are available with different-sized facepieces (Figure 5.33). Nosecups, if used, must also properly fit the firefighter. Refer to Chapter 4 for more detailed information on facepiece fit.

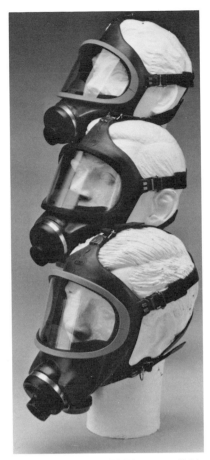

Figure 5.33 Many SCBA are available with different-sized facepieces. *Photo courtesy of MSA.*

DONNING THE FACEPIECE WITH HARNESS-MOUNTED REGULATOR

The facepiece for an SCBA with a harness-mounted regulator will have a low-pressure hose, or breathing tube, attached to the facepiece with clamps or threaded coupling nuts. The facepiece may be packed in a case or stored in a bag or coat pouch. Wherever it is stored, the straps should be left fully extended for donning ease and to keep the facepiece from becoming distorted.

The procedure for donning a facepiece having a low-pressure hose is as follows:

Step 1: Pull the protective hood back and down so that the face opening is around your neck. Turn up the collar of your turnout coat.

Step 2: If the harness is a web-type, grasp the harness with the thumbs through the straps from the inside, and spread the straps (Figure 5.34).

Figure 5.34 When donning a web-type harness, grasp the harness with the thumbs through the straps from the inside, and spread the straps.

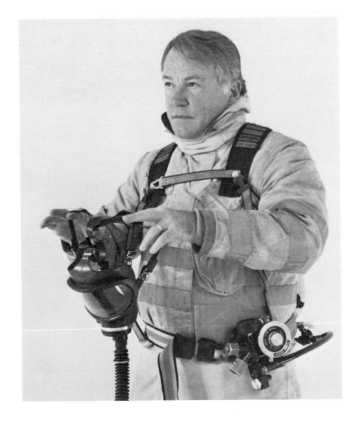

Step 3: Push the top of the harness up the forehead to remove hair that may be present between the forehead and the sealing surface of the facepiece (Figure 5.35).

Step 4: Center your chin in the chin cup and position the harness so that it is centered at the rear of your head (Figure 5.36).

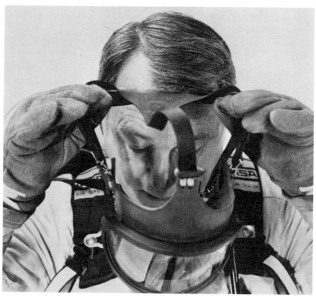

Figure 5.35 Push the top of the harness up the forehead to remove hair that may be present between the forehead and the sealing surface of the facepiece. The web is contacting the forehead.

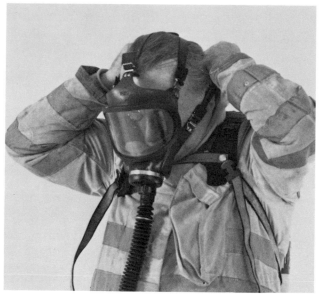

Figure 5.36 Center chin in chin cup and position harness so that it is centered at the rear of head.

Step 5: Tighten the harness straps by pulling them evenly and simultaneously to the rear. Pulling the straps outward, to the sides, may damage them and will prevent proper engagement with the adjusting buckles. Tighten the lower straps first, then the temple straps, and finally the top strap if there is one (Figures 5.37 a through c).

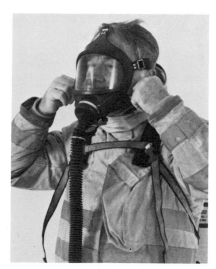

Figure 5.37a Tighten the straps evenly and simultaneously, starting with the lower straps.

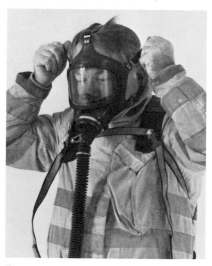

Figure 5.37b Tighten temple straps, pulling straps to the rear.

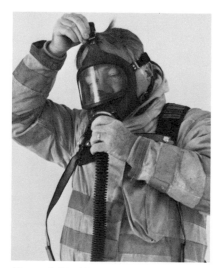

Figure 5.37c Tighten top strap last.

Step 6: Check the facepiece seal. Exhale deeply, seal the end of the low-pressure hose with a bare hand, and inhale slowly (not deeply) (Figure 5.38). Hold your breath for 10 seconds. This action allows the facepiece to collapse tightly against the face. (**NOTE:** Inhaling very quickly will temporarily seal any leak and will give a false sense of a proper seal). If there is evidence of leaking, adjust or redon the facepiece.

Step 7: Check the exhalation valve. Inhale, seal the end of the low-pressure hose, and exhale. If the exhalation does not go through the exhalation valve, keep the low-pressure hose sealed, press the facepiece against your face, and exhale to free the valve (Figure 5.39). Use caution when exhaling against a sealed facepiece in order to prevent discomfort and possible damage to the inner ear from exhaling forcefully. If you cannot get the exhalation valve free, remove the facepiece and have it checked.

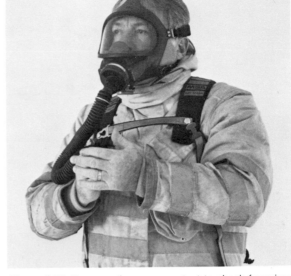

Figure 5.38 Use negative-pressure test to check facepiece seal by sealing the low-pressure hose and inhaling slowly.

Step 8: Put your helmet on, first inserting the low-pressure hose through the helmet's chin strap. The helmet should rest on your shoulder until the SCBA is completely donned (Figure 5.40). (**NOTE:** Helmets with straps that completely disconnect may be donned as a last step.)

Step 9: Connect the low-pressure hose to the regulator. If the unit has a donning switch, turn it to the PRESSURE, USE,

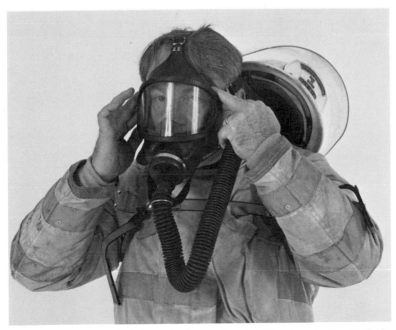

Figure 5.39 Check exhalation valve by sealing the low-pressure hose with the thumb, holding the mask near the temples, and exhaling.

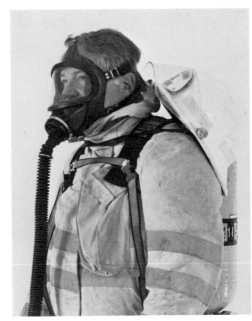

Figure 5.40 The helmet should rest on the shoulder until the SCBA is completely donned.

or ON position. If the unit does not have a donning switch, open the mainline valve.

NOTE: Positive-pressure SCBA that can supply air in a demand-type mode do not meet the requirements of NFPA 1981, 1987 edition.

Step 10: Check for positive pressure. Gently break the facepiece seal by inserting two fingers under the edge of the facepiece (Figure 5.41). You should be able to feel air moving past your fingers. If you cannot feel air movement, remove the unit and have it checked.

Step 11: Pull the protective hood into place, making sure that all exposed skin is covered and that vision is unobscured (Figure 5.42). Check to see that no portion of the hood is located between the facepiece and the face.

Step 12: Place the helmet on your head and tighten the chin strap (Figures 5.43 and 5.44).

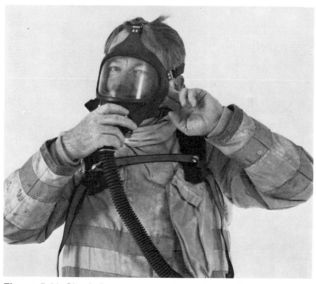

Figure 5.41 Check for positive pressure by gently breaking the facepiece seal by inserting two fingers under the edge of the facepiece.

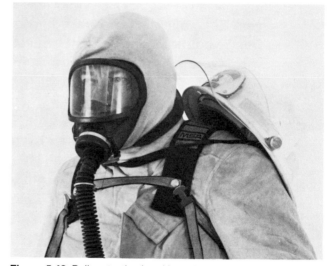

Figure 5.42 Pull protective hood into place, covering all exposed skin and being sure vision is unobscured.

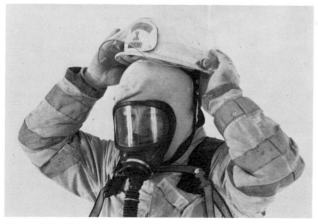

Figure 5.43 Place the helmet on the head, and assure the chin strap is under the chin and not tangled with the facepiece or hood.

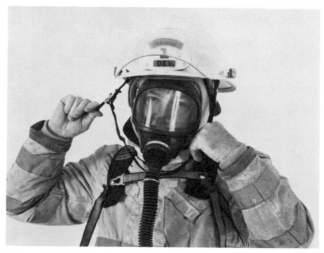

Figure 5.44 Tighten the chin strap securely.

An alternative method is to wear the helmet while donning the SCBA. After donning the backpack, loosen the chin strap, allow the helmet to rest on the air cylinder or on your shoulder, and then don the facepiece. When the facepiece straps have been tightened and the hood is on, lift the helmet back onto your head and tighten the chin strap (see Figures 5.43 and 5.44).

DONNING THE FACEPIECE WITH FACEPIECE-MOUNTED REGULATOR

Step 1: If using a protective hood, pull it back and down so that the face opening is around your neck. Turn up the collar of your turnout coat (Figure 5.45). (**NOTE:** Depending upon the style of helmet used, it may be necessary to don the helmet now and allow it to rest on the shoulder.)

Step 2: With your thumbs inserted through the straps, grasp the head harness and spread the webbing (Figure 5.46).

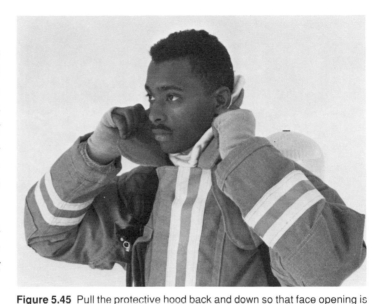

Figure 5.45 Pull the protective hood back and down so that face opening is around the neck. Turn up the collar of the turnout coat.

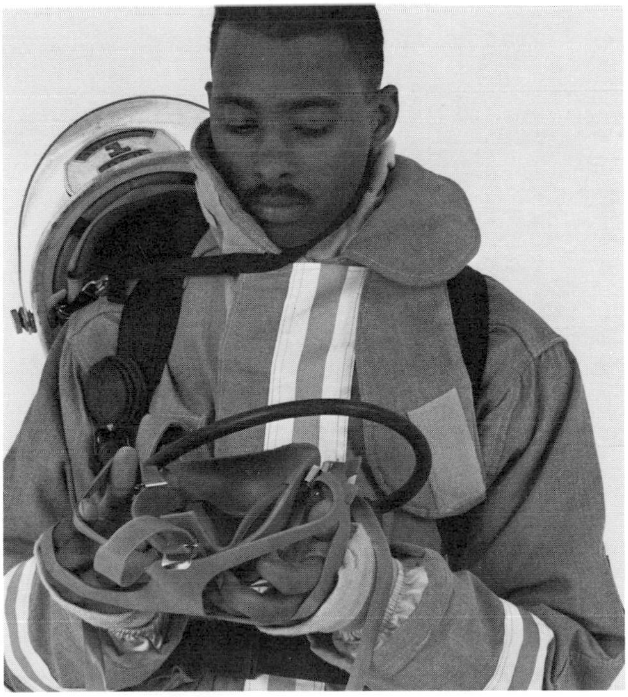

Step 3: Stabilize the facepiece with one hand, and use the other hand to remove hair that may be present between the forehead and the sealing surface of the facepiece (Figure 5.47).

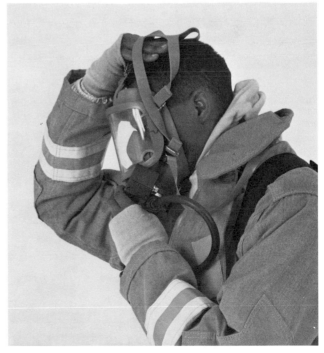

Figure 5.46 With the thumbs inserted through the straps, grasp the head harness and spread the webbing.

Figure 5.47 Stabilize facepiece with one hand. Push web strap back over the head, making sure hair does not interfere with facepiece seal.

Step 4:   Center your chin in the chin cup and position the harness so that it is centered at the rear of your head (Figures 5.48 a and b).

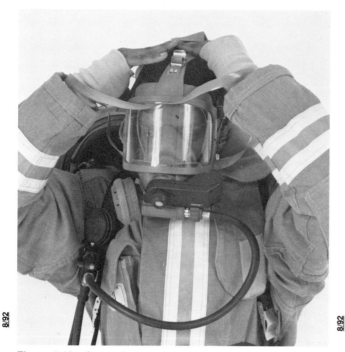

Figure 5.48a Center the harness on the head.

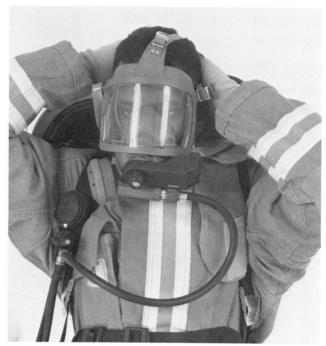

Figure 5.48b Pull the neck strap over the head and onto the neck.

Step 5:   Tighten the harness straps by pulling them backward (not outward) evenly and simultaneously. Tighten the lower straps first, then the temple straps, and finally the top strap if there is one (Figures 5.49 a through c). (**NOTE:** For 2-strap harnesses, tighten the neck straps, then stroke the harness firmly down the back of your head (Figure 5.50). Retighten the straps as necessary.)

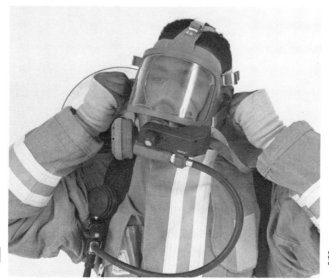

Figure 5.49a Tighten the straps starting with the lower straps, pulling backward not outward.

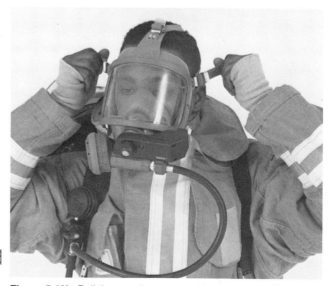

Figure 5.49b Pull the temple straps to the rear.

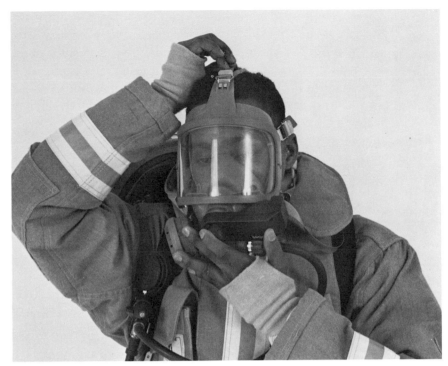

Figure 5.49c Last, tighten the center strap.

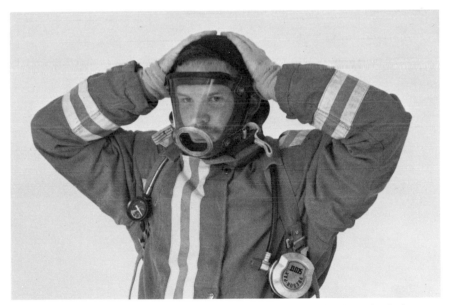

Figure 5.50 For a two-strap harness, tighten the neck straps, then firmly stroke the harness down the back of the head.

Step 6: If the SCBA is so equipped, check the regulator to ensure that the gasket is in place around the regulator outlet port.

Step 7: If the regulator is separated from the facepiece, attach it to the facepiece by positioning it firmly into the facepiece fitting. Lock it into place (Figure 5.51). (**NOTE:** This procedure will vary, depending upon the make of SCBA. Always follow the manufacturer's instructions.)

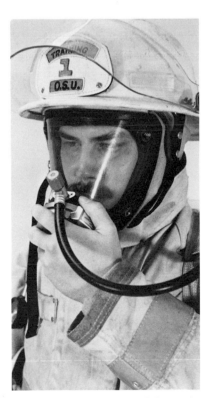

Figure 5.51 If separated from the facepiece, attach regulator to the facepiece by positioning it firmly into the facepiece fitting and locking it in place.

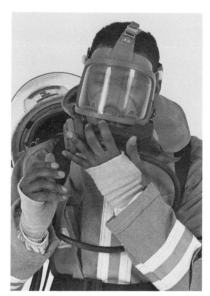

Figure 5.52 Use negative-pressure test to check the facepiece seal by inhaling slowly and deeply for 10 seconds.

Step 8: Check the facepiece seal. Make sure that the donning switch is in the DON position (positive pressure off) (Figure 5.52). Inhale slowly (not deeply), and hold your breath for 10 seconds. The mask should draw up to your face. Listen for the sound of airflow. There should be no sound and no inward leakage through the exhalation valve or around the facepiece.

Another method for checking facepiece seal is to close the cylinder valve. Continue to breathe slowly until the mask collapses against your face, and hold your breath for 10 seconds. If the mask draws up to your face and no leaks are detected, reopen the cylinder valve. Adjust or redon the facepiece if there is evidence of leaking. If leakage persists, determine and correct the cause of the leakage. If unable to eliminate the leakage, obtain another facepiece and repeat the leak-check procedure. Use care with this method because it uses up some air.

NOTE: Positive-pressure SCBA that can supply air in a demand-type mode do not meet the requirements of NFPA 1981, 1987 edition.

Step 9: Check the exhalation valve. As you exhale during Step 8, make sure that the exhalation goes through the exhalation valve. If it does not, the valve may be stuck. To free it, press your facepiece against the sides of your face, and exhale to free the valve (Figure 5.53). Use caution when exhaling against a sealed facepiece in order to prevent discomfort and possible damage to the inner ear from exhaling forcefully. If you cannot get the exhalation valve free, remove the facepiece and have it checked.

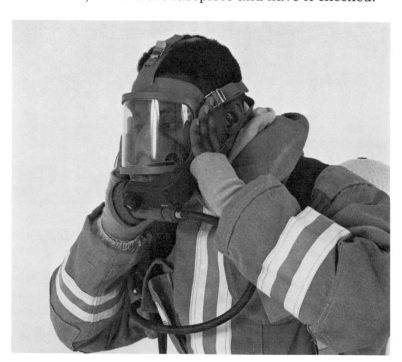

Figure 5.53 Check exhalation valve by pressing the mask against the face and exhaling sharply.

Step 10: Check for positive pressure. Gently break the facepiece seal by inserting two fingers under the edge of the facepiece (Figure 5.54). You should be able to feel air moving past your fingers. If you cannot feel air movement, remove the unit and have it checked.

Step 11: Pull the protective hood into place, making sure that all exposed skin is covered and that vision is unobscured (Figure 5.55). Check to see that no portion of the hood is located between the facepiece and the face.

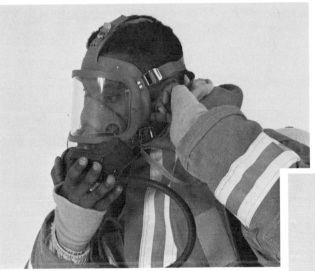

Figure 5.54 Check for positive pressure by gently breaking the facepiece seal by inserting two fingers under the edge of the facepiece. Air should be felt moving past the fingers.

Step 12: Put your helmet back on your head and tighten the chin strap (Figure 5.56). Be sure to get the helmet strap under your chin. (**NOTE:** Helmets with a breakaway strap can be donned at this point.)

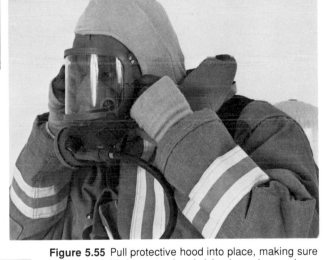

Figure 5.55 Pull protective hood into place, making sure all exposed skin is covered and vision is unobscured.

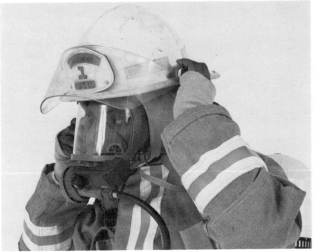

Figure 5.56 Put the helmet back on and tighten chin strap.

An alternative method is to leave the helmet on while donning the backpack, then loosen the chin strap and allow the helmet to rest on the air cylinder while donning the facepiece (Figure 5.57).

DOFFING THE OPEN-CIRCUIT SCBA
Doffing With Harness-Mounted Regulator

When you are in a safe atmosphere, take the following steps to remove SCBA having a harness-mounted regulator:

Step 1: Close the mainline valve and disconnect the low-pressure hose from the regulator. (**NOTE:** If the unit has a donning switch, make sure that it is in the donning mode.)

Step 2: Take off your helmet or loosen it and push it and your hood back off your head.

Step 3: Loosen the facepiece harness strap buckles. Either rub them toward your face or lift the buckles slightly to loosen them and to disentangle them from your hair (Figures 5.58 a and b). Take off the facepiece (Figure 5.59), extend the harness straps fully, and prepare it for inspection, cleaning, sanitizing, and storage (Figure 5.60).

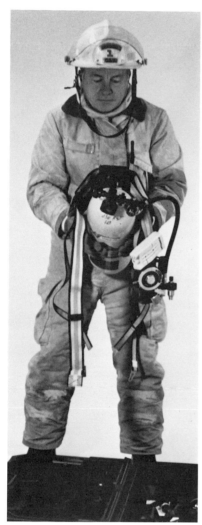

Figure 5.57 Leave helmet on while donning the backpack, then loosen the chin strap and allow helmet to rest on air cylinder or shoulder while donning facepiece.

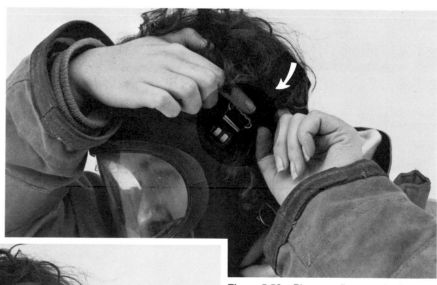

Figure 5.58a Place one finger under the strap and use the other finger to rub or flip the buckle toward the face.

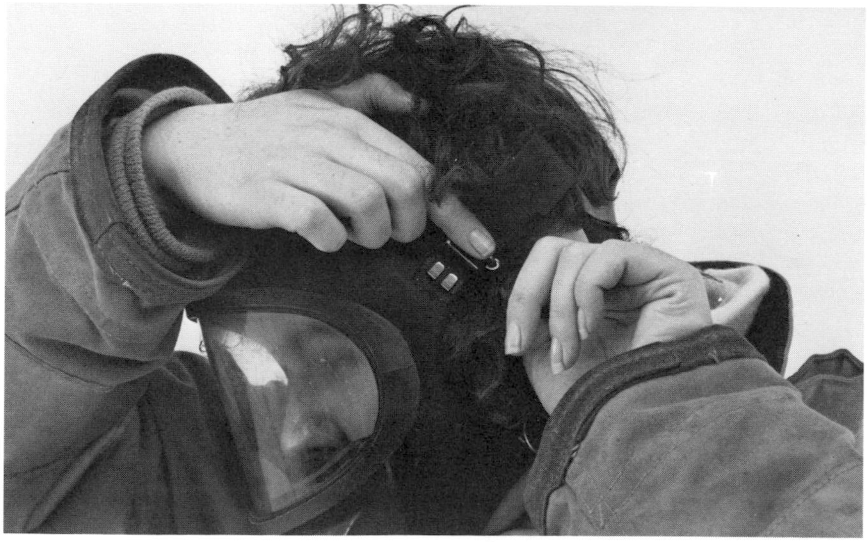

Figure 5.58b Using the finger under the strap to maintain tension on the buckle, continue to rub the buckle using a scratching motion.

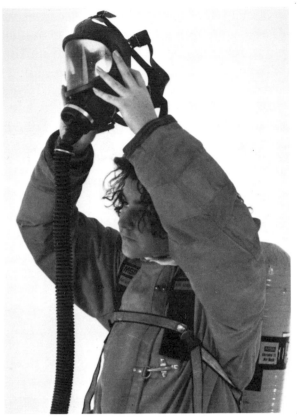

Figure 5.59 Once all of the straps have been loosened, lift the facepiece from the head.

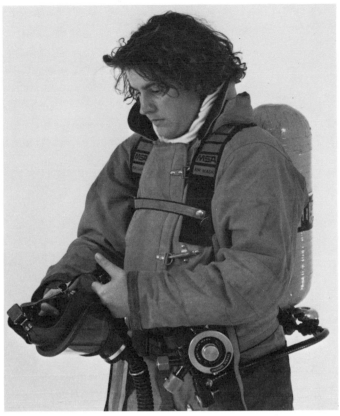

Figure 5.60 Extend harness straps completely and prepare facepiece for inspection, cleaning, and storage.

Step 4: Unbuckle the waist belt and fully extend the adjustment (Figure 5.61).

Step 5: Disconnect the chest buckle if the unit has a chest strap.

Step 6: Lean forward; release shoulder strap buckles and hold them open while fully extending the straps (Figure 5.62).

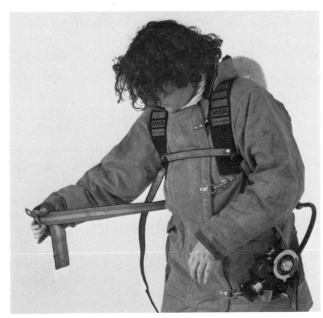

Figure 5.61 Unbuckle waist belt and fully extend.

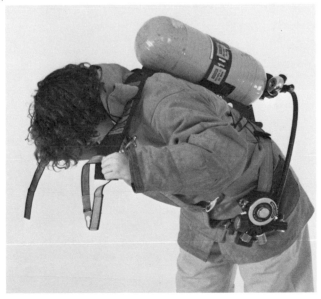

Figure 5.62 Lean forward; release shoulder strap buckles and then hold open while extending straps.

Step 7: Grasp the shoulder straps firmly with the respective hands. Slip off the shoulder strap from the shoulder opposite the regulator, and remove your arm from the shoulder strap. Grasp the regulator with your free hand, allow the other strap to slide off your shoulder, and lower the SCBA to the ground (Figures 5.63 a through c). As you remove the unit, do not drop the regulator or allow it to strike anything.

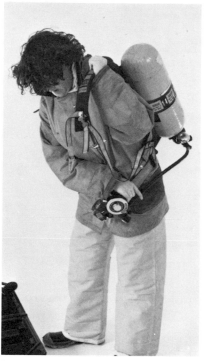

Figure 5.63a Slip the shoulder strap from the shoulder opposite the regulator, and reach around to grasp the regulator with free hand.

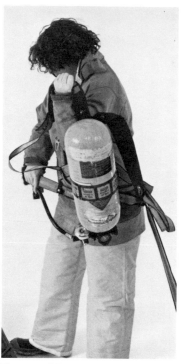

Figure 5.63b Holding the regulator and backpack harness, allow the SCBA to slip from the shoulder.

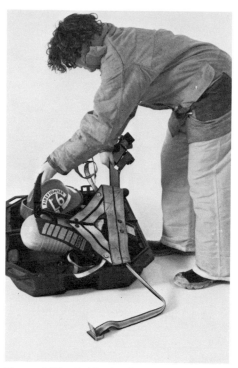

Figure 5.63c Guide the SCBA to the ground while controlling the regulator.

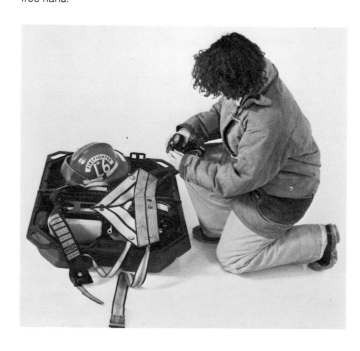

Figure 5.64 Open mainline valve to depressurize the system.

Step 8: Close the cylinder valve, then relieve the excess pressure from the regulator. If the low-pressure hose has been removed from the regulator, recouple it, hold the facepiece against your face, and breathe until the remaining pressure is depleted. Another method is to open the mainline valve and allow the excess pressure to vent (Figure 5.64). (**NOTE:** Do not use the bypass valve to relieve excess pressure.)

Step 9: Remove the facepiece from the regulator and make sure that the straps are extended fully. The facepiece should be ready for inspection, cleaning, sanitizing, and storage.

Doffing With Facepiece-Mounted Regulator

When you are in a safe atmosphere, take the following steps to remove SCBA having a facepiece-mounted regulator:

Step 1: Take off your helmet or loosen it and push it and your hood back off your head.

Step 2: If the unit has a donning switch, turn the positive pressure off or place it in donning mode (Figure 5.65).

Step 3: Depending upon the make of SCBA and manufacturer's instructions, disconnect the regulator from the facepiece (Figure 5.66).

Step 4: Loosen the facepiece harness strap buckles. Either rub them toward your face or lift the buckles slightly to loosen them. Take off the facepiece and prepare it for inspection, cleaning, sanitizing, and storage. Extend the harness straps fully (Figures 5.67 a and b).

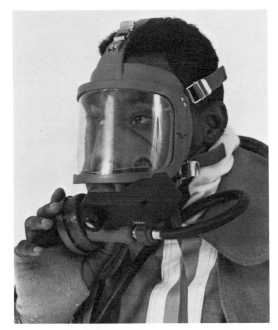

Figure 5.65 Place unit in donning mode (turn positive pressure off).

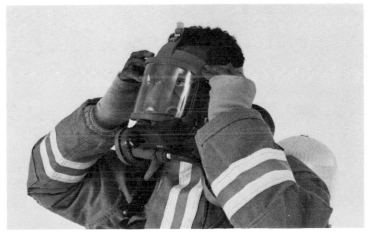

Figure 5.67a Loosen the straps by briskly rubbing the buckles toward the face.

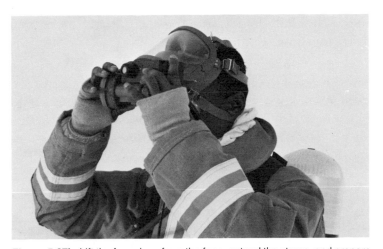

Figure 5.67b Lift the facepiece from the face, extend the straps, and prepare for cleaning and inspection.

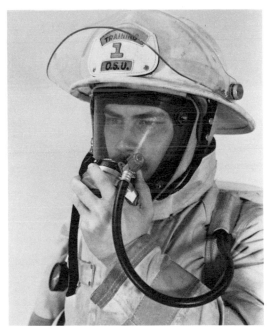

Figure 5.66 Disconnect regulator from facepiece, if required.

Step 5: Unbuckle the waist belt and fully extend the adjustment (Figure 5.68).

Step 6: Disconnect the chest buckle if the unit has a chest strap.

Step 7: If the unit is so equipped, attach the regulator to the harness clip, or control the regulator by holding it while performing the next steps.

Step 8: Lean forward; release shoulder strap buckles and hold them open while fully extending the straps (Figure 5.69).

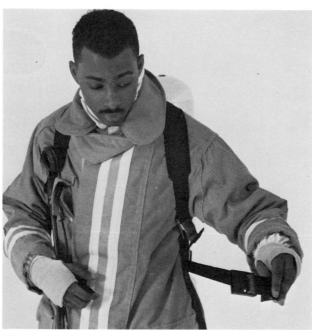

Figure 5.68 Unbuckle waist belt and fully extend the adjustment.

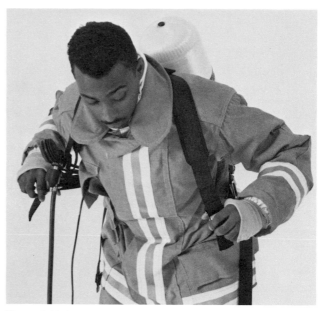

Figure 5.69 Lean forward; release shoulder strap buckles and then hold open while extending straps.

Step 9: Grasp the shoulder straps firmly with the respective hands. Slip off the shoulder strap from the shoulder opposite the regulator, and remove your arm from the shoulder strap (Figures 5.70 a and b). Grasp the regulator with your free hand, allow the other strap to slide off your shoulder, and lower the SCBA to the ground. As you remove the unit, do not drop the regulator or allow it to strike anything (Figure 5.71).

Step 10: Close the cylinder valve and breathe down the pressure from the regulator by reconnecting the regulator to the facepiece holding the facepiece against your face and breathing until the pressure is depleted (Figures 5.72 a and b). (**NOTE:** Do not bleed off air by operating the bypass valve.)

DONNING THE CLOSED-CIRCUIT SCBA

Donning a closed-circuit SCBA is basically the same as donning standard open-circuit models. However, there are differences in donning and using closed-circuit SCBA with which firefighters must be familiar.

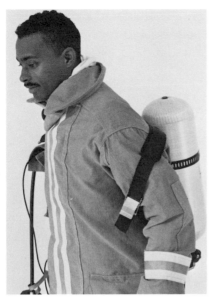

Figure 5.70a Slip shoulder strap from the shoulder opposite the regulator.

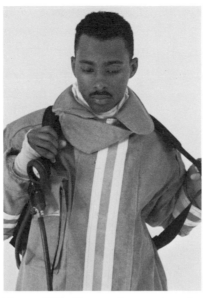

Figure 5.70b Remove the arm from the strap, and with free hand grasp the regulator.

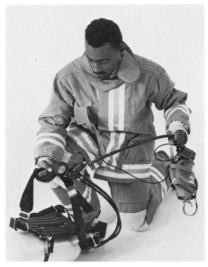

Figure 5.71 Lower SCBA to the ground while controlling the regulator.

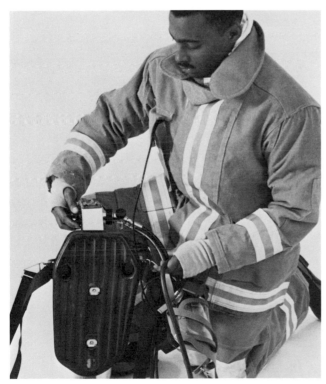

Figure 5.72a Close the cylinder valve.

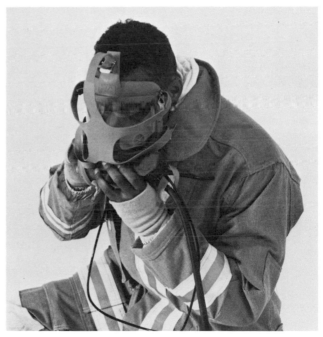

Figure 5.72b Place the facepiece against the face and breathe until the excess pressure is depleted.

NOTE: These steps may need to be adapted to the specific type of closed-circuit apparatus being used. Always refer to the manufacturer's instructions when donning and using SCBA. The inhalation and exhalation hoses must be kept sealed while the unit is stored. It is acceptable to store the unit with the facepiece hoses connected to the backpack hoses or with the hoses on the backpack connected to each other.

Step 1: If using a protective hood, pull it back and down so that the face opening is around your neck (Figure 5.73). Turn up the collar of your turnout coat.

Step 2: Check the turnaround maintenance tag. Never use a unit that does not have a completed maintenance tag attached (Figure 5.74). Tear the turnaround maintenance tag from the oxygen cylinder and begin donning procedures.

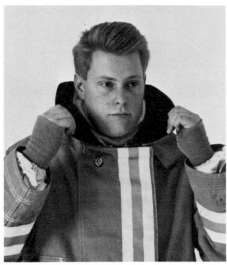

Figure 5.73 Pull protective hood back and down so that face opening is around the neck; turn up collar.

Figure 5.74 Check turnaround maintenance tag.

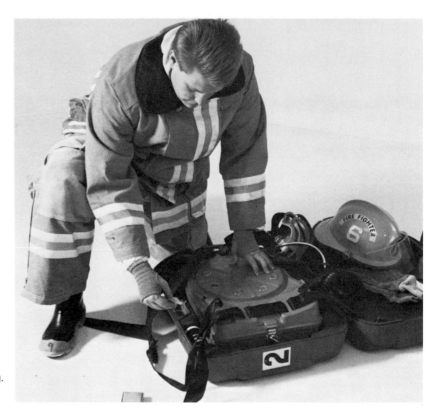

Step 3: Place the unit on the ground, with the harness side up. Crouch or kneel so that the top is toward you, and fully extend the shoulder straps. (**NOTE:** If the unit has been stored with the low-pressure hoses connected to each other, they should be separated and attached to the facepiece at this time (Figures 5.75 a and b).

Step 4: Spread out the shoulder straps.

Step 5: Grasp the body of the unit about 6 inches (150 mm) from its bottom and lift it, with the harness toward you and the top down (Figure 5.76).

Step 6: Raise the unit over your head, and allow it to slide slowly down your back (Figures 5.77 a and b). Place your arms through their respective straps. (**NOTE:** This donning sequence is shown using the over-the-head method. The other methods described earlier in this chapter are also acceptable.)

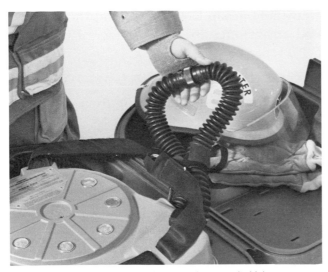

Figure 5.75a Closed-circuit SCBA may be stored with low-pressure hoses connected to each other.

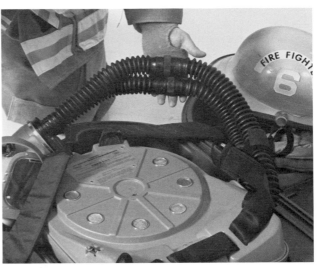

Figure 5.75b Closed-circuit SCBA also may be stored with low-pressure hoses connected to facepiece hoses.

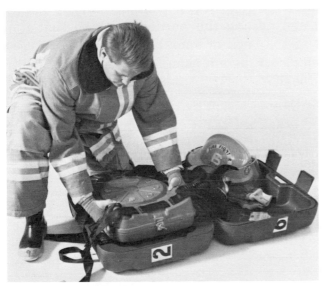

Figure 5.76 With the harness toward the user and the top of the unit down, grasp the body of the unit about 6 inches (150 mm) from the bottom and lift.

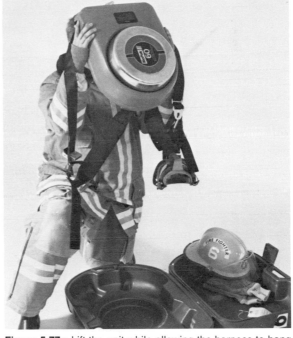

Figure 5.77a Lift the unit while allowing the harness to hang freely.

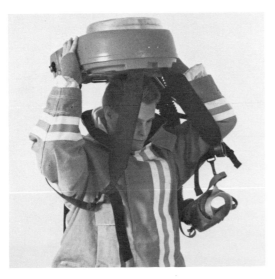

Figure 5.77b With elbows through the shoulder straps, allow the unit to slide down the back while firmly grasping the shoulder straps.

Step 7: Bend forward and grasp the free ends of the shoulder straps. Pull straps outward and downward to tighten (Figure 5.78).

Step 8: Secure the chest strap (Figure 5.79).

Step 9: Fasten and adjust the waist strap (Figure 5.80).

Step 10: Place your helmet over your head and let it drop onto your back, hanging by the chin strap. The helmet can then be placed back on your head after the facepiece has been donned.

Step 11: Hold the facepiece about 1 inch (25 mm) from your face.

Step 12: Open the oxygen cylinder valve all the way and then turn the valve knob back one-half turn. (**NOTE:** This floods the facepiece with oxygen.) Listen for a short chirp from the alarm whistle.

Step 13: Don the facepiece by holding the facepiece snugly against the chin and pulling the harness back so that it is centered at the back of your head. Tighten the chin straps, temple straps, and then the center strap (Figures 5.81 a through e).

Step 14: Check the facepiece seal by tightly pinching the hoses closed and exhaling. (**NOTE:** This may require some effort.) You should not be able to hear or feel air escaping (Figure 5.82).

Step 15: Momentarily open and close the bypass valve to be sure that it works. Close the bypass valve fully.

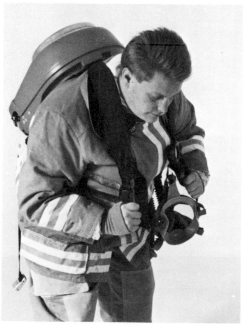

Figure 5.78 Bend forward and grasp free ends of the shoulder straps. Pull the straps outward and downward to tighten.

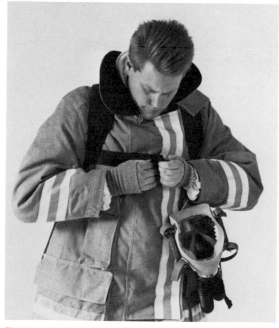

Figure 5.79 Secure chest strap.

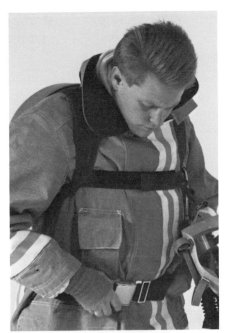

Figure 5.80 Fasten and adjust waist strap.

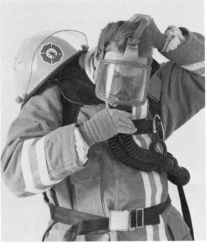

Figure 5.81a Center chin in chin cup and position harness so that it is centered at the rear of head.

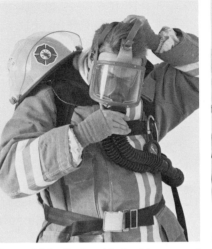

Figure 5.81b Stabilize facepiece and tighten one of the chin straps.

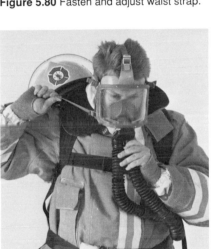

Figure 5.81c Tighten the other chin strap.

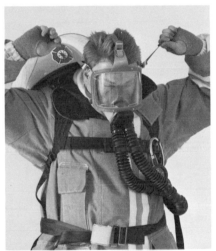

Figure 5.81d Tighten temple straps.

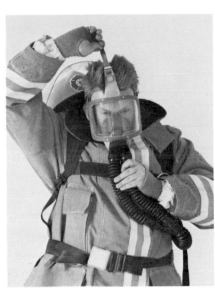

Figure 5.81e Tighten the center strap.

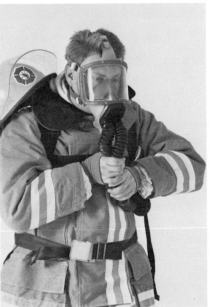

Figure 5.82 Check facepiece seal by pinching hoses closed, inhaling, and exhaling. The user should not be able to hear or feel air escaping. Pinching the hoses on some models may require a lot of effort.

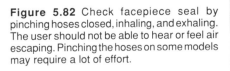

Step 16: Pull the protective hood into place, making sure that all exposed skin is covered and that vision is unobscured (Figure 5.83).

Step 17: Place the helmet on your head and secure the chin strap under your chin (Figure 5.84).

Step 18: Check the chest-mounted pressure gauge to verify cylinder pressure (Figure 5.85).

An alternative method is to wear the helmet while donning the SCBA. After donning the backpack, loosen the chin strap, allow the helmet to rest on the unit or on your shoulder, and then don the facepiece. When the facepiece straps have been tightened and the hood is on, lift the helmet back onto your head and tighten the chin strap.

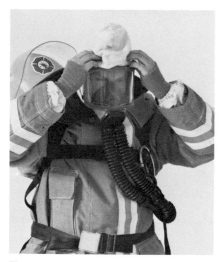

Figure 5.83 Pull protective hood into place, covering all exposed skin and making sure vision is unobscured.

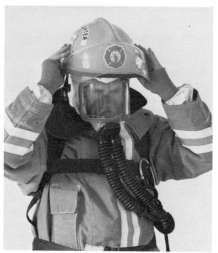

Figure 5.84 Place helmet on head and secure chin strap.

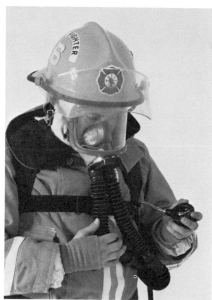

Figure 5.85 Check chest-mounted pressure gauge to verify cylinder pressure.

DOFFING THE CLOSED-CIRCUIT SCBA

The steps for removing the closed-circuit SCBA are as follows:

Step 1: Reach back with the right hand and close the oxygen cylinder valve.

Step 2: Remove your helmet and hood, loosen the facepiece straps, and remove the facepiece. Clip the facepiece D-ring to the shoulder harness (Figure 5.86).

Step 3: Release the chest strap. Loosen, unsnap, and fully extend the waist strap (Figures 5.87 a and b).

Step 4: Fully extend the shoulder straps (Figure 5.88).

Step 5: Grasp the left shoulder strap and allow the right shoulder strap to fall from your shoulder. Swing the unit around to the front and grasp the other shoulder strap; lower unit to the ground (Figures 5.89 a and b).

Step 6: Fully extend all straps before storing the unit (Figure 5.90).

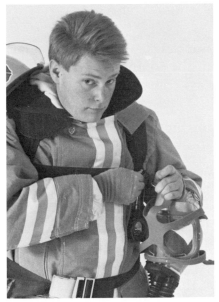

Figure 5.86 Clip the facepiece D-ring to the shoulder harness.

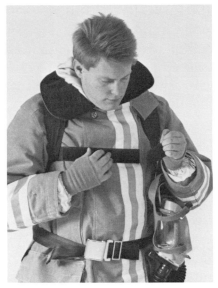

Figure 5.87a Release the chest strap.

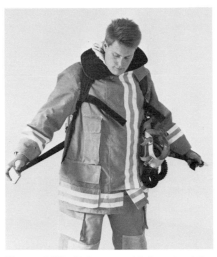

Figure 5.87b Release and fully extend the waist strap.

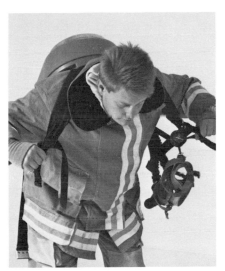

Figure 5.88 Fully extend the shoulder straps.

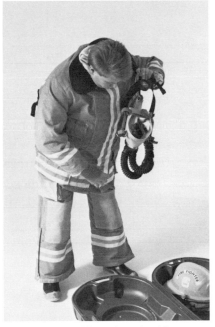

Figure 5.89a Allow the shoulder strap opposite the facepiece to fall from the shoulder, then swing the unit around to the front.

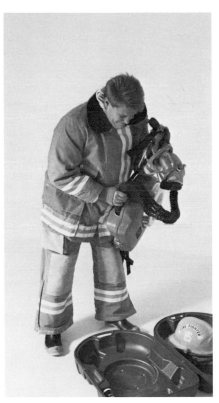

Figure 5.89b Grasp the unit where the low-pressure hoses are attached, and gently guide the unit to the ground.

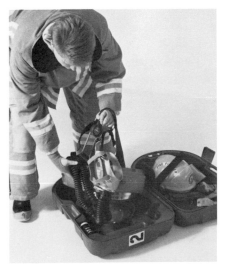

Figure 5.90 Place the unit in the box, and fully extend all straps before storing.

CHANGING CYLINDERS
Open-Circuit SCBA

With care and caution, a firefighter can change an air cylinder at the scene of an emergency so that the equipment can be used again as soon as possible. Changing cylinders can be either a one- or two-person job.

The one-person method for changing an air cylinder is described in detail as follows:

Step 1: Doff the unit using the procedures described earlier.

Step 2: Obtain a full air cylinder and have it ready.

Step 3: Disconnect the regulator from the facepiece or disconnect the low-pressure hose from the regulator (Figure 5.91).

Step 4: Close the cylinder valve on the *used* bottle and release the pressure from the high-pressure hose. On some units, the pressure must be released by breathing down the regulator or opening the mainline valve. Refer to the manufacturer's instructions for the correct method for the particular unit.

NOTE: If the pressure is not released, the high-pressure coupling will be difficult to disconnect.

Step 5: Disconnect the high-pressure coupling from the cylinder (Figure 5.92). (**NOTE:** If more than hand force is required to disconnect the coupling, repeat Step 4 and then again attempt to disconnect the coupling.) Lay the hose coupling on the ground, directly in line with the cylinder outlet, as a reminder so that the replacement cylinder can be aligned correctly and easily. Be sure that grit or

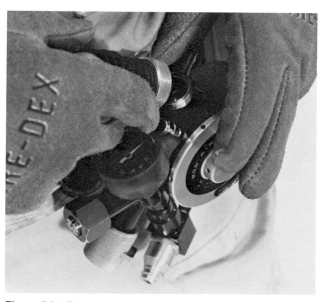

Figure 5.91 Disconnect the low-pressure hose from the regulator.

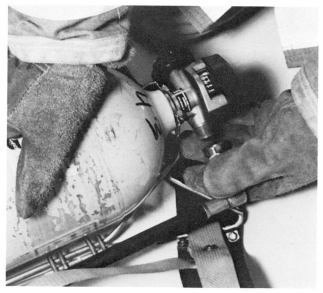

Figure 5.92 Disconnect the high-pressure coupling from the cylinder.

liquids will not enter the end of the unprotected high-pressure hose prior to attaching it to the cylinder outlet valve.

Step 6: Release the cylinder clamp and remove the empty cylinder (Figures 5.93 and 5.94).

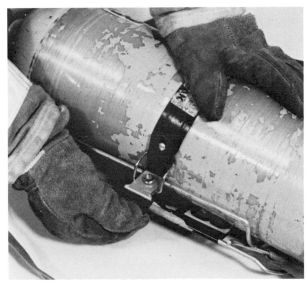

Figure 5.93 Release the cylinder clamp.

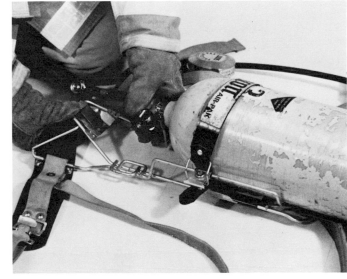

Figure 5.94 Remove the cylinder from the backpack.

Step 7: Place the new cylinder into the backpack, position the cylinder outlet, and lock the cylinder into place (Figure 5.95). (**NOTE:** For some cylinders, it may be necessary to rotate the cylinder one-eighth turn to the left; this protects the high-pressure hose by lessening the angle of the hose and preventing twisting.)

Step 8: Check the cylinder valve opening and the high-pressure hose fitting for debris and the condition of the O-ring (Figure 5.96). Clear any debris from the cylinder valve

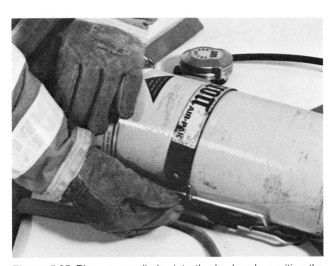

Figure 5.95 Place new cylinder into the backpack, position the cylinder outlet, and lock the cylinder into place.

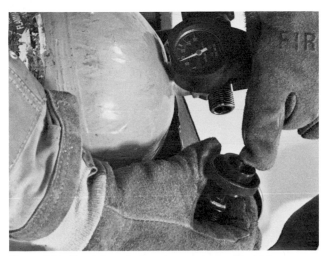

Figure 5.96 Check the cylinder valve opening and the high-pressure hose fitting for debris, and check the condition of the O-ring.

opening by quickly opening and closing the cylinder valve or by wiping the debris away. If the O-ring is distorted or damaged, replace it.

Step 9: Connect the high-pressure hose to the cylinder valve opening. (**NOTE:** Do not overtighten; hand tightening is sufficient.)

Step 10: Open the cylinder valve and check the gauges on the cylinder and the regulator (Figure 5.97). Both gauges should register within 100 psi of each other — if increments are in psi — when the cylinder is pressurized to its rated capacity. If increments are in other measurements, such as fractions or minutes, they should correspond.

NOTE: Some units require that the mainline valve on the regulator be opened in order to obtain a gauge reading. Seal the regulator outlet port by placing one hand over it. On a positive-pressure regulator, the port must be sealed for an accurate regulator gauge reading.

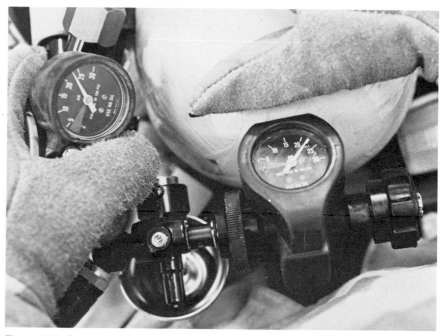

Figure 5.97 Open the cylinder valve and check the gauges on the cylinder and the regulator.

When there are two people, the firefighter with an empty cylinder simply positions the cylinder so that it can be easily changed by the other firefighter. Two methods for two people are shown in Figures 5.98 and 5.99.

Closed-Circuit SCBA

When the oxygen supply of a closed-circuit SCBA is depleted, the empty oxygen cylinder cannot simply be exchanged with a full cylinder. The chemical scrubber unit as well as the oxygen

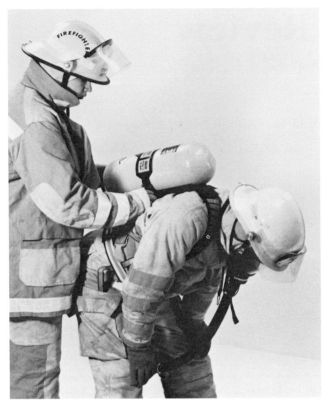

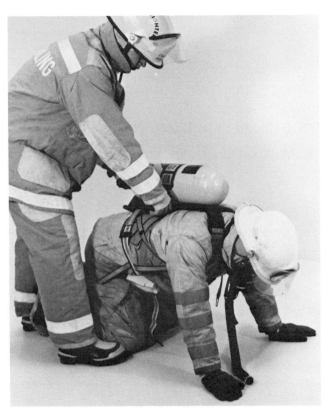

Figure 5.98 One firefighter slides a full cylinder into the backpack assembly while the other firefighter braces to remain steady.

Figure 5.99 The firefighter receiving a full cylinder may choose to kneel while the cylinder is being replaced.

cylinder must be changed. In other words, a complete inspection and turnaround maintenance must be performed before the closed-circuit SCBA can again be used. Refer to the manufacturer's instructions for recharging and maintenance procedures for closed-circuit SCBA.

SUMMARY

Firefighters must be able to don SCBA quickly and correctly. The different methods for donning the backpack include the over-the-head method, the cross-arm coat method, the regular coat method, the seat mount, the side or rear mount, and the compartment mount. The facepieces for most SCBA are donned in a similar manner. Two differences in donning facepieces are the number of straps on the head harness and whether the regulator mounts into the facepiece or is mounted on the harness. The procedures for donning closed-circuit SCBA are different than those for donning open-circuit apparatus. Regardless of the type of SCBA used or the method of donning, firefighters must be thoroughly skilled in donning the SCBA, using it safely in the prescribed manner, doffing it without damaging it, and changing cylinders.

Chapter 5 Review

Answers on page 350

TRUE-FALSE: Mark each statement true or false. If false, explain why.

1. Methods for donning the facepiece are the same, regardless of whether the regulator is harness-mounted or is facepiece-mounted.

   ☐ T ☐ F _____

   _____

2. When preparing to don the backpack using the over-the-head method, the firefighter should crouch or kneel at the valve end of the cylinder.

   ☐ T ☐ F _____

   _____

3. When using the regular coat method for donning the SCBA backpack (with the regulator on the left side), the firefighter should grasp the left shoulder strap high on the harness with the left hand and grasp the lower portion of the same strap with the right hand.

   ☐ T ☐ F _____

   _____

4. Side- or rear-mount SCBA does not permit donning en route.

   ☐ T ☐ F _____

   _____

5. Facepiece harness straps should be tightened by pulling them evenly and simultaneously to the sides, out from the face.

   ☐ T ☐ F _____

   _____

6. The protective hood should be pulled into place after the facepiece has been donned.

   ☐ T ☐ F _____

   _____

MULTIPLE CHOICE: Circle the correct answer.

7. When using the over-the-head method to don an SCBA, which of the following should you do first?

   A. Grasp the backplate or cylinder with both hands, one at each side.

   B. Adjust the shoulder straps to ensure that the SCBA harness will fit comfortably.

   C. Check the unit, including the cylinder gauge.

   D. Fasten the regulator to the harness, if the regulator is harness-mounted.

8. Firefighter A says that before donning SCBA, you should always check the cylinder pressure. Firefighter B says that you should open the cylinder valve and check the regulator gauge. Who is correct?

   A. Firefighter A

   B. Firefighter B

   C. Both A and B

   D. Neither A nor B

9. When donning the backpack using the crossed-arm coat method, the firefighter should _____.

   A. lean backward slightly to balance the cylinder, fasten and adjust the waist strap, and then tighten the shoulder straps

   B. lean forward slightly to balance the cylinder, fasten and adjust the waist strap, fasten the chest buckle if the unit has a chest strap, and then tighten the shoulder straps

   C. straighten body so that the backpack rides low on the back, fasten the chest buckle if the unit has a chest strap, fasten and adjust the waist strap, and then tighten the shoulder straps

   D. lean forward slightly to balance the cylinder, tighten shoulder straps, fasten the chest buckle if the unit has a chest strap, fasten and adjust the waist strap, and then recheck all straps to see that they are adjusted correctly

10. Firefighter A says that if the waist straps do not fit properly, they should be removed so that the firefighter will not experience any discomfort. Firefighter B disagrees and says that the waist straps prevent the firefighter from experiencing undue stress from side-to-side shifting of the SCBA. Who is correct?

    A. Firefighter A

    B. Firefighter B

    C. Both A and B

    D. Neither A nor B

11. Firefighters A and B are discussing checking the facepiece seal after donning the facepiece. Firefighter A says that the end of the low-pressure hose must be covered before inhaling. Firefighter B says that if the SCBA has a facepiece-mounted regulator, the opening on the facepiece for the regulator should be covered with one hand before inhaling. Who is correct?

   A. Firefighter A

   B. Firefighter B

   C. Both A and B

   D. Neither A nor B

LISTING

12. Seat mounting hardware comes in three main types. What are these?

   A. _____

   B. _____

   C. _____

SELECT: Circle the correct response.

13. When preparing to don SCBA using the regular coat method, the SCBA should be arranged so that (the left, the right, either) shoulder strap can be grasped for lifting.

14. While en route and donning SCBA from a seat mount, the firefighter's seat belt should be (fastened/unfastened).

15. When donning the SCBA backpack from a backup mount, the firefighter should fasten and adjust the waist strap (before/after) stepping forward to clear the unit from the mount.

SHORT ANSWER: Answer each item briefly.

16. If, after donning the facepiece, the exhalation valve seems to be stuck, what can the firefighter do to attempt to free the valve?

   _____

   _____

   _____

17. After spreading out the straps, how should the firefighter grasp the harness to don the backpack (with the regulator on the left side) using the cross-armed coat method?

   _____

   _____

   _____

18. What are the two main differences in facepiece design that affect the manner in which facepieces are donned?

_____

_____

_____

_____

19. Is tightening the facepiece harness straps as tight as possible the proper way to ensure proper facepiece fit and seal? Explain.

_____

_____

_____

_____

_____

20. After donning the facepiece, how can the firefighter check for positive pressure?

_____

_____

_____

_____

_____

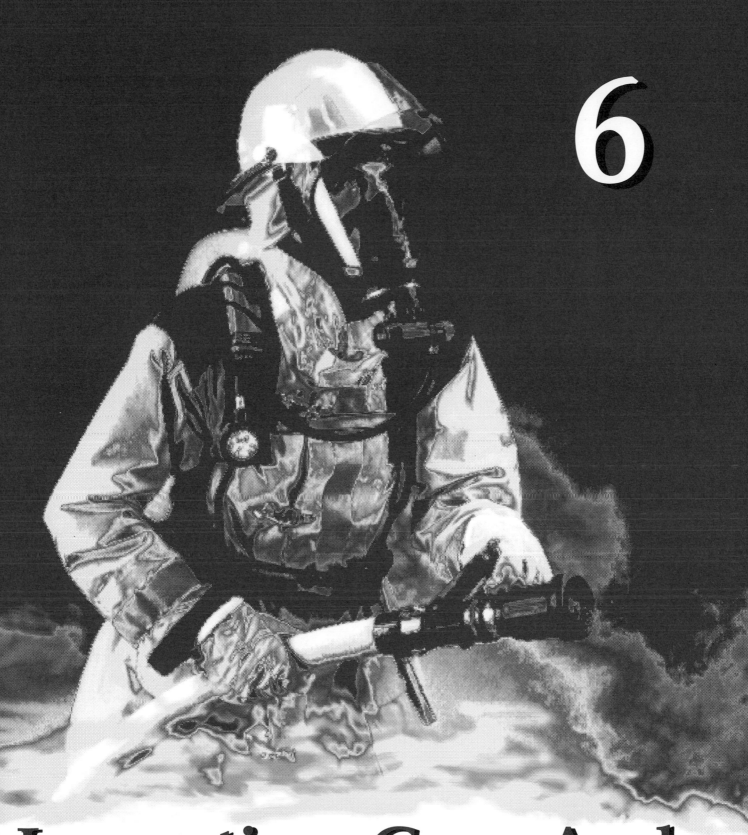

Inspection, Care, And Testing Of SCBA

This chapter provides information that addresses the following standards:

NFPA STANDARD 1001
Fire Fighter Professional Qualifications
1987 Edition

Chapter 3—Fire Fighter I
3-6.5
3-6.6

Chapter 4—Fire Fighter II
4-6.1

NFPA STANDARD 1404
Fire Department Self-Contained Breathing Apparatus Program
1989 Edition

Chapter 1—Introduction
1-4.7
1-4.7.1

Chapter 2—Provisions of SCBA
2-1.4
2-1.5
2-2.2
2-2.3
2-2.4
2-2.5
2-3.2
4-13
4-14

Chapter 5—SCBA Inservice Inspection
5-1.1
5-1.2
5-1.3
5-1.4

Chapter 6—SCBA Maintenance
6-1.1
6-1.2
6-1.3
6-2.1
6-2.2
6-2.3
6-2.4
6-3.1
6-3.2
6-3.3
6-3.4

NFPA STANDARD 1500
Fire Department Occupational Safety and Health Program
1987 Edition

Chapter 5—Protective Clothing and Protective Equipment
5-3.4.3
5-3.5

ANSI STANDARD Z88.5-1981
Practices for Respiratory Protection for the Fire Service

Section 3—SCBA Program
3.1.5
3.2.3
3.2.4

Section 5—Use of SCBA
5.2

Section 6—Maintenance of SCBA
6.1.1
6.1.2
6.2.2
6.2.3
6.2.4
6.2.4.1
6.2.4.3
6.3.1
6.3.3
6.3.3.1
6.3.3.2
6.3.3.4
6.4.1
6.4.2

Section 8—Training and Education in Proper Use of SCBA
8.1.4 (4)

Chapter 6
Inspection, Care, and Testing of SCBA

INTRODUCTION

Firefighters should take an active role in ensuring that their self-contained breathing apparatus is in proper working condition. To do this, they must be trained to use the correct procedures for inspection, care, and testing of SCBA. Regular preventive maintenance, which includes regular inspection, care, testing, and repair of SCBA, provides a margin of safety. As the name implies, preventive maintenance can prevent or minimize problems such as malfunctioning components and leaking cylinders. Because proper inspection and care of SCBA help prevent equipment malfunction, injuries or even fatalities to firefighters can be avoided. SCBA should be inspected daily or weekly (depending on its use), inspected and cleaned after each use, and inspected again monthly.

The information in this chapter applies to the inspection, care, and testing of self-contained breathing apparatus. Regardless of the type of apparatus used, firefighters should *always* follow the manufacturer's recommendations and consult appropriate personnel when they have questions about SCBA operation, maintenance, or repair. Refer to Appendix E for information regarding different manufacturers of SCBA.

The inspection procedures outlined in the following sections pertain to open-circuit SCBA. Closed-circuit SCBA inspection and maintenance procedures differ. Some of the steps, such as inspecting hoses or other parts for wear or damage or checking to see that alarms work properly, are similar. In addition, records and inspection intervals for closed-circuit SCBA are the same as those for open-circuit SCBA. However, because of the different types of components used in a closed-circuit SCBA, the overall cleaning and inspection procedures are very different from those procedures for open-circuit SCBA; the manufacturer's maintenance procedures should be strictly followed.

> **Always follow the directions and specifications given by the SCBA manufacturer whether caring for open- or closed-circuit SCBA.**

DEPARTMENT RESPONSIBILITY

Each fire department must have written SOPs for using SCBA. Included in the SOPs must be procedures that follow SCBA manufacturer's recommendations for inspecting, cleaning, testing, storing, maintaining, and repairing SCBA, along with procedures for keeping records on such. The department's SOPs must also include provisions for instructing, training, and evaluating fire department personnel in the use of these written procedures.

The fire department is responsible for establishing a preventive maintenance program and for training firefighters to properly care for their SCBA. It is also responsible for ensuring that only manufacturer-approved technicians test and repair SCBA. The department may choose to select certain personnel from the department to attend special manufacturer's repair schools to become factory-certified in certain testing and maintenance procedures.

SCBA must be properly maintained so that it is always ready for use. Therefore, each SCBA should be inspected and tested at regular intervals. The amount of time between regular inspections is determined by several factors. These factors include how often equipment is used (several times a day, once a day, once a week, and so on), the number of personnel using the equipment, whether there are several shifts of on-duty firefighters or only volunteer firefighters, and the environments in which the equipment is used. Considering these factors, fire departments must determine inspection schedules. In addition to being cleaned and inspected after each use, SCBA should be inspected each time a new shift of firefighters begins, and it should be inspected weekly if the department is volunteer. Monthly inspection of all SCBA, which includes testing of certain parts, is also required.

The particular personnel responsible for inspecting the department's SCBA will depend upon the department's written policy. One or more properly trained individuals — generally firefighters — may be assigned to perform the monthly inspections. However, the regular users are usually responsible for inspecting their own SCBA daily or weekly and after each use.

DAILY OR WEEKLY INSPECTION

To ensure that SCBA equipment is in proper working condition, it must be thoroughly inspected and then properly stored.

The procedure for inspection involves checking all of the following assemblies:

- Facepiece assembly, including low-pressure hose and exhalation valve (for SCBA with harness-mounted regulator), and head harness
- Cylinder assembly, including cylinder, valve, and pressure gauge
- Regulator assembly, including high-pressure hose and alarm
- Harness and backpack assembly

One important consideration during inspection is the compatibility of the parts of each SCBA. Therefore, it is necessary during inspection to check that parts from one manufacturer are not interchanged with parts from another manufacturer. If an SCBA contains parts from a manufacturer other than the original equipment manufacturer, the NIOSH certification of the equipment is void.

Facepiece Assembly

The procedure for inspecting the facepiece assembly is as follows:

Step 1: If the SCBA has a harness-mounted regulator, check the low-pressure hose and the exhalation valve to see that they are intact.

    a. Check the low-pressure hose and the exhalation valve for visible signs of wear, broken parts, hardening, or deterioration.

    b. Pull or stretch the low-pressure hose to check for cracking (Figure 6.1).

    c. Inspect O-rings, gaskets, and screens at low-pressure connections.

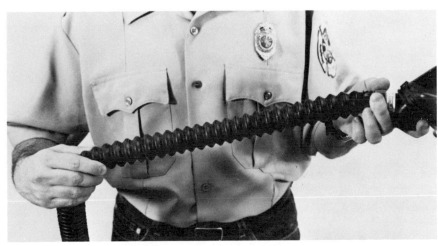

Figure 6.1 Stretch the low-pressure hose and check for holes or cracks between the corrugations.

Step 2: If the SCBA has a harness-mounted regulator, check the exhalation valve to see that it is free of foreign matter that could hold it open and check the valve seat (Figure 6.2).

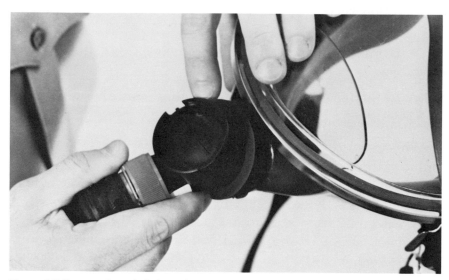

Figure 6.2 Remove the exhalation valve covering and examine the exhalation valve.

Step 3: If the SCBA has a harness-mounted regulator, hold the facepiece against the face and check the speaking diaphragm for proper operation.

Step 4: If the SCBA has a facepiece-mounted regulator, check the intermediate pressure hose for visible signs of wear, hardening, bulging, or deterioration.

Step 5: Check to see that all gaskets are intact.

Step 6: Check the facepiece elastomer to see that it is not cracked as a result of dry-rotting or exposure to chemicals (Figure 6.3).

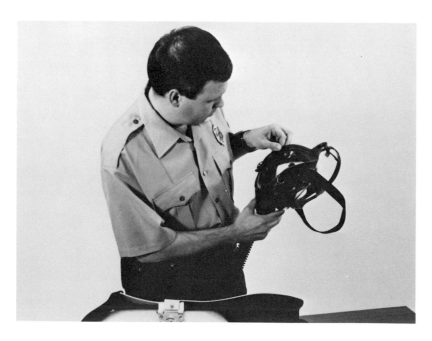

Figure 6.3 Carefully examine the facepiece sealing surface. Excessive cracking can result in an improper face-to-facepiece seal.

Step 7: Don facepiece and check face-to-facepiece seal. Remove facepiece.

Step 8: Check to see that all connection areas and threads are clean.

Step 9: Check to see that the facepiece straps are adjusted out fully.

Step 10: Check to see that the lens is clean and undamaged. If the lens is damaged beyond manufacturer's specifications, tag the facepiece and remove it from service.

Step 11: Check the head harness to see that it is not torn or excessively worn. If the harness is damaged, tag it and remove it from service.

Step 12: Set aside facepiece assembly.

Cylinder Assembly

The procedure for inspecting the cylinder assembly is as follows:

Step 1: Check to see that cylinder pressure is correct (Figure 6.4). If the cylinder is filled to less than 90 percent capacity, replace the cylinder with a fully charged cylinder.

Step 2: If replacing the cylinder, inspect any seals, gaskets, or screens at the high-pressure hose connection.

Step 3: Check cylinders for gouges, corrosion, chipping, and cracking. Remove cylinder from service if it no longer meets manufacturer's specifications.

Step 4: Check to see that the cylinder valve knob is in the correct position—it should be closed hand-tight.

Step 5: Check the high-pressure hose for bulges, wrinkles, wear, or tears (Figure 6.5).

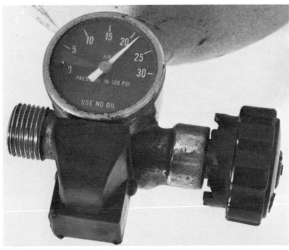

Figure 6.4 Cylinder inspection must include checking the cylinder pressure.

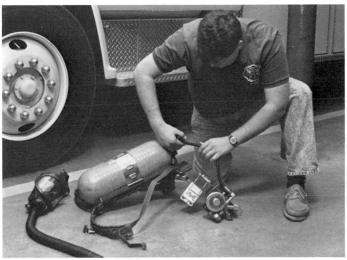

Figure 6.5 Inspect the high-pressure hose for any signs of wear or damage.

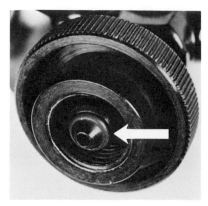

Figure 6.6 Thoroughly inspect high-pressure hose connections, including threads and any gaskets or seals.

Step 6: Check to see that the high-pressure hose is connected properly and has not been overly tightened.

    a. Disconnect the high-pressure hose from the cylinder valve and inspect any seals, gaskets, or screens (Figure 6.6).

    b. Reconnect the high-pressure hose to the cylinder valve outlet, tightening by hand only — do not use a wrench.

Step 7: Verify that the hydrostatic test date is still valid.

Regulator Assembly

The procedure for inspecting the regulator assembly is as follows:

Step 1: Check to see that the regulator controls are in the proper position.

- If the regulator is harness-mounted and has a donning or positive-pressure switch, turn off the switch. Check to see that the bypass valve is closed and the mainline valve is open.

- If the regulator is harness-mounted and *does not* have a donning or positive-pressure switch, check to see that the bypass valve is closed. Keep the mainline valve closed until ready to breathe.

- If the regulator is facepiece-mounted, check to see that the bypass valve is closed and the positive-pressure release button is depressed.

Step 2: If the regulator is facepiece-mounted, check the exhalation valve/opening on the regulator to see that it is free of debris or other foreign matter.

Step 3: Check to see that the regulator functions properly.

    a. Open the cylinder valve.

    b. Don the facepiece.

    c. Attach the facepiece assembly to the regulator assembly:

- If the regulator is harness-mounted and has a donning or positive-pressure switch, connect the low-pressure hose to the regulator and turn ON the positive-pressure switch.

- If the regulator is harness-mounted and *does not* have a donning or positive-pressure switch, connect the low-pressure hose to the regulator and open the mainline valve.

- If the regulator is facepiece-mounted, attach it to the facepiece.

d. Inhale and exhale several times to see that the regulator is functioning properly. If excessive or abnormal noises from the regulator can be heard, or if it is difficult to breathe through the regulator, remove the equipment from service and tag it for repair.

e. Compare the regulator pressure with the cylinder pressure; they should have approximately the same reading, or their pressure readings should correspond. If they do not, remove the unit from service and tag for repair.

   NOTE: Cylinder gauges indicate the cylinder air pressure in psi. However, some regulator gauges indicate the amount of air remaining in the cylinder with **FULL**, ½, ¼, and **EMPTY**; others indicate this amount as a percentage.

f. Check for positive pressure by lifting the facepiece away from the face just enough to break the facepiece-to-face seal. You should be able to hear the sound of air rushing out through the unsealed areas.

Step 4: If the SCBA has a facepiece-mounted regulator, exhale through the exhalation valve to ensure that it works properly.

Step 5: Check to see that the low-pressure alarm works properly.

a. Close the cylinder valve and *slowly* bleed excess pressure from the regulator by breathing down the remaining air or by opening the bypass valve as recommended by the manufacturer.

b. When the excess pressure has bled down, check to see that the low-pressure alarm sounds. Also note at what pressure the alarm sounds and check to see if it is within the manufacturer's specifications. If the alarm does not sound or does not sound at the pressure specified, refer to the manufacturer's instructions to see if further inspection is recommended, or remove the regulator from service and tag it for repair.

Step 6: If the regulator is harness-mounted, disconnect the low-pressure hose from the regulator. If the regulator is facepiece-mounted, disconnect the regulator from the facepiece.

Step 7: Remove the facepiece.

Step 8: If the SCBA regulator is equipped with a donning or positive-pressure switch, turn OFF the switch so that the regulator is in the demand mode.

Step 9: Inspect the regulator diaphragm as recommended by the manufacturer.

Harness And Backpack Assembly

The procedure for inspecting the harness and backpack assembly is as follows:

Step 1: Check to see that all straps are adjusted out fully.

Step 2: Check to see that the straps are untwisted and smooth (Figure 6.7).

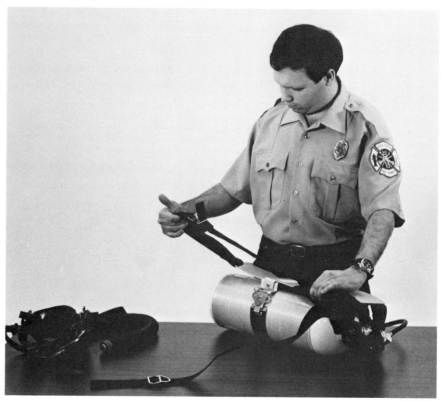

Figure 6.7 Straighten and smooth harness straps and inspect straps for wear.

Step 3: Check to see that the harness is in good working condition.

    a. Check all buckles to see that they readily clasp and unclasp.

    b. Check the harness for worn or torn areas.

    c. Remove the harness assembly from service if it is excessively damaged or worn or if the buckles do not operate properly.

Step 4: Check the backpack to see that it is in good condition.

    a. Check for damaged or worn parts.

    b. Check the cylinder strap that holds the cylinder in place to see that the locking mechanism works properly. If it does not, remove the backpack from service and tag it for repair.

    c. Check the backpack to see that it is adjusted properly.

Storage

After SCBA is inspected, it must be stored correctly. The procedure for storing SCBA is as follows:

Step 1: Put those units that pass inspection in their appropriate storage locations.

Step 2: Check to see that units are stored so that they are protected from dust, sunlight, heat, extreme cold, excessive moisture, or damaging chemicals. Also make sure that SCBA are stored so that they are not susceptible to damage from rough handling or from road shock. Units should be secured in brackets or carrying cases on fire apparatus or secured properly in specified storage locations within the fire department station.

Step 3: If not previously done, tag defective units and remove them from service until they can be repaired.

INSPECTION AND CARE AFTER EACH USE

Self-contained breathing apparatus is routinely subjected to rough handling, excessive moisture, and temperature extremes. Inspection and care after each use is very important.

This section addresses routine inspection and care. It does not include procedures for inspecting and cleaning SCBA used by firefighters working in areas exposed to toxic chemicals or radioactive materials. SCBA contaminated with hazardous materials should be segregated from other equipment and should be inspected and cleaned by individuals who are skilled in cleaning such contaminated equipment.

SCBA should be thoroughly cleaned and disinfected after every use. Strong cleaning and disinfecting agents or vigorous agitation should not be used. Solvents other than water should be used with caution. For instance, alcohol may damage rubber or elastomer parts. Manufacturers' recommendations should be followed when choosing cleaning and disinfecting agents. Also, SCBA components should be thoroughly rinsed to remove such agents in order to avoid damaging any parts and to prevent the user from experiencing dermatitis (skin rash).

The procedure for inspecting and cleaning SCBA after each use is as follows:

Step 1: Disconnect the facepiece assembly from the regulator and if the SCBA is equipped with a harness-mounted regulator, disconnect the low-pressure hose from the facepiece.

Step 2: Clean the facepiece assembly.

    a. Rinse the facepiece under a hose or faucet.

    b. Use a manufacturer-approved cleaner/disinfectant and, if necessary, a soft-bristle brush or sponge to thoroughly wash the facepiece. For facepieces without facepiece-mounted regulators, also wash the low-pressure hose and exhalation valve (Figure 6.8).

NOTE: An alternate means for cleaning/disinfecting the facepiece is to follow the guidelines from the Center for Disease Control. These guidelines call for the use of household bleach mixed in a solution of 1 part bleach to 10 parts water.

   c. Submerge and rinse completely in clean, warm water.

   d. Stretch the low-pressure hose to allow water trapped in the corrugations to drain.

   e. Allow the facepiece and the low-pressure hose to air dry in a clean area (Figure 6.9).

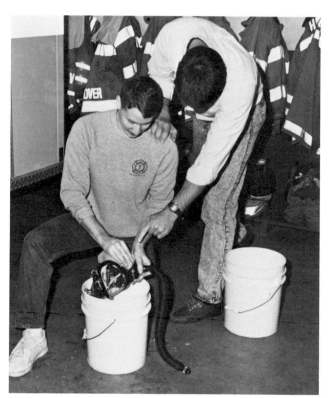

Figure 6.8 Submerge and wash the entire facepiece and rinse it thoroughly.

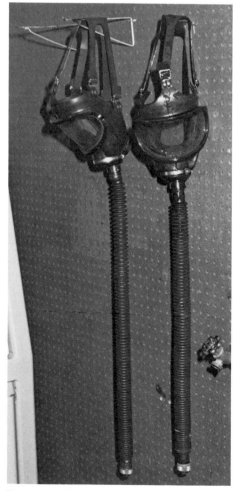

Figure 6.9 Carefully hang the facepiece and allow it to air dry.

Step 3: Wipe off the entire SCBA unit — including any components not previously cleaned — using a soft cloth and an approved cleaner/disinfectant to help deodorize it and to remove any loose dirt or debris. Also wipe the carrying case or mounting area.

Step 4: Check the harness for dirt; clean the harness if necessary.

    a. Wash the harness with a mild soap or commercial cleaning agent.

    b. Rinse thoroughly.

    c. Allow to air dry.

Step 5: Inspect SCBA components following procedures outlined in "Daily or Weekly Inspection." If any part needs to be repaired or replaced, tag the unit and remove it from service.

Step 6: If the SCBA passes inspection, reassemble and don it; check the operation of the entire system.

Step 7: Return the SCBA to proper storage.

MONTHLY INSPECTION

Whether a fire department requires SCBA inspection weekly or at the beginning of each new shift, it must also require that SCBA be inspected and that certain tests be performed monthly. Monthly inspection of SCBA includes not only those procedures in the daily or weekly inspection but also other inspection and testing procedures.

Fire department personnel must be familiar with the procedures used to test SCBA and must be able to perform certain tests. After every unit has been inspected and tested, defective units must be removed from service and sent for repair. Repairs performed on SCBA must be done only by qualified people, following the manufacturer's recommendations.

Some companies make test equipment available for qualified operators to test SCBA regulators. This equipment, which is very sensitive, measures static pressure, airflow rates, and exhalation resistance. Personnel using this equipment must be specially trained.

The bypass valve, the mainline valve, and the cylinder valve should be tested for leakage during monthly inspection or whenever leakage is suspected. Whether fire department personnel or specially trained technicians perform these tests depends upon the manufacturer's recommendations. The steps for leak-testing in the following monthly inspection procedure can be used with most SCBA. However, always check with the manufacturer's instructions before performing such tests. A typical monthly inspection procedure is as follows:

Step 1: Inspect the SCBA components following procedures outlined in "Daily or Weekly Inspection."

Step 2: Thoroughly inspect all rubber/elastomer parts and stretch and massage them so that they do not become set in a distorted shape during storage.

Step 3: Test the mainline valve for leaks.

    a. Close the regulator mainline valve and bypass valve hand-tight.

    b. Open the cylinder valve.

    c. If the SCBA is equipped with a harness-mounted regulator, cover the low-pressure hose connection on the regulator with your hand. If the SCBA is equipped with a facepiece-mounted regulator, cover the regulator opening for low-pressure air.

    d. Check the regulator gauge for about one minute to determine whether the pressure rises. If it does, the mainline valve may be defective; tag the unit and remove it from service.

Step 4: Test the bypass valve for leaks.

    a. Check to see that the regulator mainline valve and the bypass valve are closed hand-tight and that the cylinder valve is open.

    b. Apply a solution of mild soap and water across the hose connection fitting on the regulator, and check for bubbles (Figure 6.10).

    c. If soap solution bubbles, the bypass valve is leaking; tag the unit and remove it from service.

    d. Close the cylinder valve.

Step 5: Check the manufacturer's recommendations to see whether any additional regulator-functioning tests are required.

NOTE: Some of these tests can be performed by qualified fire department personnel. Other tests may be performed only by specially trained personnel or only by manufacturer-certified personnel.

Step 6: Check the date of the last hydrostatic test performed on the cylinder (Figure 6.11). Cylinders must be hydrostatically tested every three or five years, whichever is applicable for the particular cylinder: steel and aluminum cylinders must be retested every five years; composite cylinders, every three years.

Step 7: Test the cylinder valve connection at the cylinder pressure gauge, and test the safety plug for leaks.

    a. Check to see that the cylinder is fully charged and that the high-pressure hose is attached to the cylinder valve.

    b. Apply a solution of mild soap and water across the gauge assembly, hose connection, safety plug, and valve stem (Figure 6.12).

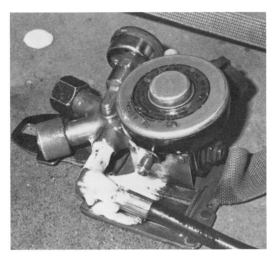

Figure 6.10 To check for leakage, apply soap solution to the hose connection fitting on the regulator and watch for bubbling.

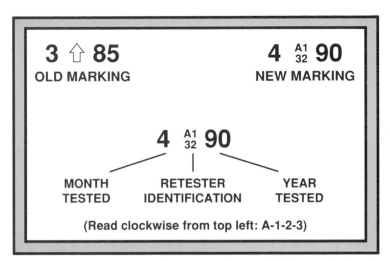

3 ⇧ 85
OLD MARKING

4 A1/32 90
NEW MARKING

4 A1/32 90

MONTH TESTED

RETESTER IDENTIFICATION

YEAR TESTED

(Read clockwise from top left: A-1-2-3)

Figure 6.11 The old markings and the new markings provide the same hydrostatic testing information. The older marking shows a retest date of March 1985; the newer marking shows a retest date of April 1990.

   c. Open the cylinder valve and check for bubbles.

   d. If the soap solution bubbles around the valve stem, gauge assembly, or safety plug, the unit should be repaired by a qualified technician; tag the unit and remove it from service.

   e. Close the cylinder valve.

Step 8: Test the cylinder valve outlet connection for leaks.

   a. Disconnect the high-pressure hose.

   b. Apply a soap solution to the valve outlet seat, and check for bubbles (Figure 6.13).

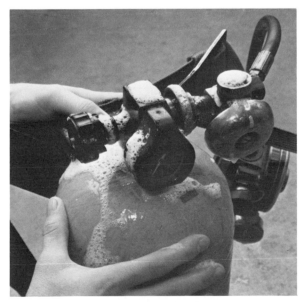

Figure 6.12 Apply soap solution to the cylinder pressure gauge, hose connection, safety plug, and valve stem to check for leakage at cylinder valve connection.

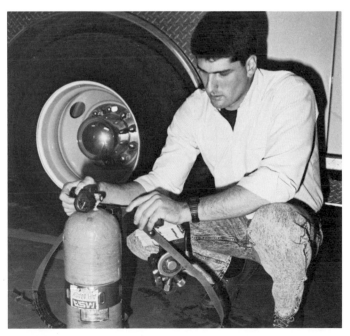

Figure 6.13 To check for leakage at the cylinder valve outlet, disconnect the high-pressure hose, apply soap solution to valve outlet seat, and watch for the presence of bubbles.

c. If soap solution bubbles around the cylinder valve outlet seat, the valve seat is leaking.

d. Attempt to clear the valve seat by quickly opening and closing the cylinder valve several times to allow pressurized air to blow through.

NOTE: Allowing air to pass through the valve in this manner may clear the valve seat of dirt that could be causing the valve to leak.

e. Close the valve and reapply the soap solution.

f. If the soap solution bubbles, the valve seat is still leaking, and the cylinder should be repaired by a qualified technician; tag the cylinder and remove it from service.

g. Rinse the soap solution from all cylinder connections. Momentarily open the cylinder valve to blow out remaining moisture from the valve seat.

Step 9: When complete air tightness is verified, assemble and don the SCBA and check for operational readiness.

Step 10: Return the SCBA to proper storage.

RECORDS AND MAINTENANCE

Adequate records must be kept on the maintenance and use of SCBA. A good record-keeping system is the only reliable way of keeping track of the regular inspection, maintenance, and use of the equipment. An example of an inspection and maintenance checklist can be found in Appendix F.

Records

It is important to keep three sets of SCBA records: one set for the facepieces, one set for the regulator-and-harness assemblies, and one set for the cylinders.

Identification numbers need to be fixed on the respective units for ready identification. These numbers may be the equipment serial numbers or they may be numbers assigned by the fire department to each cylinder, to each facepiece, and to each regulator-and-harness assembly. Records for the facepiece assemblies and records for the regulator-and-harness assemblies must include the following information for each assembly:

- Identification number

- Date of purchase

- Date of manufacture (regulator-and-harness assemblies only)

- Date placed in service (regulator-and-harness assemblies only)

- Location
- Dates and descriptions of maintenance and repairs
- Replacement parts and upgrading
- Test performance

Newly acquired SCBA must be tested and inspected by factory-certified personnel before placing the SCBA in service. So, in addition to the previously listed items, documentation of such testing and inspection also must be included in SCBA records.

The department must also keep records for each cylinder. Information contained in these records is similar to that in regulator-and-harness assembly records. The following information must be included in cylinder records:

- Identification number
- Date of purchase
- Date of manufacture
- Date placed in service
- Location
- Date of hydrostatic pressure test
- Hydrostatic test pressure
- Inspections
- Dates and descriptions of repairs

Many fire departments are now using or developing computerized record-keeping systems. These systems are used to record information on use, maintenance, updates of components, function tests, and other related data on each particular unit. Fire service software vendors have a variety of packages available to develop record-keeping systems for SCBA maintenance records. These computer programs offer the advantage of tracking large numbers of SCBA units easily. If you elect to use computerized record keeping, be sure that the product meets previously listed criteria as a minimum.

Several available testing devices — some of which produce records — could be called computerized systems. One such device, the Posicheck™, allows a qualified maintenance technician to perform flow and pressure tests on complete SCBA. These tests are critical in determining whether an SCBA still meets minimum flow requirements annually or after extensive repair. The Posicheck™ will produce a printed report, including identification number, pressures, and flows for every unit tested. This information can be entered into the computerized records or the maintenance files for SCBA.

Storage

Methods of storing SCBA differ among fire departments. Each department should use the method most appropriate to facilitate quick and easy donning. The SCBA storage areas, however, must offer the equipment protection from dust, sunlight, heat, extreme cold, and excessive moisture. Also, SCBA must be properly secured in the storage locations so they will not be damaged during transportation, either while moving carrying cases containing the equipment or while the fire apparatus on which the equipment is stored is in transit. In addition, the SCBA should be positioned so that the shape of certain components, mainly the facepiece, will not become distorted. (**NOTE:** Proper storage for different donning methods is described in Chapter 5, Donning and Doffing.)

Attention should also be given to correct storage of reserve cylinders. Such cylinders should be stored in cool, dry areas and should be secured properly so that they cannot be upset. Additionally, reserve cylinders should be stored so that they are not in contact with electrical wiring or outlets.

Repair And Reconditioning

Fire department personnel, unless trained and certified by the SCBA manufacturer, must not attempt to repair an SCBA. Unqualified repairs could cause serious injury or death and also void the warranty. Any nonfunctioning, damaged, or worn parts or components must be repaired or replaced following the manufacturer's instructions. Only qualified personnel using proper tools and testing equipment should be allowed to repair defective SCBA (Figure 6.14).

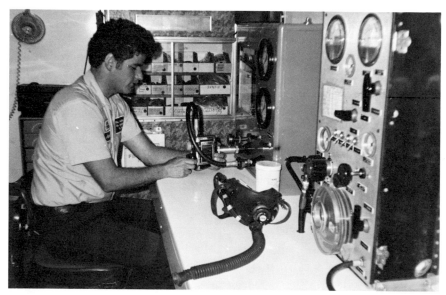

Figure 6.14 Special testing equipment can be used by factory-trained personnel to test regulator operation. *Courtesy of Weis American Fire Equipment Company.*

In many areas, mobile maintenance and repair services are available to local departments (Figure 6.15). These services, normally provided by companies who sell and maintain breathing apparatus, are done either on an as-needed basis or on a fixed

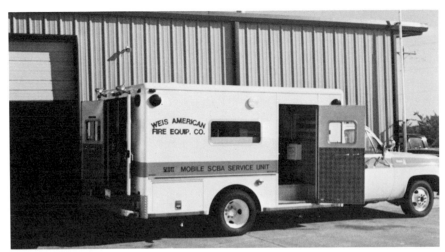

Figure 6.15 Many fire departments have their SCBA repaired by mobile service units. *Courtesy of Weis American Fire Equipment Company.*

schedule. The advantages that make this maintenance option very attractive are factory-certified technicians and parts availability. Such maintenance and repair services can also perform total reconditioning of breathing apparatus as well as function tests and equipment updates without causing major downtime of the units.

Rebuilding

According to ANSI Z88.5-1981, SCBA must be rebuilt by authorized personnel whenever necessary and at intervals specified by the manufacturer. If the manufacturer makes no such specification, the apparatus should be rebuilt every five years. All rubber/elastomer parts should be replaced every five years.

Cylinder Testing

Steel cylinders and aluminum cylinders must be hydrostatically tested every five years. Composite cylinders must be tested every three years. (**NOTE:** Composite cylinders have a 15-year life span.) To meet DOT requirements, the following information must be clearly shown on the cylinder:

- The month and year of manufacture

- The original test date

- The manufacturer's identification number

- The month and year of the last retest

- The tester's identification

This information is stamped directly on the neck of steel and aluminum cylinders (Figure 6.6). A label with this information is epoxied to composite bottles (see Figure 6.17 on next page).

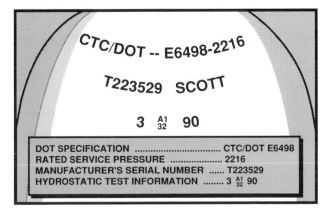

Figure 6.16 In addition to hydrostatic retesting information, cylinder markings also indicate the manufacturer, the date of manufacture, and the original test date.

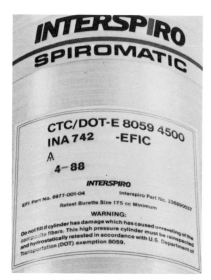

Figure 6.17 The label on a composite cylinder must include the same information that is stamped on steel or aluminum cylinders.

Additional hydrostatic test dates are represented by foil labels epoxied to the cylinder (Figure 6.18).

Cylinders must also be inspected internally and externally. Internal inspection should be done at the same time intervals as for hydrostatic testing. External inspection procedures should include those steps previously described and should be performed at time intervals recommended by the manufacturer of the cylinder.

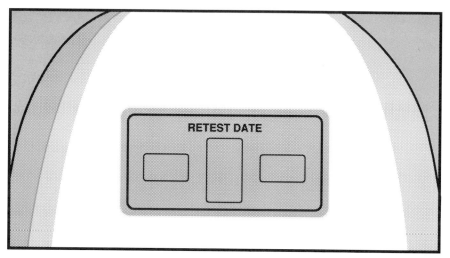

Figure 6.18 The latest hydrostatic test date and the retester's identification number are shown on the small foil label.

SCBA Advisories

At times, SCBA users or manufacturers become aware of problems with a particular model of SCBA. Such problems must be identified and corrected. Sometimes the SCBA manufacturer works with NIOSH to do this. When it becomes apparent that there is a problem with a particular model, NIOSH issues a warning or advisory that identifies the specific model and defective parts. For example, NIOSH has issued warnings regarding certain fiberglass-wrapped aluminum cylinders that developed cracks around the neck and were leaking breathing air during use and storage. Advisories may also be issued by the SCBA manufacturer and are usually published in trade journals.

Firefighters and departments should keep up to date on such information from NIOSH or SCBA manufacturers by routinely reviewing trade journals or other publications that publish such advisories and warnings. Departments owning SCBA that have been found to be defective by NIOSH or the manufacturer should heed any warnings and immediately see that the problem is corrected.

Modification

SCBA should not be modified in any way without the manufacturer's approval. This modification includes removing straps or installing communication devices that interfere with the functioning of the regulator. Any type of modification will void NIOSH approval and manufacturers' warranties. In addition, parts of SCBA manufactured by different companies should not be interchanged. This policy also applies to cylinder components.

SUMMARY

SCBA must be properly maintained so that the equipment will be ready to use. Proper maintenance includes daily or weekly inspection, inspection and cleaning after each use, and monthly inspection and testing. Other important elements in proper maintenance are following manufacturer's cleaning, inspection, and testing recommendations; maintaining proper records; and having SCBA repaired by qualified technicians.

Chapter 6 Review
Answers on page 350

TRUE-FALSE: Mark each statement true or false. If false, explain why.

1. The number of personnel using a department's SCBA and how often the SCBA equipment is used are two factors used to determine whether equipment inspections should be performed daily or weekly.

   ☐ T ☐ F _____

   _____

2. All cylinders must be hydrostatically tested every year.

   ☐ T ☐ F _____

   _____

3. After the cylinder valve has been closed, bleeding excess pressure from the regulator should cause the low-pressure alarm to sound.

   ☐ T ☐ F _____

   _____

4. To ensure disinfection, alcohol should be used to clean all rubber areas of the facepiece.

   ☐ T ☐ F _____

   _____

5. SCBA should be thoroughly cleaned and disinfected at every inspection.

   ☐ T ☐ F _____

   _____

6. The regulator diaphragm should be inspected as recommended by the manufacturer.

   ☐ T ☐ F _____

   _____

7. The bypass valve and the cylinder valve outlet on some models of SCBA can be tested for leaks by applying a solution of mild soap and water and observing to see whether or not bubbles appear.

   ☐ T ☐ F _____

   _____

8. It is required that SCBAs be reconditioned by authorized personnel at intervals specified by the fire department.

☐ T ☐ F _____

_____

MULTIPLE CHOICE: Circle the correct answer.

9. To check the face-to-facepiece seal when inspecting an SCBA with a harness-mounted regulator, hold facepiece against face, and _____.

A. cover end of high-pressure hose, exhale, and hold breath for several seconds

B. slightly rotate facepiece until facepiece is positioned so that it feels snug against face, inhale, and hold breath for several seconds

C. cover end of low-pressure hose, inhale, and hold breath for several seconds

D. disconnect regulator and check to see that pressure does not change

10. The high-pressure hose should be connected to the cylinder valve outlet and _____.

A. tightened with a torque wrench to 20 ft-lbs (27.1 Nm)

B. tightened with an appropriate-sized open-end wrench

C. tightened by hand

D. none of the above should be done

11. SCBA equipment should be stored in areas where they can be protected against _____.

A. damaging chemicals

B. sunlight

C. dust

D. all of the above

12. Firefighter A says that it is important to check the compatibility of SCBA components when inspecting each SCBA and that one manufacturer's parts should not be used on an SCBA from another manufacturer. Firefighter B disagrees and says that parts can be interchanged as long as the connections are the same. Who is correct?

A. Firefighter A

B. Firefighter B

C. Both A and B

D. Neither A nor B

13. Firefighters A and B are discussing inspecting the cylinder assembly during monthly inspection. Firefighter A says that if the cylinder is not full, it should not be replaced until just before it is actually used and says that air could leak from a fully charged cylinder, anyway, before it may ever be used. Firefighter B says that cylinders less than 90 percent full should be replaced at the time of inspection. Who is correct?

   A. Firefighter A

   B. Firefighter B

   C. Both A and B

   D. Neither A nor B

LISTING

14. The procedure for daily, weekly, or monthly inspection involves checking what four assemblies?

   A. _____

   B. _____

   C. _____

   D. _____

FILL IN THE BLANK: Fill in the blanks with the correct response.

15. During inspection, check cylinder pressure and replace the cylinder if it is filled to less than _____ percent of cylinder capacity.

16. When inspecting the regulator, you should check to be sure that the mainline valve is _____ and the bypass valve is _____.

SHORT ANSWER: Answer each item briefly.

17. One part of SCBA inspection is checking the low-pressure hose and the exhalation valve. For what conditions must these be checked?

   _____

   _____

   _____

18. When comparing the regulator pressure with the cylinder pressure, you find that the readings are not the same. What does this fact indicate?

   _____

   _____

   _____

   _____

19. What checks should be included when inspecting the harness assembly?

_____

_____

_____

_____

_____

_____

20. What is the difference between the procedures for daily/weekly inspection and the procedures for monthly inspection?

_____

_____

_____

_____

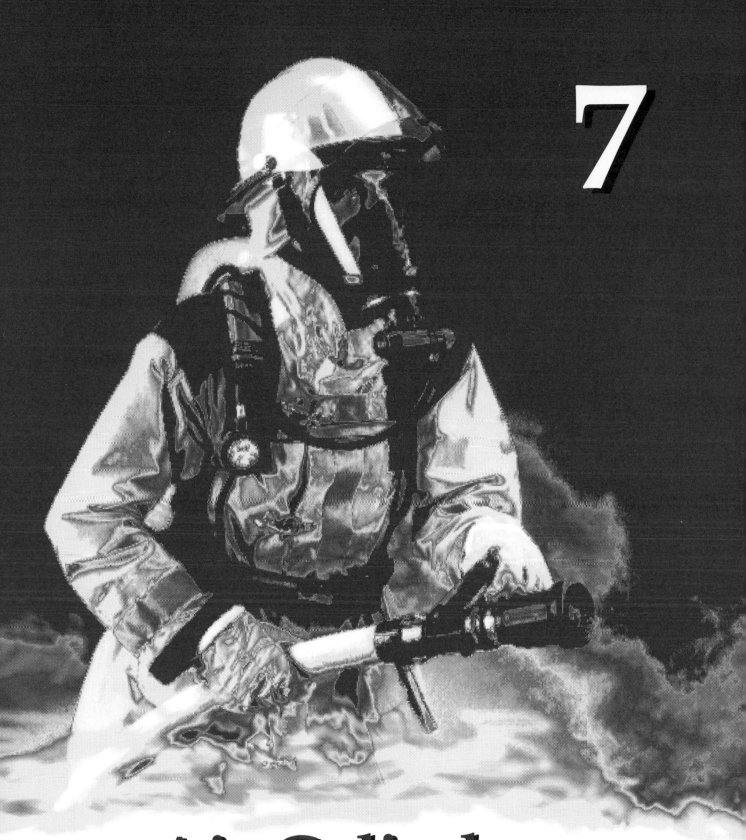

Air Cylinder
Recharging Systems

7

This chapter provides information that addresses the following standards:

NFPA STANDARD 1404
Fire Department Self-Contained Breathing Apparatus Program
1989 Edition

Chapter 2—Provisions of SCBA
2-1.3

Chapter 7—Breathing Air Program
7-1.1
7-1.2
7-1.3
7-1.4
7-2.1
7-2.2
7-2.3
7-2.4
7-2.5
7-2.6
7.2.7
7-2.8
7-2.9
7-2.10
7-2.11
7-2.12
7-2.13
7-2.14

NFPA STANDARD 1500
Fire Department Occupational Safety and Health Program
1987 Edition

Protective Clothing and Protective Equipment
5-3.4
5-3.4.1

ANSI STANDARD Z88.5-1981
Practices for Respiratory Protection for the Fire Service

Section 6—Maintenance of SCBA
6.5

ANSI STANDARD Z88.2-1980
Practices for Respiratory Protection

Section 5—Classification, Description, and Limitations of Respirators
5.2

Chapter 7
Air Cylinder Recharging Systems

INTRODUCTION

"Be prepared" is an excellent motto for firefighters to remember when dealing with air supplies for the modern fire service. Extra cylinders must be available to ensure adequate air supplies for lengthy or numerous emergencies when in-service cylinders cannot be refilled conveniently.

Fire departments handle air supply problems in several ways. Some departments contract with commercial firms to refill department-owned air cylinders. This is an economical method if the department does not use self-contained breathing apparatus often and the firm is conveniently located. Other departments buy air in large storage cylinders from commercial firms and then use the stored air to do their own recharging. Departments with a medium-pressure compressor (2,000 psi to 2,800 psi [13 800 kPa to 19 320 kPa]) can purchase a booster pump to convert the medium-pressure air to the high-pressure air (3,000 psi to 5,000 psi [20 700 kPa to 34 500 kPa]) needed to fill department air cylinders. When the air cylinders are depleted many times every month for training or fire fighting, it is a distinct advantage for a department to recharge its cylinders using its own compressor.

How a department maintains its air supply should be included in the department's SOPs. It is important that breathing air be obtained from a source that meets NFPA requirements, and this should also be included in a department's written policies. Each department must also keep records of the various components of its air supply systems. These records must include such information as dates of purchase, locations, inspection and maintenance, and testing.

A complete air supply system is composed of four elements: a compressor, a purification system, a cascade (storage) system, and a charging station (Figures 7.1 a through d). This chapter explores these four elements of an air supply system and explains how they function to recharge SCBA air cylinders.

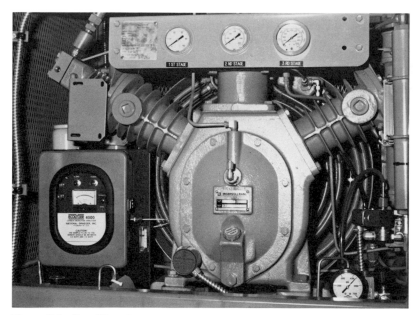

Figure 7.1a Breathing-air compressor.

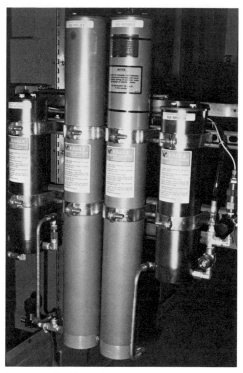

Figure 7.1b Air purification system.

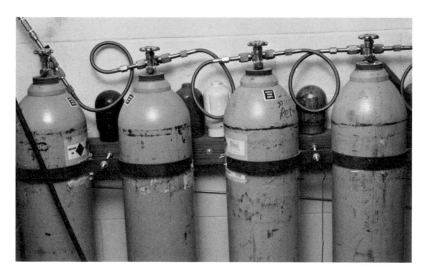

Figure 7.1c Cascade system.

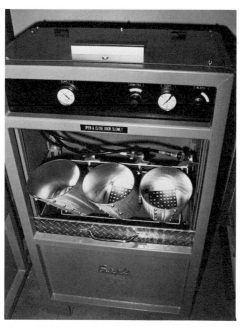

Figure 7.1d Charging station.

COMPRESSORS

Most fire department compressors used for breathing air are three- or four-stage piston compressors. Electric compressors are preferred because gasoline- or diesel-powered engines introduce additional sources of contamination to the air that fills the cylinders. Piston compressors are usually oil lubricated. If a compressor is oil lubricated, only oil recommended by the manufacturer should be used. Some firms use piston rings made of Teflon™ or carbon that require no lubrication. The compressors of several manufacturers are shown in Figures 7.2 through 7.4.

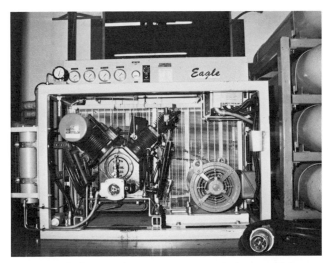

Figure 7.2 A closeup of a compressor mounted on a vehicle.

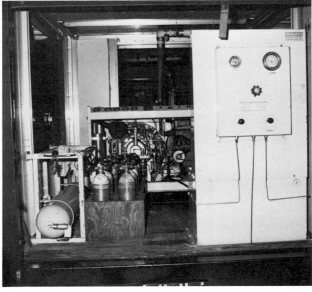

Figure 7.3 A closeup of an air supply system mounted on a trailer.

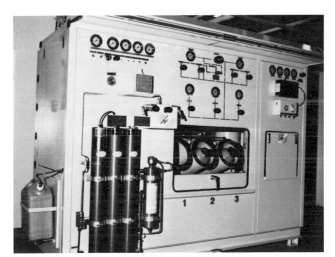

Figure 7.4 The four units of an air supply system may be combined all in one unit. *Courtesy of Champaign (Illinois) Fire Department.*

There are several factors a department should consider when deciding what kind of compressor to buy:

Quantity of air needed by the department. Generally, a compressor will deliver 1 cubic foot of air per minute at 3,000 psi (28 L/min at 20 700 kPa) for every horsepower of its rating. One expert has warned that departments buying their first compressor should expect their needs to double because of training demands. So, a department should determine what horsepower rating a compressor must have in order to meet the department's refilling needs. For example, using a 15-hp compressor, a firefighter could refill a 45-cubic-foot air cylinder in 3 minutes. Table 7.1 on the next page shows how many 45-cubic-foot (1 275 L) air cylinders can be filled in an hour with compressors of different outputs. It should be noted that using a cascade system in conjunction with an air compressor would provide adequate air supplies for fast filling without requiring a large air compressor.

TABLE 7.1
NUMBER OF 45 FT³ (1 275 L) CYLINDERS FILLED IN ONE HOUR BY COMPRESSORS OF DIFFERENT OUTPUT

Compressor Output Per Minute		Compressor Output Per Hour		Cylinders Filled
ft³	L	ft³	L	
2.5	70.8	150	4 245	3
4.0	113.2	240	6 792	5
8.0	226.4	480	13 584	10
12.0	339.6	720	20 376	15
15.0	424.5	900	25 470	20
20.0	566.0	1,200	33 960	26
25.0	707.5	1,500	42 450	33
30.0	849.0	1,800	50 940	39

Metric conversion factor: 1 ft³ = 28.3 L
Source (customary units): Pressure Systems, Inc.

Space availability. The size of different types of compressors varies, so the space limitations of a particular department must be considered when choosing a particular type of compressor.

Water availability. Water bath filling stations require an adequate supply of water for cooling cylinders.

Air purity at compressor installation. How pure the air is at this location will affect the kind of filtering system needed at the air compressor intake.

Cost of maintenance. Each fire department must consider how much time, money, and effort it has available for maintenance. The oil-lubricated compressor usually needs to be dismantled and have its parts inspected for wear and corrosion every 1,000 operating hours. The unlubricated-piston type and the diaphragm type are the easiest to maintain.

Location Of Compressor

The compressor takes in air from the surrounding atmosphere, so the air intake can be installed either outside or inside in the cleanest possible surroundings (Figures 7.5 a and b). The air intake should have a filter that can be cleaned or replaced and that can trap particles measuring 15 microns or larger. Despite the filter, the air intake should be installed away from contamination

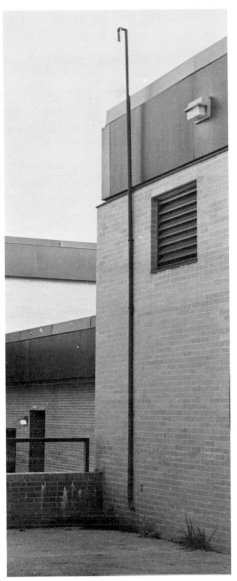

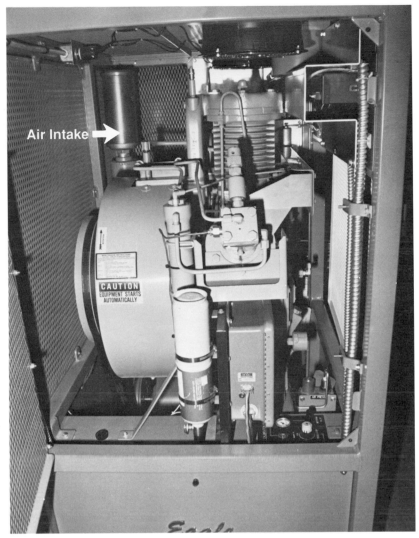

Air Intake ➡

Figure 7.5b Compressors having an interior air intake should be located in an area free from contaminants.

Figure 7.5a Placement and configuration of an exterior air intake for an air compressor is very important.

sources such as motor vehicle exhaust, furnaces, smoke, fumes, sewers, chimneys, and from operations such as sandblasting, painting, welding, and fire extinguisher refilling. Outside intake pipes should be made of a noncorrodible material such as plastic, copper, or stainless steel. Galvanized pipe should not be used for outdoor piping because zinc oxide deposits, which can contaminate the air, can form in the pipe. In addition, the piping and air intake should be installed so that birds cannot roost or nest on or in them.

If the outside air is contaminated, the intake can be installed inside the building in a relatively clean atmosphere. The intake should not be placed in rooms with hot or uncirculated air or in rooms where people congregate or smoke. Rooms where solvents are used or kept or rooms containing combustion equipment, such as water heaters, boilers, or internal-combustion engines (engine room), are not suitable installation areas, either. In addition, the air intake should be 2 or 3 feet (0.6 m or 1 m) above the floor.

Safety Factors

Compressors *must* be placed in a room containing a clean atmosphere. Ideally, the room should be separate from high-use areas (because of noise emitted by the compressor) and should be used only for compressing and purifying air for SCBA cylinders and for storing cylinders (Figure 7.6). Compressors used for breathing air cannot be treated as if they are shop compressors. Dust, dirt, and moisture will impair their function and contaminate the breathing air or overload the purification system.

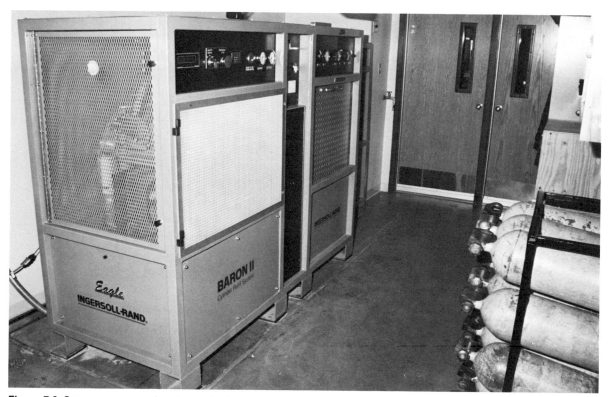

Figure 7.6 Compressors must be situated in clean surroundings and away from all possible sources of air contaminants.

Personnel operating the compressor must carefully observe the compressor during operation to ensure that it is working correctly and safely. Each stage of the compression cycle must have a relief valve. Failure to keep compressors clean can result in relief-valve failure and explosion. There should also be a pressure gauge for each stage of the compression cycle, and the operator should monitor these gauges (Figure 7.7). Therefore, if the gauge readings are recorded in the maintenance log when the compressor is new and operated at capacity, the operator then can determine from subsequent gauge readings whether the compressor is working incorrectly and needs repair.

Compression can heat air to 300°F (149°C). This compressed, heated air is cooled after each stage of the compression cycle and

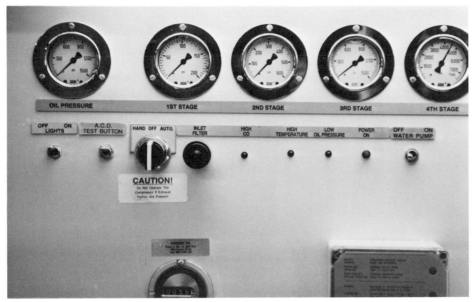

Figure 7.7 The operator should monitor the pressure gauge for each stage of compression. *Courtesy of Champaign (Illinois) Fire Department.*

again by an aftercooler before it enters the purification system. Some compressor systems use water-cooled aftercoolers to bring the heated air to within 10°F to 25°F (-12°C to -4°C) of the ambient air temperature.

WARNING

Personnel can be accidentally burned by pipes that carry hot compressed air to an aftercooler. Make sure these pipes are clearly marked in order to prevent injuries. Also, make sure that these pipes are well secured so that they will not vibrate or whip if they should break.

Teflon™ or carbon piston rings or diaphragms do not usually add contaminants to the air during compression, but an improperly cooled, unlubricated piston compressor with Teflon™ rings can produce fluorine gas. Fluorine gas cannot be removed by the typical purification system, so such a compressor should have a device to warn operators that the unit is overheating.

As air is heated during each stage of compression, water and oil vapors are forced from the air and collect in the sumps as liquids (Figure 7.8). In some compressors, these sumps are connected to a central collecting chamber. If the compressor does not have an automatic drain, the compressor operator must manually drain the sumps or collector at least once every 10 to 20 minutes during compressor operation, depending on the humidity of the air and the capacity of the sump (see Figure 7.9 on next page). Otherwise, the water and oil will be forced through each stage of

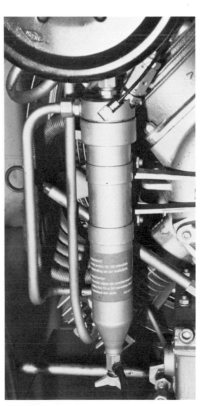

Figure 7.8 Compressor sumps collect water and oil vapors.

the compressor and through the components of the air purification system; and there is a good chance that the breathing air in the cascade cylinders and SCBA cylinders will be contaminated with water vapor mixed with oil, or worse, with air that is toxic.

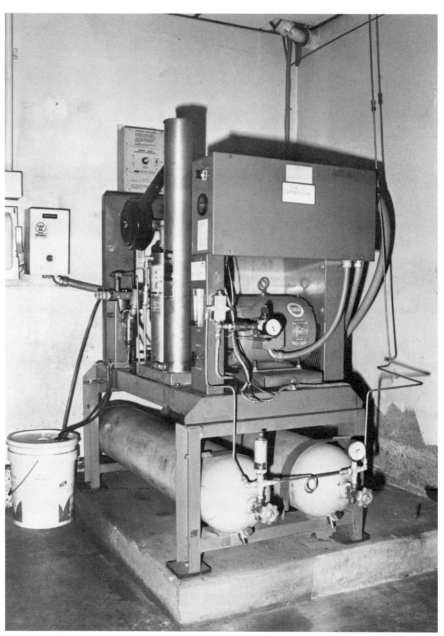

Figure 7.9 Sumps should be drained regularly, either manually or automatically, and the liquid drained from the sumps should be disposed of properly.

Oil used in compressors is specially formulated to reduce the possibility of toxic air developing during compressor use. Only the type of oil recommended by the manufacturer should be used in a compressor.

Other safety features that the compressor should have include the following:

- A wall-mounted power-shutoff switch

- A starter with a circuit breaker that can be reset by hand

- A certified motor

- Alarms and/or shut-down switches to warn operators when the high-pressure air is too hot (high-temperature shut-down switch)

- Gauges and alarms to monitor the crankcase oil level and oil pressure and an automatic device to shut down the compressor when the oil pressure gets too low

- An operating-hour meter so that operators will know how long the compressor has been in use

- A belt guard to protect operators in the event that the drive belt breaks

- Detectors to indicate when carbon monoxide (CO) levels are too high — above levels permitted for Grade D breathing air

Shop-Built Compressors

Compressors built in the shop, with surplus parts and home-built or scavenged filters, are *not* adequate for generating breathing air used to fill SCBA cylinders. In addition, *they are dangerous because the parts are not compatible and will not long withstand the pressures necessary to fill breathing-air cylinders.* Fire departments should use *only* those compressors designed specifically to supply compressed breathing air.

AIR PURIFICATION SYSTEMS

The air intake filter on the compressor removes only solid particles and suspended liquids; it does *not* remove oil vapors, gaseous hydrocarbons, toxic gases, or enough water. To remove these contaminants, an air purification system must be installed downstream from the compressor. After the air is compressed, it passes through the purification system before it is stored. Most purification systems use both permanent filtering systems for preliminary removal of larger solid and liquid contaminants, and replaceable, disposable cartridges for removal of oil and water vapors, other gaseous contaminants, and odors. Disposable cartridges contain desiccants (drying agents), adsorbents, or catalysts, depending on their purpose. Typical purification units are shown in Figures 7.10 through 7.12.

The air purification system is composed of four basic components, each of which filters out or absorbs water and other contaminants (Figure 7.13 on next page). In some systems, the functions of two or more of these components may be combined and performed in a single component. The basic components of an

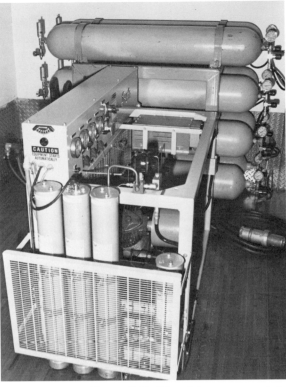

Figure 7.10 After air is compressed, it must pass through the air purification system.

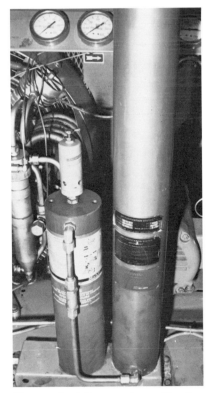

Figure 7.11 Some air purification systems contain only two different purifying cartridges.

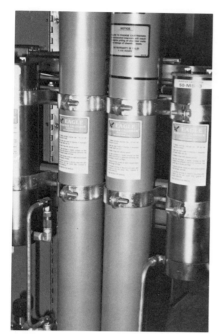

Figure 7.12 The basic components of an air purification system absorb water and filter out other contaminants from the compressed air.

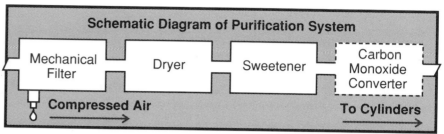

Figure 7.13 An air purification system includes a mechanical filter, dryer, air sweetener, and carbon monoxide converter.

air purification system are the mechanical filter, the dryer, the air sweetener, and the carbon monoxide converter.

Mechanical Filter. The first component in an air purification system, this permanent filter accepts the air from the compressor and removes oil and water mixtures and particulate matter of sizes of at least 10 microns. Contaminants that are removed by the mechanical filter drain into a sump. The sump must be emptied frequently to prevent the collected contaminants from entering the rest of the purification system.

Dryer. The next component in the purification system is the dryer. The dryer purifying cartridge, which contains a desiccant or drying compound, removes the remaining water and oil vapors, lowering the dew point to -100°F (-73°C). It also reduces noxious gases to extremely low levels. Contaminants that are strongly absorbed include carbon dioxide, hydrogen sulfide, sulfur dioxide, ammonia, oil vapors, alcohols, ketones, ethers, esters, olefins, acetylenes, and halogenated hydrocarbons. Most reputable manufacturers use a desiccant called a molecular sieve, which removes water and oil vapors from the air.

Air Sweetener. After it passes through the dryer, the compressed air passes through the air sweetener. This is a cartridge containing activated carbon (another type of adsorbent), which is effective in removing odors and tastes from the compressed air. Such a cartridge is often called an "air purifier." However, this term is misleading because activated carbon will neither absorb toxic gases such as carbon monoxide nor convert them to inert gas.

Carbon Monoxide Converter. This optional subsystem can consist of several cartridges. These cartridges contain a special chemical, and in the presence of this chemical, carbon monoxide (CO) combines with oxygen to form carbon dioxide (CO_2). The converter most commonly used in the fire service contains a catalyst called *Hopcalite*™.

NOTE: The chemical in the air purification system converter *must be dry* in order for the converter to function properly. Before the air reaches the converter, the compressor intercoolers and aftercoolers remove water and other liquids, the mechanical filter aids in liquid removal, and the dryer removes water and oil vapor and other harmful substances. If sufficient amounts of water and oil are not first removed at the compressor, the water and oil will be forced through each stage of the compressor, the mechanical filter, and the dryer/purifier. The water will reduce the life of the dryer and destroy the ability of the purifier to function properly.

Recommended Dew Point Levels

Even with an air purification system, some water will always make it through the compressor-purification system and into the air cylinder or cascade cylinders. Water affects the purification chemicals, can damage interior surfaces of the air cylinders, and causes problems for SCBA regulators (Figures 7.14 and 7.15).

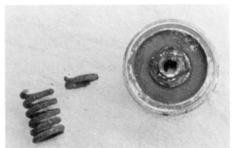

Figure 7.15 Moisture within the regulator can result in corroded and broken parts. *Courtesy of Joe McDonagh.*

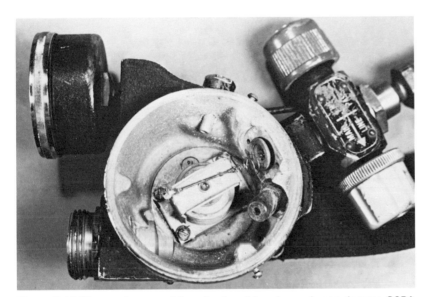

Figure 7.14 Water not removed from the breathing-air supply can damage SCBA regulators. *Courtesy of Joe McDonagh.*

NFPA 1500, *Standard on Fire Department Occupational Safety and Health Program*, sets the standard for dryness at a water vapor level of less than 25 parts per million (ppm). Dryness of breathing air can also be expressed as dew point, or mg/L, as shown in Table 7.2 on the next page. Of these two measurement units, dew point is the more meaningful. Dew point is the temperature at which the water vapor in air begins to condense as droplets of liquid.

It is extremely important that the air has the correct dew point level. If air has too high a dew point, and especially if the temperature is low, small crystals of ice can form in the regulator when this air flows through. These crystals can impede breathing and can even freeze the regulator. Repeated freezing and melting of ice crystals over a period of time can cause the brass and aluminum parts of the regulator to weld together by electrolysis.

When purchasing a purification system, specify the desired dew point. NFPA's requirement of less than 25 ppm water vapor corresponds with a dew point of -64°F (-53°C). The Compressed

TABLE 7.2
AIR QUALITY STANDARDS

CONTAMINANT	CGA Grade D (1)	CGA Grade E (1)	NFPA 1500 (3)	CSA Z180.1 (4)
Carbon Monoxide, ppm/v	10	10	5	5
Carbon Dioxide, ppm/v	1,000	500	500	500
Condensed Hydrocarbons, mg/m³	5	5	--	1
Gaseous Hydrocarbons, as methane, ppm/v	--	--	10	
Water Vapor, ppm/v, dew point	(2)	(2)	25 ppm	-63°F
Objectionable Odors	None	None	None	None
Nitrogen Dioxide (NO$_2$), ppm/v	--	--	0.5	0.2
Nitrous Oxide (N$_2$O), ppm/v	--	--	--	5
Sulfur Dioxide (SO$_2$), ppm/v	--	--	0.5	--
Halogenated solvents, ppm/v	--	--	1	--
Other gaseous contaminants	--	--	--	(5)
Inorganic particulates, mg/m³	--	--	--	1

-- indicates that the standard shows no limiting characteristics

(1) Compressed Gas Association Pamphlet G-7 1989, Compressed Air for Human Respiration, and Compressed Gas Association Pamphlet G-7.1, Commodity Specification for Air.

Pamphlet G-7 specifies Grade D as the minimum grade for routine use in self-contained or supplied-air protective breathing equipment, as used in industry, fire fighting, for general respiratory use.

Pamphlet G-7 specifies Grade E as the minimum grade to be used for sports diving to 125 feet.

(2) For breathing air used in conjunction with self-contained breathing apparatus in extreme cold where moisture can condense and freeze, causing the breathing apparatus to malfunction, a dew point not to exceed -50°F (63 ppm v/v) or 10 degrees lower than the coldest temperature expected in the area is required.

(3) National Fire Protection Association Standard 1500, Fire Department Occupational Safety and Health Program, requires a water vapor level of less than 25 ppm.

(4) Canadian Standards Association, Rexdale, Ontario, Standard CAN3-Z180.1-M85, Compressed Breathing Air and Systems.

(5) Maximum allowable content of tricholotrifluorethane, dichlorodifluoromethane, and chlorodifluoromethane is 2 ppm/v for each. Unlisted contaminants shall not exceed one-tenth of the Threshold Limit Values (TLV's) for Chemical Substances in Workroom Air adopted by the American Conference of Governmental Industrial Hygienists (ACGIH).

This table is reprinted with permission from the Compressed Gas Association Pamphlet G-7.1-1989 (Commodity Specification for Air), Copyright, 1989, Compressed Gas Association, Inc.

Gas Association's (CGA) recommended dew point of -50°F (-46°C) corresponds with a water vapor level of 63 ppm — a level that is 38 ppm higher than that allowed by NFPA. See Table 7.3 for a comparison of dew point recommendations.

Computing Air Purification Cartridge Life

Most air purification systems require very little maintenance; however, the purifying cartridges must be replaced when the desiccants and chemicals that they contain become ineffective. Manufacturers specify the volume of air that a particular car-

TABLE 7.3
MOISTURE CONVERSION DATA
(All referred to 70°F and 14.7 psia)

Dew Point (F)	Dew Point (C)	PPM (v/v)	Mg/liter
-100	-73.3	1.5	.0011
-90	-67.8	3.5	.0026
-80	-62.2	7.8	.0058
-75	-59.4	11.4	.0085
-70	-56.7	16.2	.012
-65	-53.9	23.0	.017
-60	-51.1	32.0	.024
-55	-48.3	45.0	.034
-50	-45.6	63.0	.047
-45	-42.8	87.0	.065
-40	-40.0	120.0	.089
-30	-34.4	225.0	.17
-20	-28.9	400.0	.30
-10	-23.3	690.0	.51
0	-17.8	1180.0	.88

The table is reprinted with permission from the Compressed Gas Association Pamphlet G-7.1-1989 (Commodity Specification for Air), Copyright, 1989, Compressed Gas Association, Inc.

tridge will treat. However, it is advisable for fire department personnel to also know the service life of a cartridge if a limit has been set by the manufacturer. Because moisture can collect within a cartridge in an infrequently used purification system — causing the cartridge to function ineffectively or even damaging the cartridge — the cartridge may need to be replaced even before it has treated the volume of air it was designed to treat. Cartridge replacement on most types of purification systems is a simple and quick operation.

Air testing results that do not meet specifications may also indicate that one or more of the cartridges in the system needs replacing. Another means of checking the air cartridge life is to mathematically compute it. Thus, knowing *when* to replace the cartridge requires good record keeping, routine air quality testing, and some mathematical calculation.

To mathematically compute cartridge life, the firefighter must know the given volume of air that the cartridge is designed to treat. Using this total treatment volume, the following formula can be used to determine cartridge life in hours:

$$t = \frac{volume}{(x \text{ cu ft/min}) (60 \text{ min/hr})}$$

where:
t = hours of life for cartridge
volume = volume cartridge will treat (in cu ft)
x = airflow rate from compressor (in cu ft/min)
60 min/hr = constant

EXAMPLE: Given a compressor with an airflow rate of 10 cu ft/min and a cartridge designed to treat 40,000 cu ft, figure the life of the cartridge in hours.

$$t = \frac{40,000 \text{ cu ft}}{(10 \text{ cu ft/min})(60 \text{ min/hr})}$$

Step 1: Multiply (10 cu ft/min) by (60 min/hr):

$$\left(\frac{10 \text{ cu ft}}{\text{min}}\right)\left(\frac{60 \text{ min}}{\text{hr}}\right) = 600 \text{ cu ft/hr}$$

Step 2: Divide 600 cu ft/hr into 40,000 cu ft to find hours of life for cartridge:

$$t = \frac{40,000 \text{ cu ft}}{600 \text{ cu ft/hr}} = 66 \text{ hours}$$

TESTING AIR QUALITY

Even with a good compressor and purification system, the quality of the cylinder air cannot be taken for granted. Breathing air must be tested for purity. NFPA 1500 states that the breathing air that comes from the compressor-purifier must be tested quarterly by a qualified laboratory to be sure that the system is working properly. Many testing laboratories also recommend that compressed air be tested quarterly.

Testing must be done routinely, and the department must keep accurate, up-to-date records (Figure 7.16). This routine testing is a necessary part of maintenance. The testing results indicate when compressor repair is needed and when purification system cartridges need replacement. If testing results indicate that breathing air does not meet standards, any cylinders filled with such air should be emptied and purged.

Only a well-equipped, reputable testing laboratory should test the purity of the breathing air. Such a laboratory could be at the local health department or a university or could be a private firm whose only business is testing. A reputable company will be able to complete a laboratory analysis within 24 hours of receipt of the air sample and advise the department immediately if a sample is found to be outside the acceptable range. A detailed written analysis should accompany the results of the testing and be maintained on file. *When choosing a testing laboratory, consider the types of reports the department needs and select a laboratory that will provide such reports.* Specify that the reports contain data concerning the contaminants listed in Tables 7.4 and 7.5, as well as the dew point of the air. If no nearby laboratory can determine the dew point, an approximation can be made by converting ppm of water content of the air to dew point, using Table 7.2. Make sure that the laboratory gives actual ppm. Some

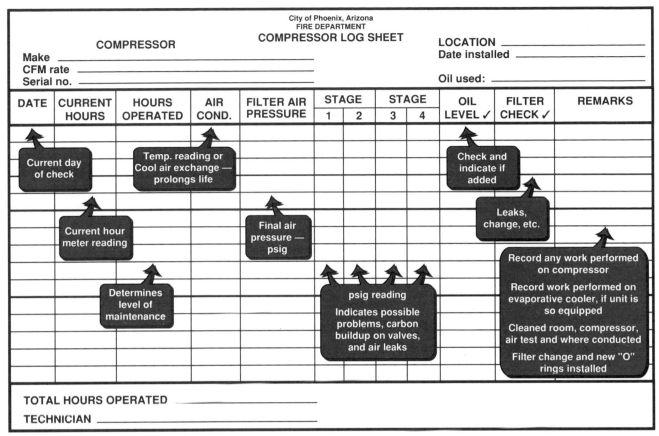

Figure 7.16 Information about compressor operation and maintenance is recorded on compressor log sheets. *Courtesy of Phoenix (Arizona) Fire Department.*

TABLE 7.4
ALLOWABLE BREATHING-AIR CONTAMINATION LEVELS
(CANADIAN STANDARDS ASSOCIATION)

Contaminant	Maximum Allowable Level (by volume unless shown otherwise)
Carbon monoxide	5 (ppm)
Carbon dioxide	500 ± 25 (ppm)
Total Volatile Nonsubstituted Hydrocarbons*	5 (ppm)
Moisture	Pressure dewpoint 10°C (122°F) below lowest airline temperature
Odor	Free from any detectable odor
Particulates, Including Oil	1 mg/m³

*For substituted hydrocarbons, see CSA standard 180.1-M

TABLE 7.5
ALLOWABLE BREATHING-AIR CONTAMINATION LEVELS
(OSHA and U.S. Navy Standards))

| Contaminant | Maximum Allowable Level (by volume unless shown otherwise) | |
	Compressed Gas Assoc.	U.S. Navy
Carbon monoxide	20 ppm	20 ppm
Carbon dioxide	1,000 ppm	500 ppm
Oil Vapor	5 mg/m³	5 mg/m³

will consider a fractional ppm as zero, which is not accurate enough.

If an independent testing firm is chosen for the testing of breathing air, the firm will require that air samples be taken and sent to them for analysis. These sampling kits should have very specific instructions for obtaining air samples, a data sheet for recording test information, and a reliable method of tracking the test sample (Figure 7.17).

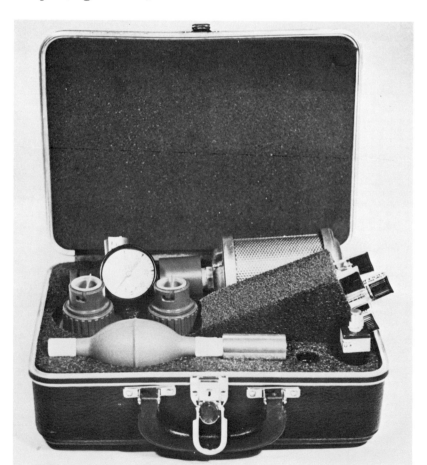

Figure 7.17 Air-testing firms provide kits that fire department personnel use to obtain air samples. *Courtesy of TRI.*

Some companies make available test kits that are used for testing air at the fire department or compressor site (Figure 7.18). Such test kits can provide an immediate reference to the quality of the breathing air. They can be used by the technician to draw samples from either a compressor or an air cylinder, and they provide immediate feedback on the test results. If the sample test results fall outside of the recommended range, the test can be repeated to verify the results.

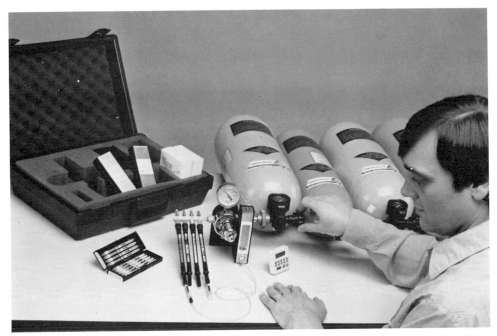

Figure 7.18 Air can be tested with a special test kit at the fire department or at the compressor site. *Photo courtesy of MSA.*

MOBILE AIR CASCADE AND/OR COMPRESSOR UNITS

Many fire departments and county organizations are placing mobile air units in service. These units may simply carry a large number of air cylinders for replacement, may be a single or multiple cascade of three to five or more large cylinders, or may include an air compressor to refill a series of storage cylinders. The types of vehicles used range from pickup trucks with trailers to larger vans or custom-designed apparatus. These units

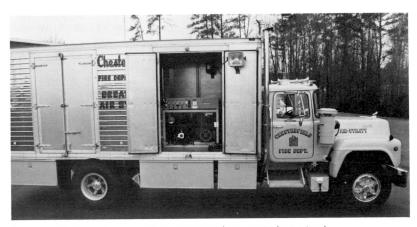

Figure 7.19 A mobile air supply system may be mounted on a truck.

may be combined with other operations such as light apparatus and rescue. Figures 7.19 though 7.21 on the next page show mobile air units with compressors.

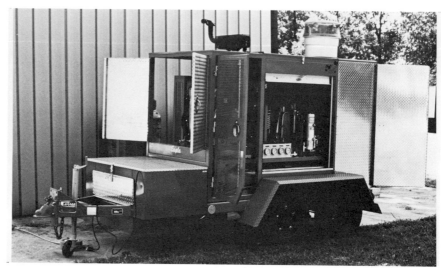

Figure 7.20 Some mobile air units are mounted on trailers and can easily be moved from one location to another.

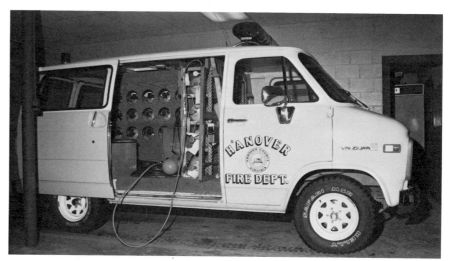

Figure 7.21 Air cascade systems can be mounted in vans.

For safety, the mobile unit should have an adequate refilling station. With sufficient storage cylinders (more than six) and proper planning, several SCBA cylinders can be filled simultaneously (Figure 7.22). Each mobile air unit should meet the following safety standards.

- Those units with a compressor must position the air intake at a high level.
- All vehicle exhaust piping should discharge at a maximum practical distance from the air compressor intake.
- Each unit must have carbon monoxide monitoring equipment with an automatic shutoff switch that is activated when carbon monoxide exceeds acceptable limits.
- An air purification system must be installed and properly maintained on the discharge side of the compressor.
- Proper training must be given to all personnel operating these units.

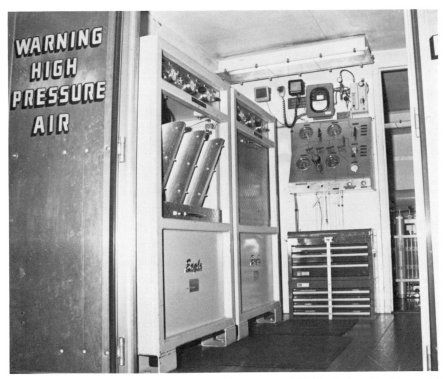

Figure 7.22 A well-equipped mobile unit can recharge several SCBA cylinders simultaneously.

RECHARGING SCBA CYLINDERS

Air cylinders for open-circuit SCBA are filled from either a cascade system — a series of at least three, 300-cubic-foot (8 490 L) cylinders (Figures 7.23 and 7.24) — or directly from a compressor purification system. No matter how the cylinders are filled, the following two safety precautions always apply: Put the cylinders into a shielded charging station to prevent injury to the operator in case of cylinder or hose rupture, and be sure that the cylinder is fully charged but not overpressurized.

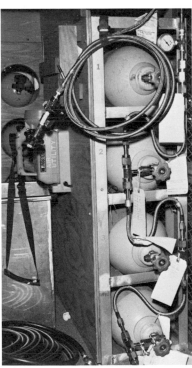

Figure 7.23 A cascade system is composed of three or more storage cylinders.

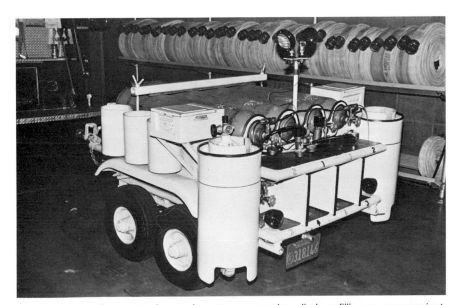

Figure 7.24 A trailer-mounted cascade system may make cylinder refilling more convenient.
Courtesy of David Grimes, Chico (California) Fire Department.

It is important that cylinders be filled correctly. An air cylinder should be filled to at least 90 percent of its rated pressure; any cylinders having less than this amount need to be recharged and should be separated from fully charged cylinders until they are recharged. Although all refilling safety precautions and operating instructions should be posted at every fill station, SCBA cylinders should be filled by trained personnel using proper equipment and should be filled only with *approved* breathing air.

Cylinders can be filled at a rate of 300 to 600 psi/minute (2 070 kPa/minute to 4 140 kPa/minute) in order to reduce the amount of cylinder heating that occurs during the compression of air in cylinder refilling. By filling a cylinder at this lower rate, the amount of heating that takes place is reduced. When air in a cylinder is heated, it expands and causes a higher gauge pressure reading. Once the air in the cylinder has cooled, the pressure gauge will have a lower pressure reading than when the cylinder was initially filled. With a slower fill rate, heating during refilling is reduced; and the change in gauge pressure can be kept at a minimum, enabling the cylinder to be charged fully.

Closed-circuit SCBA cylinders should be recharged by specially trained personnel. These systems contain compressed oxygen, not compressed air. Empty oxygen cylinders should be refilled by an approved charging agency and should be refilled by fire department personnel only if they are specially trained and only if the department has the necessary equipment for refilling breathing-oxygen cylinders. During routine use and maintenance, however, empty breathing-oxygen cylinders of closed-circuit SCBA are usually replaced with fully charged cylinders.

The following two sections outline typical cylinder refilling procedures. However, always follow manufacturer's instructions whenever refilling air cylinders.

Filling From A Cascade System

Step 1: Check the hydrostatic test date, and inspect the SCBA cylinder for damage such as deep nicks, cuts, gouges, or discoloration from heat. If the cylinder is damaged or is out of hydrostatic test date, remove the cylinder from service and tag it for further inspection and hydrostatic testing. (**CAUTION:** *Never* attempt to fill a cylinder that is damaged or is out of hydrostatic test date.)

Step 2: Place the SCBA cylinder in a fragment-proof charging station and connect the charging hose to the cylinder. If the charging hose has a bleed valve, make sure that the bleed valve is closed (Figure 7.25).

Step 3: Open the SCBA cylinder valve.

Step 4: Open valve at charging hose, at cascade system manifold, or valves at both locations, if system is so equipped.

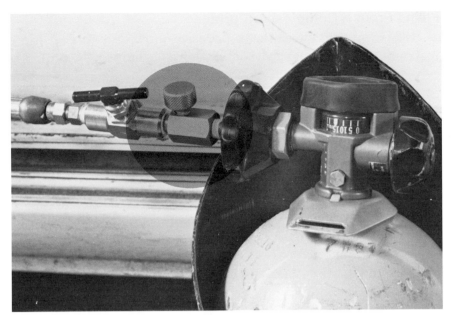

Figure 7.25 Make sure bleed valve is closed before filling the SCBA cylinder; after filling, be sure to open bleed valve before disconnecting the charging hose from the SCBA cylinder.

(**NOTE:** Some cascade systems may have a valve at the charging hose, at the manifold, or at both places.)

Step 5: Open the valve of the cascade cylinder that has the least pressure but that has more pressure than the SCBA cylinder. The airflow from the cascade cylinder must be slow enough to avoid "chatter" or excessive heating of the cylinder being filled. Watch to see that the cascade system gauge needle rises slowly by about 300 to 600 psi (2 070 to 4 140 kPa) per minute. A person's hand should be able to rest on the SCBA cylinder without undue discomfort from the heating of the cylinder.

Step 6: When the pressures of the SCBA and cascade cylinder equalize, close the cascade cylinder valve. If the SCBA cylinder is not yet fully charged, open the valve on the cascade cylinder with the next highest pressure.

Step 7: Repeat Step 6 until the SCBA cylinder is fully charged.

Step 8: Close the valve or valves at the cascade system manifold and/or charging line if the system is so equipped.

Step 9: Close the SCBA cylinder valve.

Step 10: Open the hose bleed valve to bleed off excess pressure between the cylinder valve and the valve on the charging hose. (**CAUTION:** Failure to do so could result in O-ring damage.)

Step 11: Disconnect the charging hose from the SCBA cylinder.

Step 12: Remove the SCBA cylinder from the charging stand and return the cylinder to proper storage.

Filling From A Compressor/Purifier

NOTE: Always check the compressor/purifier manufacturer's instructions for filling cylinders before attempting to fill any cylinders.

Step 1: Check the hydrostatic test date, and inspect the SCBA cylinder for damage such as deep nicks, cuts, gouges, or discoloration from heat. If the cylinder is damaged or out of hydrostatic test date, remove the cylinder from service and tag it for further inspection and hydrostatic testing. (**CAUTION:** *Never* attempt to fill a cylinder that is damaged or is out of hydrostatic test date.)

Step 2: Place the SCBA cylinder in a fragment-proof charging station and connect the charging hose to the cylinder. Make sure the hose bleed valve is closed (see Figure 7.25).

Step 3: Open the SCBA cylinder valve.

Step 4: Set the cylinder pressure adjustment on the compressor (if applicable) to the desired full-cylinder pressure (Figure 7.26). (**NOTE:** If there is no cylinder pressure adjustment, you must watch the pressure gauge on the cylinder during charging to determine when it is full.)

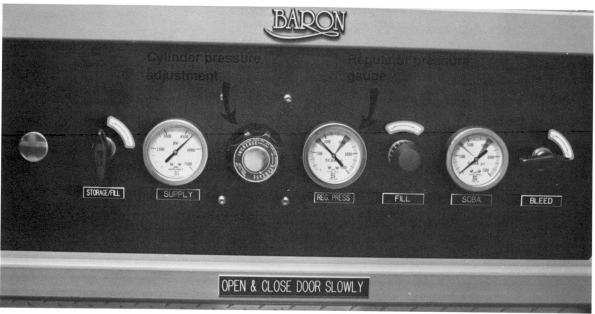

Figure 7.26 Compressor/purifier units have adjustments to preset the desired SCBA cylinder filling pressure. On this unit, the regulator pressure gauge indicates maximum pressure for filling SCBA cylinders.

Step 5: Open the fill valve on the compressor/purifier unit. Airflow should be slow (300 to 600 psi [2 070 to 4 140 kPa] per minute) to avoid excessive heating of the cylinder.

Step 6: When the cylinder is full, close the fill valve on the compressor/purifier.

Step 7: Close the SCBA cylinder valve.

Step 8: Open the hose bleed valve to bleed off excess pressure between the cylinder valve and valve on the charging hose. (**CAUTION:** Failure to do so could result in O-ring damage.)

Step 9: Disconnect the charging hose from the SCBA cylinder.

Step 10: Remove the SCBA cylinder from the charging stand, and return cylinder to proper storage.

Rapid Refilling Of Cylinder While Wearing SCBA

Step 1: Remove the protective caps from refill connection on the SCBA and from refill hose connected to cascade system (Figure 7.27).

Step 2: Connect the refill hose to the SCBA refill connection (Figure 7.28).

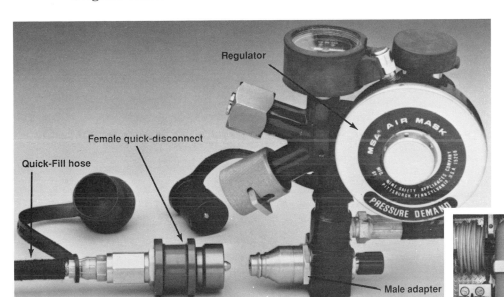

Figure 7.27 The Quick-Fill™ System has special connections that allow the SCBA cylinder to be filled without removing the cylinder from the backpack. *Photo courtesy of MSA.*

Step 3: Fill the cylinder, following SCBA manufacturer's instructions, and monitor refilling pressure until the cylinder is charged.

Step 4: Disconnect the refill hose from the SCBA refill connection.

Step 5: Replace the protective caps on the SCBA refill connection and on the refill hose.

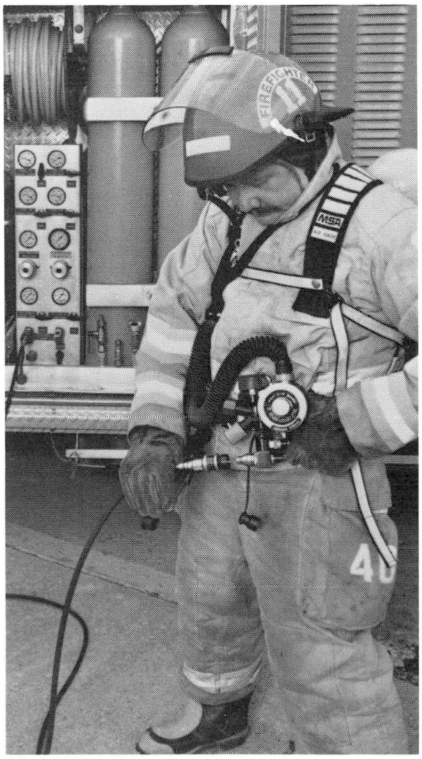

Figure 7.28 The MSA Quick-Fill™ System allows the firefighter the convenience of filling the SCBA cylinder without removing the cylinder or doffing the apparatus. *Photo courtesy of MSA.*

SUMMARY OF BREATHING-AIR COMPRESSOR AND PURIFIER GUIDELINES

Equipment And Operating Safety

- Investigate all system components before purchase; observe actual operation, if possible, and read instruction book thoroughly.

- Be sure that the intake pipe is made of noncorrodible material.

- Verify that all components are for breathing-air system use and are properly rated.

- Verify that the compressor motor is properly rated.

- Be sure that valves are properly rated.

- Secure the system adequately to prevent toppling.

- Install a compressor belt guard.

- Take precautions to prevent the operator from touching the compressor hot-air lines. Clearly mark hot pipes and other hot surfaces.

Equipment Setup

- Be sure that inlet air supply is drawn from a contamination-free area.

- If the air intake line is located inside, keep it away from rooms with high temperatures or little air circulation.

- Install the air intake 2 to 3 feet (0.6 m to 1 m) above floor level.

- Raise the system above floor.

- Anchor piping.

- Secure piping with pressure-rated fittings.

Operation And Charging

- Place cylinders in fragmentation deflector before filling.

- Shield the filling stand in case the cylinder ruptures.

- Design the filling station base so that the operator does not lean directly over the cylinder.

- Locate the filling controls away from the filling area.

Maintenance

- Follow manufacturer's recommendations for inspecting and maintaining equipment used to produce compressed breathing air.

- Follow manufacturer's instructions when inspecting and changing filters and other air purification system components.

- Check filling hoses and hose bleed valves periodically.
- Do not allow manual drain valves to remain open.

SUMMARY

There are several methods fire departments can use for obtaining air supplies for their SCBA cylinders. Some departments contract with commercial firms to refill cylinders; others buy air in large storage cylinders from commercial firms and use the stored air to do their own recharging. When air cylinders are depleted many times every month, a department may need to recharge its cylinders with its own air supply system — compressor, purification system, cascade system, and charging station.

Fire department personnel should understand the operation and function of the various components of the air supply system and the importance of component operations, dew point levels, frequent air quality testing processes, and contamination levels. Safety considerations include the need for contamination-free areas for equipment, intake, and charging stations. Shielding for belts and filling stands is needed, along with clearly marked hot-air lines and other surfaces for operator safety. Properly rated motors and valves are also necessary.

Many fire departments use mobile air supply units to fill air cylinders from a cascade system; others fill cylinders directly from a compressor-purification system. Important precautions to observe, regardless of the method used, include shielding and taking care to not overpressurize when filling breathing air cylinders.

Chapter 7 Review

Answers on page 351

TRUE-FALSE: Mark each statement true or false. If false, explain why.

1. For air cylinder recharging systems, electric compressors are preferred over gasoline- or diesel-powered engines.

   ☐ T   ☐ F _____

   _____

2. Closed-circuit SCBA oxygen cylinders cannot be filled by fire department personnel using a breathing-air recharging system.

   ☐ T   ☐ F _____

   _____

3. A fire department can use its breathing-air compressor for operating shop power tools and for producing breathing air used to recharge cylinders.

   ☐ T   ☐ F _____

   _____

4. The compressor for an air cylinder recharging system may be located either indoors or outdoors.

   ☐ T   ☐ F _____

   _____

5. The air intake filter on the compressor removes solid particles, suspended liquids, oil vapors, gaseous hydrocarbons, toxic gases, and water vapor.

   ☐ T   ☐ F _____

   _____

MULTIPLE CHOICE: Circle the correct answer.

6. Which of the following types of information about air cylinder recharging systems should be included in fire department SOPs?

   A. Inspection and maintenance procedures

   B. Dates of equipment purchase

   C. Location of equipment

   D. All of the above

7. A complete air supply system is composed of four elements. These four elements are _____.

    A. compressor, purification system, carbon monoxide converter, and charging station

    B. compressor, purification cartridge, aftercooler, and charging station

    C. compressor, purification system, storage system, and charging station

    D. compressor, purification cartridge, carbon monoxide converter, and mobile recharging unit

8. Generally, a compressor will deliver 1 cubic foot of air per minute at 3,000 psi (28 L/min at 20 700 kPa) for every horsepower of its rating. What can this information tell fire department personnel?

    A. A department should determine what horsepower rating a compressor must have in order for it to meet the department's refilling needs.

    B. A department rarely will be able to meet its air supply needs by using only one compressor.

    C. A department with a higher-than-normal usage of breathing air should contract with commercial air suppliers rather than purchase a compressor.

    D. None of the above gives the desired information.

9. Firefighter A says that an improperly cooled, unlubricated piston compressor with Teflon™ rings can produce fluorine gas. Firefighter B says that fluorine gas cannot be removed by a typical purification system. Who is correct?

    A. Firefighter A

    B. Firefighter B

    C. Both A and B

    D. Neither A nor B

10. According to NFPA 1500, how often must breathing air that comes from a compressor-purifier be tested?

    A. Annually

    B. Semiannually

    C. Quarterly

    D. Semimonthly

LISTING

11. List five factors that a fire department should consider when deciding what kind of compressor to buy.

    A. _____

    B. _____

    C. _____

    D. _____

    E. _____

12. The air purification system is composed of four basic components. List these components.

A. _____

B. _____

C. _____

D. _____

FILL IN THE BLANK: Fill in the blanks with the correct response.

13. Compression can heat air to _____°F (_____°C). This compressed, heated air is cooled after each stage of the compression cycle and again by an _____ before it enters the purification system.

14. In an air purification system, the component called the _____ contains a desiccant and removes water and oil vapors from the air, lowering the dew point.

15. According to NFPA 1500, the water vapor level of breathing air should be less than _____ ppm, which corresponds to a dew point of _____°F (_____°C).

16. Cylinders can be filled at a rate of _____ to _____ psi/minute in order to reduce the amount of cylinder heating that occurs during the compression of air in cylinder refilling.

SHORT ANSWER: Answer each item briefly.

17. Outside intake pipes should be made of what type of material?

_____

_____

18. If a compressor does not have an automatic drain, why must the sumps or collector be manually drained at least once every 10 to 20 minutes during compressor operation?

_____

_____

_____

_____

19. What is important for fire department personnel who operate and maintain breathing-air compressors to remember about the oil used in the compressors?

_____

_____

_____

_____

_____

20. What is dew point?

_____

_____

_____

_____

_____

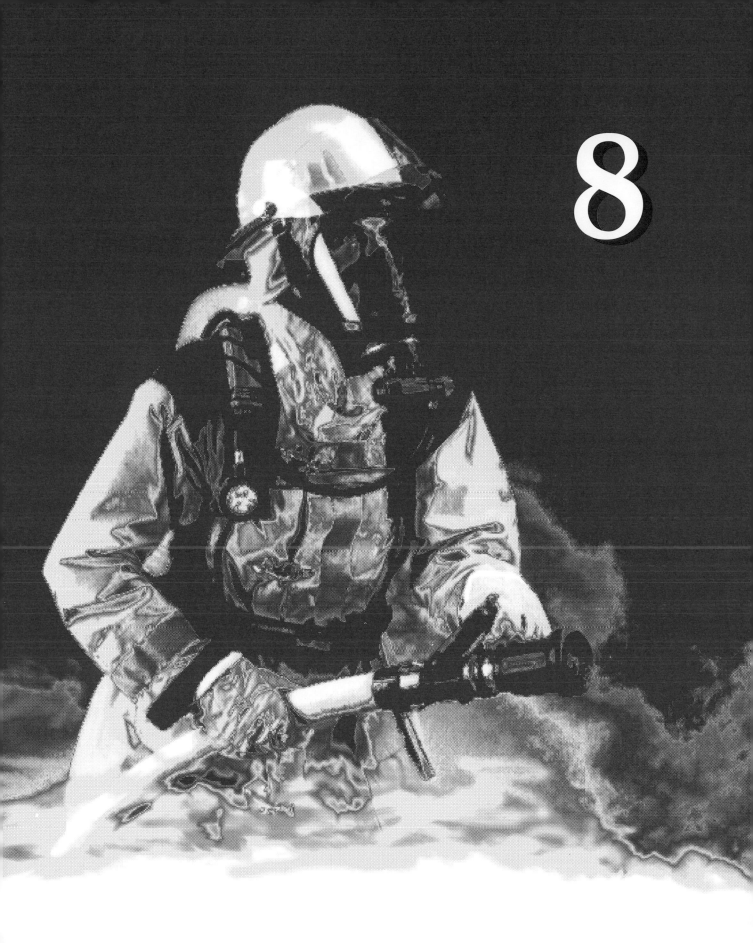

8

Using SCBA

This chapter provides information that addresses the following standards:

NFPA STANDARD 1404
Fire Department Self-Contained Breathing Apparatus Program
1989 Edition

Emergency Scene Use
3-1.3
3-1.6
3-1.7

Chapter 4—SCBA Training
4-12.1

NFPA STANDARD 1500
Fire Department Occupational Safety and Health Program
1987 Edition

Chapter 3—Training and Education
3-3.7
3-5.1
3-5.2

Chapter 5—Protective Clothing and Protective Equipment
5-3.1
5-3.4
5-3.7
5-3.8

Chapter 6—Emergency Operations
6-3.1
6-3.2

ANSI STANDARD Z88.5-1981
Practices for Respiratory Protection for the Fire Service

Section 5—Use of SCBA
5.1
5.2

Section 9—Special Problems
9.1
9.2
9.3
9.4
9.5
9.8
9.9
9.10

ANSI STANDARD Z88.2-1980
Practices for Respiratory Protection

Section 3—Respirator Program Requirements
3.5.5

Section 6—Selection of Respirators

6.4

6.5

6.6

6.7

6.8

6.9

6.10

Section 9—Special Problems

9.3

9.4

9.5

9.6

Code of Federal Regulations
Title 29, Part 1910

Section 146—Permit Required Confined Spaces*

*This is a proposed regulation that may be effective as early as 1991.

Chapter 8
Using SCBA

INTRODUCTION

The preceding chapters of this manual discussed why and how to operate self-contained breathing apparatus. This chapter covers SCBA use on the fireground, at hazardous materials incidents, and during confined space rescues.

As with any type of emergency incident, proper size-up is a key factor in achieving a successful outcome. The nature of the incident, its scope, weather and environmental conditions, the likely duration of the incident, personnel and equipment available, and the degree of hazard to which firefighters will be exposed are all essential considerations.

NFPA 1500, *Standard on Fire Department Occupational Safety and Health Program*, is very specific as it pertains to the use of SCBA. In Section 5-3.1, it states that SCBA shall be provided for and be used by all personnel working in areas where:

- the atmosphere is hazardous.
- the atmosphere is suspected of being hazardous.
- the atmosphere may rapidly become hazardous.

It is in the best interests of all fire service personnel to follow these guidelines when making decisions concerning the use of SCBA during emergency operations. Failing to do so can result in injury or death during an emergency situation. The following account reinforces the importance of wearing SCBA:

> *A tragic incident in Tennessee, in which one firefighter and two workmen were killed, reinforces the need to use SCBA in rescues from covered wells. The incident involved a 50-foot well covered with cement, except for a 24-inch opening. The well apparently had been pumped out the day before the incident with a gas-operated pump that had been lowered*

down through the opening and then removed. On the day of the incident, the first workman lowered into the well passed out. His co-worker called the fire department and then proceeded to attempt a rescue. He also was overcome. When the fire department arrived, firefighters lowered hoses into the well and pumped in oxygen to ventilate the shaft and force out any trapped methane. Then a firefighter was lowered into the well. He was not equipped with SCBA, principally because the well opening was so small. The firefighter was overcome by carbon monoxide fumes trapped in the well. The carbon monoxide, which is heavier than air, had been unaffected by the ventilation procedure.

Courtesy of FireFighter News, Dec/Jan 1989, p. 6.

As stated in the beginning of this manual, fire departments should have and should enforce written standard operating procedures (SOPs) regarding the use of SCBA. But it is ultimately the firefighters' responsibility to wear *all* of their personal protective equipment. Officers and senior firefighters should set the example by always wearing their own personal protective equipment and by enforcing SOPs.

FIREGROUND USES OF SCBA
Engine Company Operations

Firefighters responding to engine company alarms may don their SCBA on the way to the call if seating arrangements permit it to be done safely. Since the firefighter cannot be sure of the situation he or she is about to encounter, SCBA should always be donned. If the situation requires the use of SCBA, then it is there ready for use. If it turns out that SCBA is not needed, the firefighter has at least gained practice in donning SCBA. Situations in which firefighters should be sure to have SCBA donned include responses to the following:

- Fire or waterflow alarms
- Structure fires
- Smoke investigations
- Gas leaks and spills
- Vehicle fires
- First response at hazardous materials incidents

Since engine company operations mainly involve hose advancement and fire extinguishment, these operations should be practiced in training evolutions with SCBA (Figure 8.1). Firefighters should practice maneuvering equipment and appliances and communicating with their SCBA donned and functioning.

Truck Company Operations

Since the work of truck companies — search and rescue, ventilation, salvage and overhaul, forcible entry — is supportive

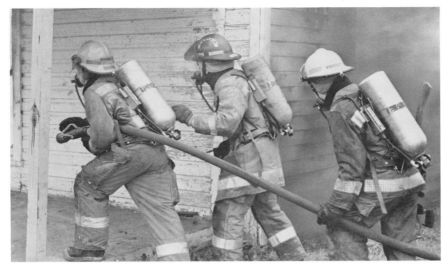

Figure 8.1 In engine company training sessions, firefighters practice hose advancement while wearing SCBA.

to engine company operations, truck company members must wear their SCBA in the same manner as outlined for engine company operations.

During ventilation operations, firefighters must wear SCBA even if they are on the roof in seemingly clean air (Figure 8.2). Winds can shift suddenly, blowing toxic smoke into the firefighters' work area. Worse yet, the firefighter could fall through a soft roof or hole and become trapped. Wearing SCBA reduces the potential of injury or even death in these situations.

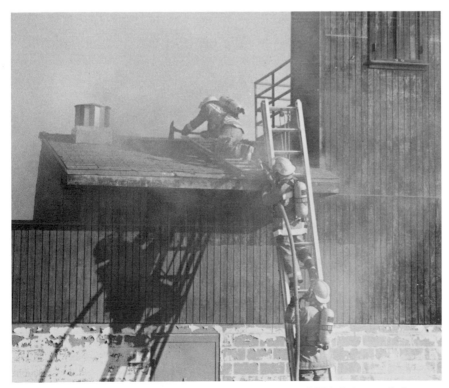

Figure 8.2 In truck company operations, firefighters must wear SCBA during ventilation even though they may seem to be in clear air.

A steady supply of breathing air can become a problem for firefighters who must work from aerial devices. Nonetheless, NFPA 1904, *Standard for Aerial Ladder and Elevating Platform Fire Apparatus*, specifies that a breathing-air system must be provided that is capable of supplying breathing air for at least two persons in the platform. Aerial apparatus manufacturers provide fixed platform connections for multiple users. These breathing-air connections are supplied from one or more 300-cubic-foot cylinders carried on the apparatus. Even with supplied air, however, it may still be advisable for firefighters to wear supplemental backpacked cylinders to provide a source of escape air if it is needed.

Firefighters involved in overhaul operations need to avoid premature removal of SCBA (Figure 8.3). Tests have proven that due to incomplete combustion, extremely high levels of carbon monoxide are present during this fire fighting stage. Firefighters also need to remember that asbestos can be encountered when pulling ceilings.

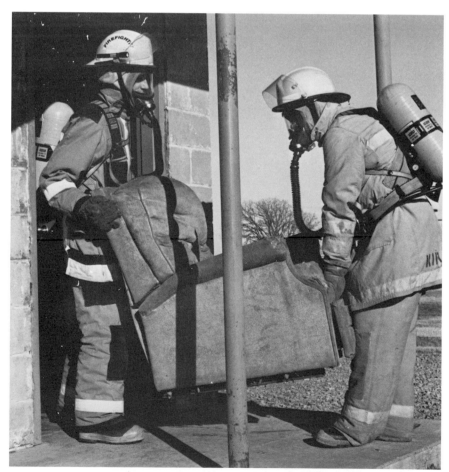

Figure 8.3 Because carbon monoxide may still be present during overhaul operations, firefighters should continue wearing their SCBA for this stage of fire fighting.

Rescue Company Operations

Rescue operations may or may not require breathing apparatus, depending on the situation found by the responding company.

In some departments, the rescue company acts as a manpower squad, working with truck and engine companies. In these cases, SCBA must be worn as dictated by the conditions of the emergency.

SPECIAL SITUATIONS INVOLVING FIREGROUND OPERATIONS

Temperature Extremes

Firefighters seldom encounter temperature extremes for very long, but they should know what can happen to their breathing apparatus in temperatures ranging from -40°F to 200°F (-40°C to 93°C). Self-contained breathing apparatus works well in naturally hot temperatures. The biggest problems with its use during high temperatures are not with the functioning of the equipment, but with the effects of heat on the firefighter. Hot temperatures commonly cause fluid loss and firefighter fatigue. Low temperature extremes, however, can adversely affect the performance of SCBA. The following information is taken from the "NIOSH Emergency Information Bulletin on the Use of SCBA in Low Temperatures."

All firefighters should exercise extreme caution while using open-circuit SCBA during freezing weather. The following precautions are particularly important:

- *Be sure that moisture in the air cylinders is kept at an absolute minimum.* Even small amounts of moisture in the air supply may freeze and result in failure of the breathing apparatus. Moisture content is controlled by the filtration system on the compressor. Regular air testing will alert the fire department if moisture content exceeds minimum requirements.

- *Always use a nosecup in the SCBA facepiece when temperatures are below freezing* (Figure 8.4). Failure to use a nosecup under such circumstances can result in facepiece fogging and severely impaired vision. Chemical antifog agents may not perform adequately in low temperatures.

- *Prepare for a cold weather response in advance* by carefully reading the approval label on the respirator to

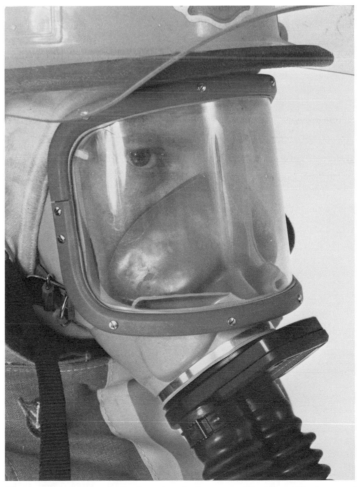

Figure 8.4 A nosecup in the facepiece helps prevent fogging of the lens and is essential in below-freezing temperatures.

determine whether it is necessary to install special accessories before use in subfreezing weather. Certain older models of SCBA approved by the U.S. Bureau of Mines prior to March 25, 1972, require such low-temperature accessories.

- *Learn in advance the procedures for coping with exhalation valves that have frozen open or closed* in low temperatures. (Contact the manufacturer or your State Fire Training Officer for specific instructions.)

- *When leaving an extremely hot environment,* such as a fire scene, and entering cold air (below or near freezing), *always place the SCBA facepiece in your turnout coat to keep it warm if it is to be quickly reused.* When not being actively breathed, SCBA can freeze due to moisture buildup.

- *Use special care to remove all moisture after washing SCBA facepieces and breathing tubes.* Water drainage can freeze in the regulator.

- *Because SCBA alarms can fail in low temperatures, make visual checks of remaining service time* when SCBA are used in freezing conditions.

- SCBAs are NIOSH laboratory approved for use in temperatures as low as -25°F (-32°C). *Use extreme caution if SCBA are used in temperatures below -25°F (-32°C).* At extremely low temperatures, metal can fatigue and crack. In addition, anything at -25°F (-32°C) will cause the skin to freeze if it comes into contact with it.

- *In addition, observe the following general precautions:*
  —Use 6-7.1, Type I, Grade D air or air of equivalent specifications.
  —Follow all information listed on the NIOSH/MSHA or Bureau of Mines approval label for the specific SCBA in use.
  —Follow the manufacturer's recommendations included in their instruction and maintenance manual accompanying the SCBA.
  —Follow all applicable federal, state, and local regulations regarding the use of SCBA.
  —Keep SCBA in a warm location between use.

Structure Types

Firefighters will have to use SCBA in different types of structures — from one-story dwellings to high-rise structures. Firefighters have two main goals when fighting structure fires: rescue and fire control. SCBA must be worn when fighting fire in any building type. Firefighters should be prepared to handle many different types of building fires. This can be accomplished through training and pre-incident planning.

Fires in high-rise buildings pose a challenge to fire departments. Rescues are difficult because most floors are above the reach of fire department aerial apparatus. A major problem with high-rise buildings is maintaining adequate support of the interior companies. This is especially important when SCBA cylinder changes are necessary. Shuttling cylinders from street level to an interior staging area on an upper floor requires the use of firefighters who may be needed more in another capacity. One alternative is to use a remote-type fill station connected to an air unit (Figure 8.5). This fill hose can be run up interior stairs to an upper floor or up the outside of the building. Another alternative is to use an aerial device to bring the airline to an upper floor where it can be run inside (Figure 8.6). Whichever method is used, planning how the operation will be performed and securing the needed materials are crucial.

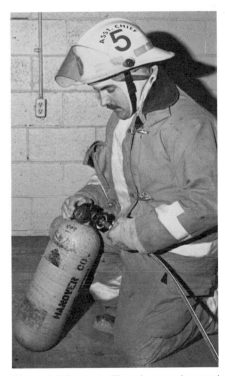

Figure 8.5 A remote fill station may be used to refill SCBA cylinders, as this firefighter is doing.

Figure 8.6 An aerial device can bring an airline to an upper floor so that firefighters can refill their SCBA cylinders. *Photo courtesy of MSA.*

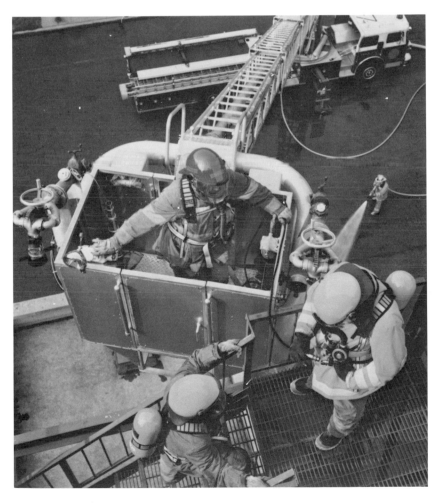

Another type of structure that presents special problems is the large open-plan building. These buildings include supermarkets, warehouses, and manufacturing concerns. Certain features make open-plan buildings problematic: absence of standard floor plan or layout, limited exits and ventilation points, varied populations, truss roofs, high ceilings, and long distances from walls to the center of rooms. It is easy for firefighters to become disoriented in these buildings. Firefighters will be better prepared to deal with incidents in open-plan buildings if they have had proper training. This training must include the use of SCBA, PASS devices, alternative search methods, calculating the point of no return, and emergency procedures in all fire fighting situations. Limited air supplies in SCBA cylinders must be monitored closely by the firefighter to allow for the return trip to safety.

SPECIAL SITUATIONS INVOLVING NONFIREGROUND OPERATIONS
Hazardous Materials Incidents

Wearing SCBA at transportation or industrial incidents involving hazardous materials is essential. But firefighters must be aware that some chemicals, as well as radiation, are absorbed through the skin; SCBA *will not protect* against absorption through the skin. In these cases, firefighters must wear special protective clothing. Firefighters who are expected to wear special protective clothing in addition to SCBA should receive special training relevant to the duties they are expected to perform.

Special Protective Clothing

Special protective clothing helps protect firefighters from the effects of hazardous materials and can also help protect against high radiant heat and flames. Proximity suits let firefighters approach fires and work close to high heat sources. Fire entry suits protect firefighters for short periods when they must enter flames. Chemical entry suits protect firefighters when they must come into contact with chemicals. Chemical entry suits worn in conjunction with a flash-protection suit additionally protect the firefighter from flash fires (Figure 8.7). The flash-protection suit should not be confused with a fire entry suit, however.

Potential problems for SCBA users wearing special protective clothing fall into four general categories:

- Wearing the unit with special protective clothing
- Having enough air to do the job
- Escaping from the hazardous atmosphere if the SCBA fails
- Changing cylinders with chemical protective suits

Sometimes SCBA can be worn over hooded protective suits and operated as usual (Figure 8.8). Generally, this is associated with Level B protection. When an encapsulated suit associated with Level A protection is used, firefighters may encounter problems wearing the SCBA facepiece under the suit hood. Unless the breathing apparatus is matched with the suit, there may not be enough clearance between the facepiece and the lens of the hood.

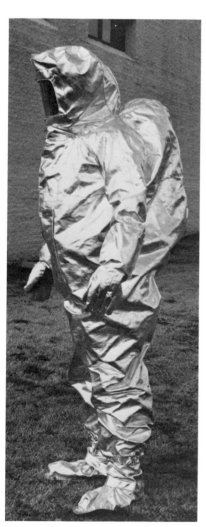

Figure 8.7 A flash-protection suit can be worn over a chemical-entry suit to protect the firefighter from flash fires.

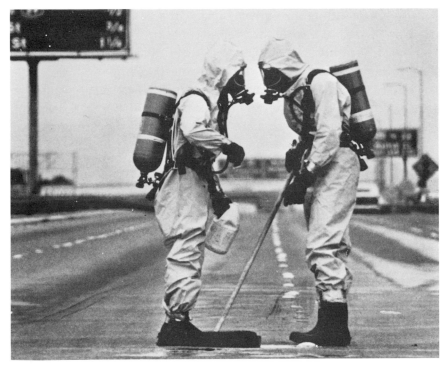

Figure 8.8 Firefighters can wear SCBA over most Level B hooded protective suits.

To accommodate breathing air cylinders, some suits have pockets the size of standard air cylinders built into the back. However, wearing SCBA with protective clothing that does not have a pocket, or with a pocket designed for a different style cylinder, may make wearing the suit more awkward and uncomfortable than usual.

Another major problem with wearing SCBA under some suits is that precious time and air can be lost while donning the breathing unit, donning the suit, or changing a depleted air cylinder because the SCBA has to be donned before the suit is donned. The firefighter must turn on the air supply before completely donning the suit and entering the hazardous atmosphere.

Air Duration

Firefighters wearing special protective clothing may find SCBA breathing duration time more of a problem than when wearing regular turnout clothing. This problem occurs because heat accumulation inside the suit is so high that the firefighter may use up the air supply more quickly. Firefighters wearing fire entry suits, however, should be able to complete their tasks while wearing a 30-minute unit. This is because the fire entry suits themselves cannot remain in contact with flame for more than 10 minutes without danger of being damaged.

Personnel using chemical entry suits often or for long periods will need more air than the standard SCBA can supply. Because of the increased air duration available, closed-circuit SCBA is often chosen for hazardous materials incidents. Even greater air duration is available through the use of airline respirators. Using an airline system, a firefighter can travel up to 300 feet (100 m) from the air supply source. If even greater mobility is needed, the firefighter can also wear a standard backpack and cylinder (Figure 8.9). Then, he or she can temporarily disconnect from the airline, turn on the cylinder to provide breathing air, and perform necessary tasks beyond the range of the airline equipment.

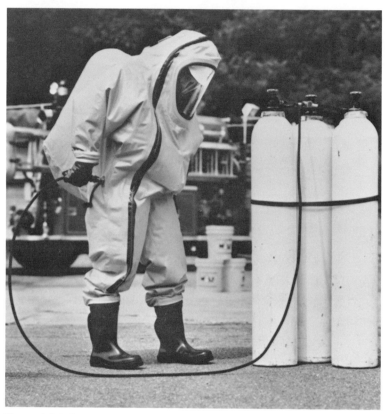

Figure 8.9 A firefighter can wear an SCBA backpack under a Level A chemical entry suit. This allows the firefighter to disconnect from the cascade source. *Photo courtesy of MSA.*

Using airline respirators in hazardous environments requires the use of a 5-minute escape cylinder—a small air cylinder worn on the hip that is part of the airline unit (Figure 8.10). Using the 5-minute escape cylinder for untethered work is not permitted. However, the worker is permitted to perform untethered tasks using a standard 30-minute SCBA with airline attachment capabilities.

When it is necessary to operate air compressors in the field, they should be operated in an area remote from the incident to guarantee that contaminated air is not drawn into the compressor pump and refilled cylinders. Personnel engaged in decontamination *should not* participate in servicing any breathing air cylinders. Normally, High-Efficiency Particulate Air (HEPA) filters are used to filter

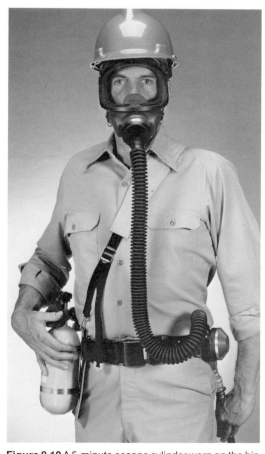

Figure 8.10 A 5-minute escape cylinder worn on the hip is required when airline respirators are used. *Photo courtesy of MSA.*

out small particulate matter of 0.03 microns or larger. These filters should not be relied upon to provide protection against all possible contaminants found in field emergencies.

Changing Air Cylinders

Changing air cylinders during a hazardous materials incident is also a complex and time-consuming procedure. The firefighter in a fully encapsulated suit first has to leave the Hot Zone, undergo primary decontamination (showering with the suit still on), partially remove the suit, have the cylinder changed, and put the suit back on before work can be resumed. It is essential that all personnel involved plan for the amount of time these procedures will take; otherwise, a firefighter may be nearly out of air with no way of safely receiving a new air supply.

When workers in Level B protection are only stopping for air cylinder changeovers and must immediately reenter the Hot Zone, it *may* be acceptable to undergo primary decontamination and simply replace the SCBA cylinder in a noncontaminated atmosphere. The contaminated cylinder must be segregated from noncontaminated equipment and should be inspected and cleaned by an individual skilled in handling contaminated equipment. For high-risk hazardous materials incidents that present respiratory hazards, long-duration apparatus or airline units should be considered.

Emergency Escape

Team Emergency Breathing Procedures (also known as *buddy breathing*) are out of the question when wearing SCBA under encapsulated suits. If the SCBA fails in some way, the firefighter would be forced to remove some of the protective suit and would be unable to undergo preliminary decontamination before another firefighter with an air supply could help. There are essentially two possibilities for the firefighter caught in such a predicament. First, the firefighter could try to remove the SCBA facepiece without removing any of the protective clothing — a difficult task — and try to escape while breathing a few minutes' worth of air trapped in the suit. The other possibility is for team members to try to get the stricken firefighter out of the hazardous atmosphere before serious injury occurs. Working in teams while wearing special protective clothing in hazardous atmospheres is essential for safety. In addition, teams are required by OSHA 29 CFR 1910.120 and by NFPA 1500 and 1404. Those fully encapsulated suits that provide the hardware necessary to connect an airline offer the advantage of an extended air supply or the possibility of refilling the air cylinder as needed.

Confined Space Entry

A confined space is an enclosure that has limited openings for entry and exit, has unfavorable natural ventilation that may contain or produce contaminants, and is not intended for continuous occupation. Confined spaces include trenches, underground utility vaults, sewers, pressure vessels, caves, silos, and rooms using toxic or flammable vapors as part of an industrial process.

Confined space entry presents special problems beyond those normally associated with the difficulty of entering with SCBA. Many confined spaces are oxygen deficient and may contain toxic gases. *Common sense and caution dictate that rescuers assume that ALL confined spaces are life-threatening.*

WARNING

Confined space entry is one of the most dangerous procedures performed by emergency responders. Only persons trained in confined space entry techniques should attempt such rescues.

OSHA (29 CFR 1910) and NIOSH have detailed confined space entry procedures. A minimum procedural outline for making a confined space entry is as follows:

- *Reason for Entry.* Fire department personnel shall perform emergency entries only to rescue people.

- *Entry Permit.* If appropriate, fire department personnel need to obtain a confined space entry permit (Figure 8.11). This permit might be obtainable from the safety engineer or supervisor responsible for the accident site.

- *Atmospheric Testing.* An evaluation of the Lower Explosive Limit (LEL), oxygen content, and the presence of any hazardous material shall be performed. If this evaluation is not possible, rescuers must wear SCBA and/or special protective clothing; and all equipment used in the confined space should be explosion proof.

- *Ventilation.* Ventilation equipment shall be used to make the entry less hazardous during any type of confined space emergency. The type of ventilation used — positive or negative — must be evaluated in order to prevent accidental explosions. Whether air is blown into or exhausted out of a confined space is dependent on the control desired and the potential for exposure of rescuers.

When ventilating a confined space, the most important considerations are the control of airflow and the potential for exposing rescuers to the vented gases. Flexible ducting is used to ventilate confined spaces with only a single opening. The ducting allows for effective air exchange. However, a confined space with two or more openings provides a continuous, unrestricted airflow and

Entry Permit Hotwork	NO. _____	
Permit Initiator	Number/pager	Emergency Number

Location of work

Type of space

Purpose of entry

Description of work being done

Hazards

Safety precautions

Date	Start m.	Finish m.
Oxygen %	Combustible gas % LEL	Toxicity measurements Agent: PPM:

Requirements:

Respiratory Protection	❏ SCBA	❏ Resp.	❏ Air Line
Skin Protection	❏ Chemical Gloves	❏ Chemical Suit	
Eye Protection	❏ Glasses	❏ Face Shield	❏ Goggles
Ear Protection	❏ Plugs	❏ Muff	❏ Combination
Portable Fire Protection	❏ Dry Chemicals	❏ CO2	❏ Halon
Hazard Control	❏ Isolation	❏ Double block and bleed	
	❏ Blinds	❏ Ventilation	❏ Disconnect/cap
	❏ Lockout	❏ Tagout	❏ Inert
Special Precautions	❏ Stand By	❏ Safety Harness/Lifeline	❏ Cover MSDS
	❏ Rope Off Area/Barricades		❏ 12 Volt GF1 Lighting
	❏ Signal Horn	❏ Danger Sign	❏ Access Ladder

Additional Special Precautions:

We (I) have reviewed the job site and are satisfied that proper safety measures are being taken. We agree to abide by these requirements on the job and to bring any job hazards to immediate attention.

Operator	Safety Dept.	Maint./Const. Supv.	Prod. Supv.

See reverse for authorized entrants and attendants.

Distribution: Canary — Control Room   Green — Safety

                Manilla — Post at Job Site   White —

Figure 8.11 A confined space entry permit is available from the safety engineer or supervisor responsible for the site.

better ventilation (Figures 8.12 a and b). *Under no circumstances should the ventilator exhaust be directed toward unprotected persons.*

- *Harnesses and Lifelines.* Firefighters entering confined spaces shall be required to use harnesses and lifelines. An attendant shall monitor these lines at all times and have knowledge of the number, identity, time of entry, and point-of-no-return figures for each firefighter.

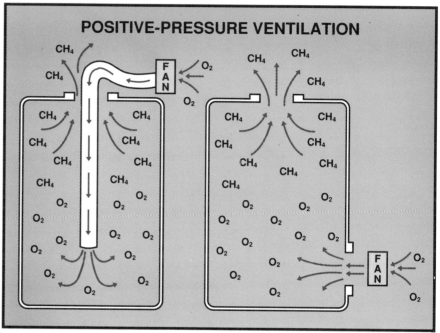

Figure 8.12a During positive-pressure ventilation, air must be ducted into a confined space having only a single opening; a confined space with two or more openings is more easily ventilated.

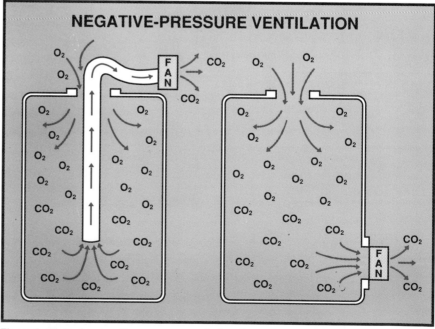

Figure 8.12b During negative-pressure ventilation of a confined space, airflow is reversed and ventilation is achieved in a manner similar to positive-pressure ventilation.

- *Standby Personnel.* At least one firefighter in full gear and SCBA shall stand by *for each rescuer* in case another rescue situation develops. (**NOTE:** This is important because one person will not likely be able to rescue two stricken rescuers.)

- *Lift Systems.* If the firefighter or victim must be lifted vertically, the appropriate hauling system needs to be in place before entry is made.

- *Buddy System.* As always, firefighters should work in teams of two or more. Some confined spaces, by their restrictive nature, will not allow a buddy team to operate effectively. In this instance, the second team member shall remain outside the area ready to enter the space if a secondary emergency arises.

- *Expert Advice.* If time permits, knowledgeable people shall be questioned as to the nature of the space (for example, type of contaminant: toxic, flammable, explosive) and whether ventilation of the space would make the entry safer.

Entering some confined places such as sewers, tanks, caissons, and silos is sometimes made more difficult because the access hatch or hole may be too small to admit a rescuer wearing an SCBA backpack. If the opening or access route is limited to the point of barring entry while wearing an SCBA backpack, an airline breathing system should be considered. The following procedures can be used for entering with an airline breathing system:

Step 1: Don an approved Class III, full-body harness (Figure 8.13).

Step 2: Don the airline unit, test for correct facepiece seal and positive pressure, and have partner inspect unit rig (Figure 8.14 on next page).

Step 3: Attach the rescue rope to the body harness D-ring (Figure 8.15 on next page).

Step 4: Enter the confined space (Figure 8.16 on next page).

Step 5: Maintain an awareness of the approximate length of time needed for a person to be removed from the confined space. The egress bottle on an airline unit is rated for approximately 5 minutes.

Step 6: Maintain an awareness of the airline to prevent entanglement and damage from sharp objects.

If an airline is not available, it will be necessary to enter the confined space with a standard SCBA cylinder and backpack. The opening of many confined spaces will not permit the entry of a

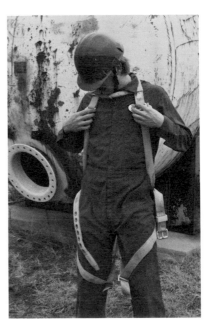

Figure 8.13 A rescuer dons a full-body harness before entering a confined space.

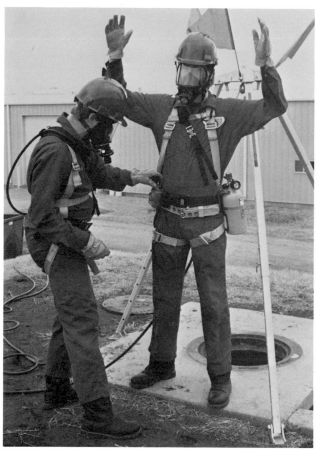

Figure 8.14 The rescuer's partner inspects the rescuer's airline unit to ensure that it has been properly donned.

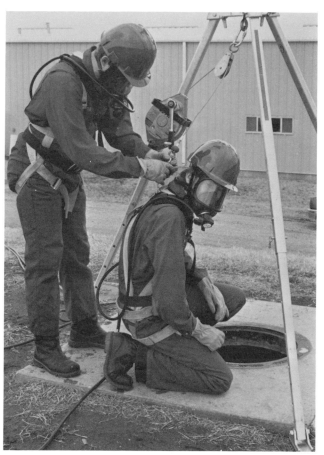

Figure 8.15 The partner attaches a rescue rope to the rescuer's body harness D-ring.

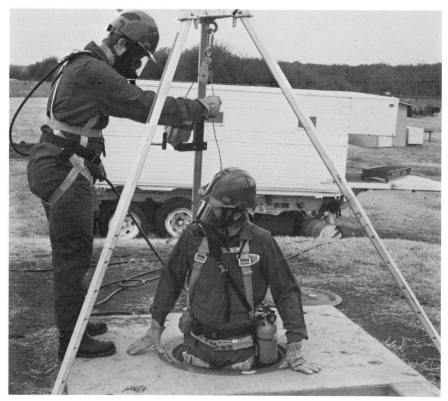

Figure 8.16 A rescuer, properly outfitted, enters the confined space.

rescuer wearing a backpack (Figure 8.17); therefore, it will be necessary to remove the backpack, enter the confined space, and redon the backpack. The following procedures can be used for making a vertical entry with SCBA:

Step 1: Don an approved Class III full-body harness.

Step 2: Don the SCBA and test for correct facepiece seal and positive pressure.

Step 3: Remove the backpack and attach it to the body harness by one of the D-rings or other hardware, using an approved knot or prepared lanyard. This procedure allows the backpack to be lowered at the same time as the rescuer and helps prevent accidental removal of the facepiece.

Step 4: Attach the rescue rope to the body harness D-ring.

Step 5: Enter the confined space, maintaining contact with the SCBA backpack (Figure 8.18).

Step 6: Once inside the confined space, redon the backpack if possible (Figure 8.19).

Step 7: If necessary, adjust the facepiece.

Step 8: At all times, maintain an awareness of the approximate length of time needed to remove a victim from the confined space, as well as the point-of-no-return figure of the rescuer.

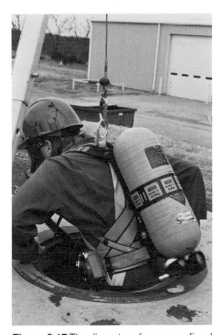

Figure 8.17 The diameter of many confined space openings prohibits the entry of a rescuer wearing a backpack.

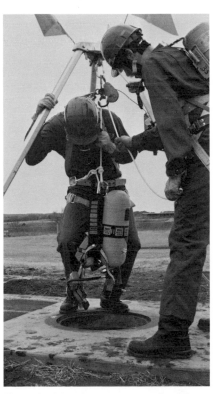

Figure 8.18 A rescuer enters a confined space with the SCBA backpack attached to the rescue harness.

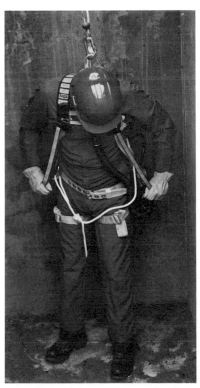

Figure 8.19 A rescuer redons the SCBA backpack inside the confined space.

For a horizontal entry with SCBA, the following procedures can be used:

Step 1: Don an approved Class III, full-body harness (Figure 8.20).

Step 2: Don the SCBA and test for correct facepiece seal and positive pressure (Figure 8.21).

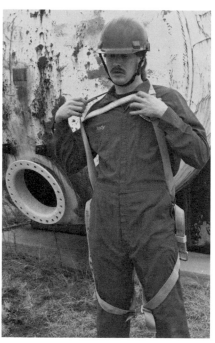

Figure 8.20 For a horizontal entry into a confined space with an SCBA, the rescuer dons a full-body harness.

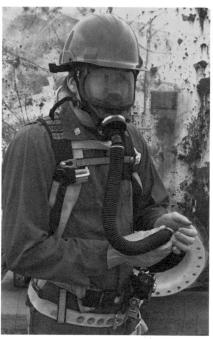

Figure 8.21 The rescuer dons the SCBA and checks for proper facepiece seal and positive pressure.

Step 3: Remove the backpack and attach a short tag line or lanyard between the backpack and the full-body harness. The tag line should be shorter than the breathing tube or regulator hose. Attaching a tag line prevents the apparatus from falling away and pulling the facepiece from the rescuer's face. (See Figure 8.22.)

Step 4: Attach the rescue line to the body harness D-ring, and enter the space while a team member or attendant maintains control of the backpack (Figure 8.22.)

Step 5: After entering the confined space, have the team member outside pass the backpack assembly to the rescuer through the opening (Figure 8.23).

Step 6: If applicable, redon the backpack, taking care not to get tangled in the rescue rope (Figure 8.24).

Step 7: Adjust the facepiece if necessary.

Step 8: At all times, maintain an awareness of the length of time needed to remove a victim from the confined space, as well as the point-of-no-return figure of the rescuer.

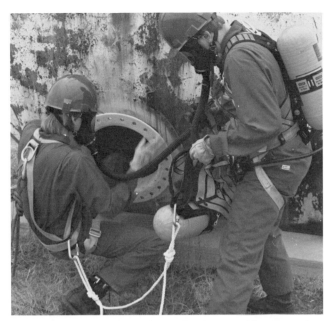

Figure 8.22 A rescuer enters the confined space while an attendant maintains control of the SCBA backpack. Note that the rescue rope is attached to the body harness D-ring and the SCBA backpack is attached to a short tag line.

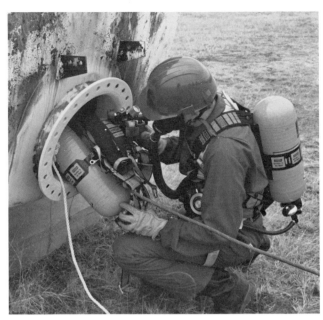

Figure 8.23 After the rescuer enters the confined space, the partner passes the SCBA backpack to the rescuer for redonning.

SUMMARY

Firefighters should always don SCBA en route to an emergency scene to be fully prepared on arrival. Firefighters should also be sure to wear SCBA during ventilation and overhaul operations. Because different types of buildings present their own fire fighting and rescue problems, firefighters must determine their own point of no return to guarantee a safe exit.

SCBA is essential for special situations involving nonfireground operations, such as hazardous materials incidents, but will not protect against absorption through the skin. Firefighters who must wear special protective suits over SCBA need special training. Some potential problems during these situations include having enough air to do the job, wearing SCBA with the protective suit, and escaping from the hazardous atmosphere if the SCBA fails. Changing air cylinders at hazardous materials incidents also requires several extra protective procedures.

Confined space rescues also require that firefighters pay particular attention to safety. Firefighters must be well trained in entry and rescue procedures to keep from becoming victims themselves. In very restricted confined spaces, there is not enough room to admit the firefighter who is wearing an SCBA backpack. In these situations, airline breathing systems provide more mobility and longer air duration.

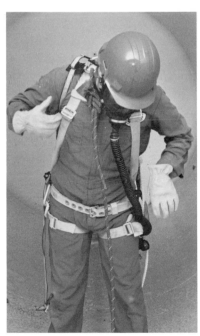

Figure 8.24 Once inside the confined space, the rescuer redons the SCBA backpack.

Chapter 8 Review

Answers on page 351

TRUE-FALSE: Mark each statement true or false. If false, explain why.

1. During ventilation operations, firefighters must wear SCBA even if they are on the roof in seemingly clean air.

   ☐ T ☐ F _____

   _____

2. Since engine company operations mainly involve hose advancement and fire extinguishment, these operations should be practiced in training evolutions by the firefighters while wearing SCBA.

   ☐ T ☐ F _____

   _____

3. Rescue operations always require breathing apparatus.

   ☐ T ☐ F _____

   _____

4. Self-contained breathing apparatus works well in naturally hot temperatures.

   ☐ T ☐ F _____

   _____

5. Low temperature extremes do not adversely affect SCBA performance.

   ☐ T ☐ F _____

   _____

6. SCBA will protect firefighters from chemicals and radiation that are absorbed through the skin.

   ☐ T ☐ F _____

   _____

MULTIPLE CHOICE: Circle the correct answer.

7. Firefighters A and B are discussing ventilation and using SCBA. Firefighter A says that SCBA should be worn during ventilation operations only if the wind is blowing smoke and toxic gases directly toward the firefighter. Firefighter B says that SCBA does not need to be worn during ventilation operations. Who is correct?

   A. Firefighter A

   B. Firefighter B

C. Both A and B

D. Neither A nor B

8. A type of suit that lets firefighters approach fires and work close to high heat sources is a _____.

A. chemical entry suit

B. fire entry suit

C. high-heat entry suit

D. none of the above is correct

9. A type of suit that protects firefighters for short periods when they must enter flames is a _____.

A. proximity suit

B. fire entry suit

C. chemical entry suit

D. special protection suit

LISTING

10. Firefighters should be sure to have SCBA donned when responding to what types of situations?

A. _____

B. _____

C. _____

D. _____

E. _____

F. _____

SELECT: Circle the correct response.

11. The biggest problems with using SCBA during high temperatures are with the (functioning of the equipment/effects of heat on the firefighter).

12. Wearing SCBA over protective suits and operating SCBA as usual is usually associated with (Level A/Level B) protection.

FILL IN THE BLANK: Fill in the blanks with the correct response.

13. SCBAs are NIOSH laboratory approved for use in temperatures as low as _____°F (_____°C).

14. _____ suits protect firefighters when they must come into contact with chemicals.

15. Using an airline system, a firefighter can travel up to _____ feet (_____ m) from the air supply source.

SHORT ANSWER: Answer each item briefly.

16. According to NFPA 1500, SCBA shall be provided for and be used by all personnel working in areas having what types of atmosphere?

_____

_____

_____

17. When working in temperatures below freezing, what can result if the firefighter does not have a facepiece equipped with a nosecup?

_____

_____

_____

18. When working in high-rise buildings, why may a remote-type fill station connected to an air unit be advantageous?

_____

_____

_____

_____

19. Why can changing an air cylinder be a complex and time-consuming procedure for the firefighter who is working at an incident involving hazardous materials?

_____

_____

_____

_____

_____

20. What is the definition of _confined space_?

_____

_____

_____

_____

_____

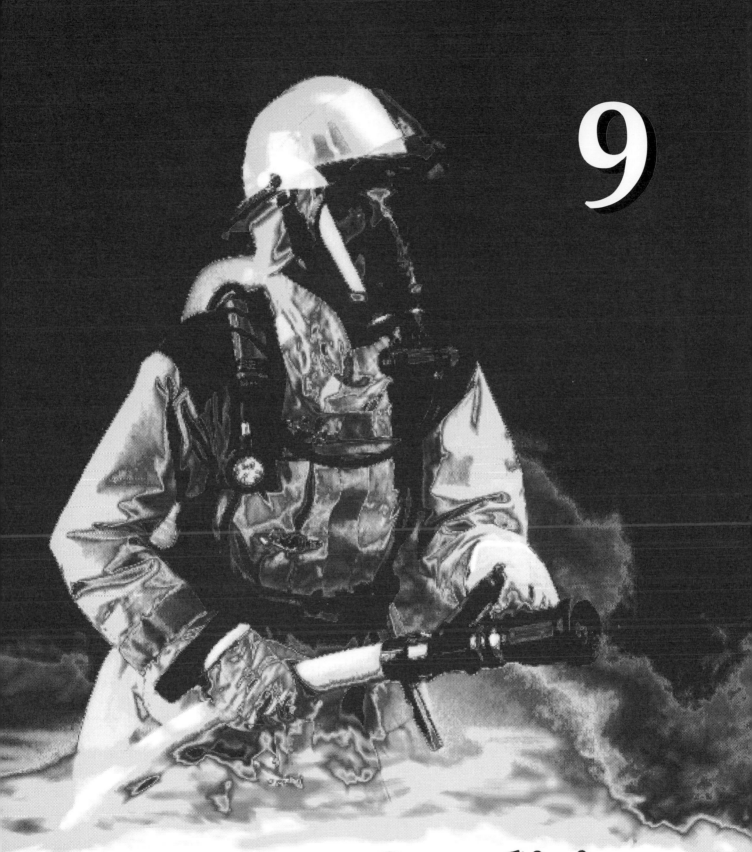

Emergency Conditions Breathing

This chapter provides information that addresses the following standards:

NFPA STANDARD 1001
Fire Fighter Professional Qualifications
1987 Edition

Fire Fighter II
4-6.3

NFPA STANDARD 1404
Fire Department Self-Contained Breathing Apparatus Program
1989 Edition

Chapter 3—Emergency Scene Use
3-1.6
3-1.7

Chapter 4—SCBA Training
4-4.1
4-4.2
4-10 (d)
4-10 (e)
4-12.1 (d)

NFPA STANDARD 1500
Fire Department Occupational Safety and Health Program
1987 Edition

Protective Clothing and Protective Equipment
5-3.7
5-3.8

ANSI STANDARD Z88.5-1981
Practices for Respiratory Protection for the Fire Service

Section 5—Use of SCBA
5.2

Section 9—Special Problems
9.11

Code of Federal Regulations
Title 29, Part 1910

Section 134—Respiratory Protection

Chapter 9

Emergency Conditions Breathing

INTRODUCTION

Firefighters may find themselves in situations in which their self-contained breathing apparatus malfunctions, they run out of air, or they become trapped. Ideally, this should never happen. Realistically, however, it does happen. With proper training, firefighters can be prepared to react appropriately when faced with such dangerous situations.

When a firefighter hears the low-pressure alarm or finds that his or her SCBA is malfunctioning, the fire fighting team should immediately leave the structure or area. There may be times, though, when retreat may not be possible or when the firefighter may not have enough air to reach an exit. In these instances, the firefighter may need to use emergency conditions breathing.

The methods for both individual emergency conditions breathing and team emergency conditions breathing (buddy breathing) are very controversial. Some particular emergency breathing techniques void NIOSH certification of SCBA equipment, and some are really very unsafe. For instance, *it is never safe nor smart to remove the facepiece or break its seal during emergencies.* SCBA users should avoid using any emergency technique that requires facepiece removal or facepiece-seal violation. Emergency conditions breathing methods are last-resort procedures. Using an emergency conditions breathing method considered unsafe may save a firefighter's life. On the other hand, using such a breathing method may cost a life. Therefore, it is easy to see why all emergency conditions breathing procedures are not acceptable to all jurisdictions. According to NFPA 1404, however, the fire department is responsible for training firefighters in the emergency operations required when SCBA fails and for evaluating firefighter performance of these operations in simulated emergency conditions.

> ## EMERGENCY CONDITIONS BREATHING METHODS ARE LAST-RESORT PROCEDURES.

This chapter discusses department and firefighter responsibilities, emergency conditions breathing methods, and other information about emergency conditions and SCBA.

DEPARTMENT RESPONSIBILITY

Departments and instructors must determine which emergency breathing procedures should be taught and the extent to which they should be taught. Whether or not the procedures are acceptable is only one factor the department must consider when planning training in this area. Although these procedures may never be used or may rarely be used, the department must consider the training time required to ensure that firefighters are skilled in these procedures.

Further, a fire department's policy on emergency conditions breathing must include provisions for training and periodic evaluation of firefighters. To comply with NFPA standards, the department must develop an evaluation process, evaluate firefighters using SCBA during simulated, but safe, emergency conditions, and determine the skill level of each firefighter.

> ## EMERGENCY BREATHING PROCEDURES CAN BE PERFORMED ONLY BY THOROUGHLY TRAINED FIREFIGHTERS.

Emergency breathing methods should also be outlined in the department's policies and procedures. The department's SOPs should include when to take these emergency measures, keeping in mind that under most circumstances, the fire fighting team should exit the area rather than attempt emergency conditions breathing. The department is also responsible for deciding which methods to include. When making this decision, the department must consider the type of SCBA used and the recommendations of the SCBA manufacturer. The department must also realize that using some methods may void the equipment's NIOSH certification.

During SCBA training, firefighters are told how important it is never to remove the facepiece. This point should be stressed again and again during emergency conditions breathing instruction. Removing facepieces for any reason can cause firefighters to become victims themselves.

FIREFIGHTER RESPONSIBILITY

Firefighters should understand the importance of being properly trained in using emergency breathing procedures. To comply with NFPA 1001 and 1404, firefighters must be able to use SCBA and emergency breathing methods to assist other firefighters, to conserve their own air supplies, and to properly use their bypass valves in emergency situations. All firefighters using SCBA should learn these skills as outlined in their fire department's SOPs.

Firefighters must also learn the department's communications system. Each department should teach its communications system—usually a set of signals—during SCBA training (Table 9.1). In emergency situations, reaction time is critical, and there must be no confusion in communications.

Learning emergency breathing skills is extremely important. However, firefighters should remember that it is better in all instances to *leave the area* when the low-pressure alarm sounds or as soon as it is evident that the air supply is low or the SCBA is malfunctioning. By doing so, firefighters themselves may not become victims. All firefighters should remember:

> ## WHEN IN TROUBLE, QUIT WORKING AND GET OUT!

TABLE 9.1
LIFELINE SIGNALS

Number of Tugs	Signal	Meaning
1	OK	When made from outside: "Is everything all right?" When made from inside: "Everying is all right."
2	Advance	When made from outside: "Advance." When made from inside: "Give me more line so I can advance."
3	Take up	When made from outside: "Turn back." When made from inside: "Take in line. I am backing out or changing position."
4	Help	When made from outside: "Get out at once!" When made from inside: "I need assistance."

The rule about leaving the facepiece on at all times also applies when rescuing victims. The firefighter should not attempt to give a victim air by sharing the facepiece. In most situations, the victim may panic, fearing that no more breathing air will be made available. Such a victim may fight or not give the mask back to the firefighter. A hazardous atmosphere is NOT the place to administer first aid. The firefighter should first remove the victim to a safe environment.

Most importantly, by taking off their facepieces, firefighters expose themselves to other dangers. Without facepieces they can inhale smoke and toxic gases and may also become victims. In addition, firefighters should keep in mind that the facepiece protects them from the surrounding superheated air. Inhaling superheated air is extremely dangerous to the firefighter and can cause death.

Even a damaged facepiece offers some protection. The main reason a damaged facepiece should not be removed is that it still provides positive pressure to the firefighter's face.

SCBA TEAMS

When using SCBA, firefighters should always work in teams of two or more. Team members should stay calm and act immediately when one member is in trouble. The members of these teams should communicate with one another to be able to work effectively and to assist each other during emergencies. Team members must be able to communicate with one another and with personnel outside the involved area. The team member designated as Breathing Apparatus Officer should remain outside the area where SCBA is used while the other SCBA team members are in the area. The Breathing Apparatus Officer is responsible for knowing the number and identity of all personnel using SCBA, their location and function in the fire building, and their entry time. Individual air consumption rates should be provided to the Breathing Apparatus Officer, who uses these rates to calculate the remaining air available for each firefighter. If the Breathing Apparatus Officer notes that a firefighter inside the structure is low on air, the officer is responsible for recalling the team and replacing it with a new team. Refer to Chapter 4, Safety and Training, for more information about SCBA team operational procedures.

Firefighters should follow departmental procedures when one team member's air supply is depleted before he or she can exit the area. In most instances, it is better for one team member to assist the other out of the area than to attempt to practice team breathing techniques. Even when a firefighter is pinned and cannot be freed, it is usually better for the uninjured team member to leave and get assistance rather than stay and share his or her air supply. These same basic rules apply to rescuing or assisting a nonfirefighter victim.

EMERGENCY CONDITIONS BREATHING

The emergency breathing methods described in this section include some methods familiar to firefighters and some newer methods that can be used with specially designed SCBA. The descriptions here are general, and firefighters must follow departmental policy regarding when and how to use these methods. The emergency conditions breathing procedures used with different equipment may be similar, or they may vary. Therefore, procedures for emergency conditions breathing should always follow the recommendations of the SCBA manufacturer.

In any emergency it is best for firefighters to remain calm. Not only will staying calm enable them to work better and to communicate more clearly, but it will also help them to use their air supplies more efficiently. Exertion and panic, of course, cause firefighters to require more air.

Skip Breathing

Firefighters should practice controlled breathing whenever using SCBA. However, when air supply is low, they may practice skip breathing. Skip breathing is an emergency breathing technique used to extend the use of the remaining air supply. To use this technique, the firefighter inhales, as during regular breathing, holds the breath as long as it would take to exhale, and then inhales once again before exhaling. The firefighter should take normal breaths and exhale slowly to keep the carbon dioxide in the lungs in proper balance.

Using The Bypass Valve

Although a regulator usually works as designed, it can malfunction, and one method of using SCBA when the regulator becomes damaged or malfunctions is to open the bypass valve. During normal SCBA operation, the mainline valve is fully open while the bypass valve is fully closed. If needed in an emergency, the firefighter can close the mainline valve and open the bypass valve to provide a flow of air into the facepiece (Figures 9.1 and 9.2). The bypass valve should be closed after the firefighter takes a breath and then opened each time the next breath is needed.

Using A Cylinder Transfilling System

Some of the newer SCBA equipment designs include additional valves or valve adapters for transfilling capabilities (Figure 9.3 on next page). With this type of system, an empty or nearly empty cylinder of one SCBA can be filled with air from another SCBA air cylinder. This is done by connecting a hose with special connections on each end to special valve connections or valve adapters on

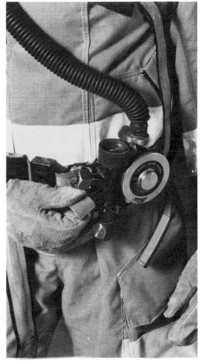

Figure 9.1 Close the mainline valve for bypass breathing.

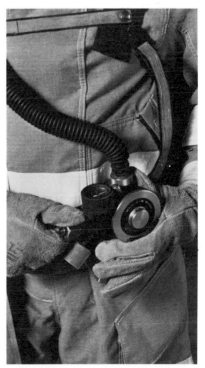

Figure 9.2 After closing the mainline valve, open and close the bypass valve momentarily each time a breath is needed.

two different SCBA (Figure 9.4). The air pressure of the two air cylinders can then equalize. When transfilling, air from one cylinder flows to another and does not flow through the regulator of either SCBA. This system should not be confused with using an airline unit.

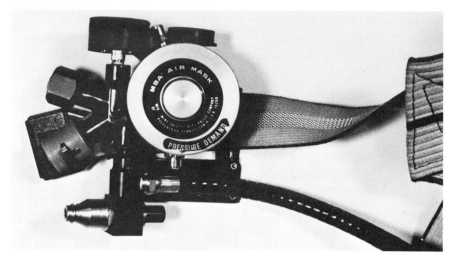

Figure 9.3 Some SCBA have connections for transfilling. A special connection on one type of SCBA system is located on the regulator.

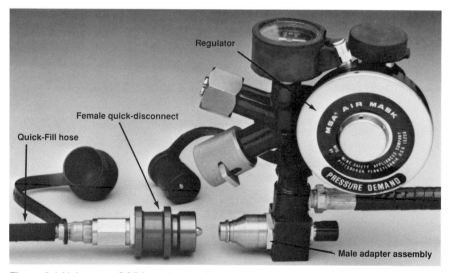

Figure 9.4 Air from one SCBA can be transferred to another through a section of hose attached to the special connections of each SCBA. *Photo courtesy of MSA.*

This system has advantages that make it desirable to use in many instances. A major advantage of using a transfilling system is that the facepiece seal is not violated. Another advantage is that firefighters outfitted with encapsulated suits can refill their air supply without exposing themselves to hazardous materials or without leaving the contaminated area. Additionally, a transfilling system can be used as an emergency escape breathing support system (EEBSS).

There are, however, some disadvantages of using a transfilling system. The air supply of the donor (firefighter supplying the air) will be greatly reduced, shortening the length of time for escape. Also, it may not be practical in some instances to use a transfilling system as an EEBSS. For instance, if the low-pressure alarm of the donor has sounded or begins to sound, transfilling should not be performed; and both firefighters should exit immediately. By attempting to transfill in such a situation, neither firefighter may have an adequate air supply for escape. Firefighters should keep in mind, too, that transfilling should be done only in emergency situations in which one firefighter has an adequate air supply. Both firefighters should immediately exit after transfilling.

Fire departments having SCBA with transfilling capabilities should address their use in the departments' SOPs. The policies should include procedures for transfilling cylinders in emergency situations, the situations in which transfilling should and should not be attempted, and any other guidelines or factors to be considered depending upon the department's particular type of SCBA.

The Mine Safety Appliances Company (MSA) has a transfilling system that can be used as an EEBSS (Figure 9.5). This system is the Quick-Fill™ system. The Quick-Fill™ system is certified by NIOSH—the system does not affect the performance of the airflow from the regulator during use, and it does not require that the two firefighters using the system be permanently attached to each other. Some older MSA self-contained breathing apparatus can be upgraded to use the Quick-Fill™ system.

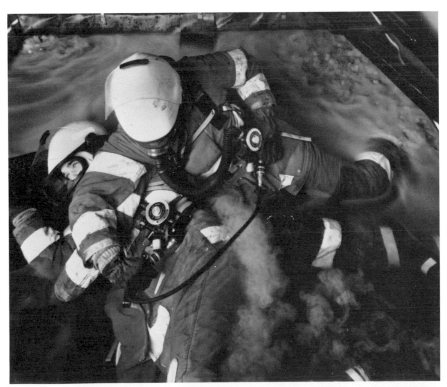

Figure 9.5 A firefighter connects his SCBA to another firefighter's SCBA to share his air supply. *Photo courtesy of MSA.*

Using Other Types Of Emergency Escape Breathing Support Systems

There are other systems that use a hose to connect two SCBA and that can be used as EEBSS. However, in these systems, air does not flow from the full cylinder into the empty cylinder; in other words, these systems do not have transfilling capabilities. Air from the full SCBA cylinder of one firefighter travels through the regulator or a pressure-reducing assembly, through a connecting hose, and then to the SCBA and facepiece of the other firefighter. The hose must remain connected to both SCBA while the firefighters escape. This type of system used as an EEBSS voids NIOSH certification of the equipment.

Nevertheless, this type of system does allow two SCBA users to share an air supply without violating the facepiece seal of either user. There are a variety of manufacturers whose SCBA are equipped with hose connections so that they can be used as an EEBSS (Figure 9.6). Also, many SCBA models can be retrofitted with these connections. Refer to Appendix E for information about different SCBA manufacturers' products.

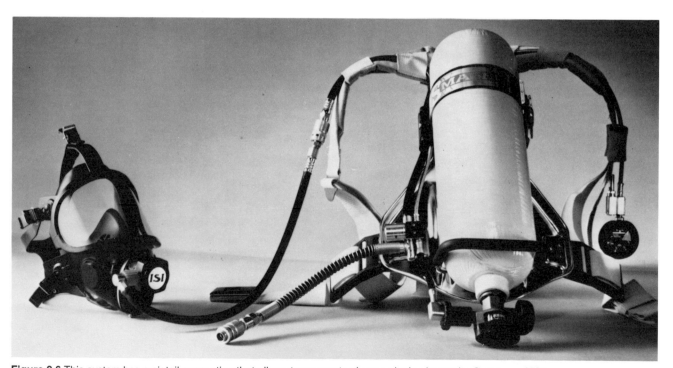

Figure 9.6 This system has a pigtail connection that allows two users to share a single air supply. *Courtesy of ISI.*

Using A Common Regulator

One method of team emergency conditions breathing involves sharing a regulator. This technique can be used only with SCBA having harness-mounted regulators. A firefighter with a depleted air supply receives air by connecting his or her low-pressure hose to another team member's regulator (Figure 9.7). Both firefighters disconnect their low-pressure hoses from their regulators and take turns connecting their low-pressure hoses to the regulator of the SCBA having the adequate air supply. After one firefighter takes two or three breaths, the other takes two or three breaths. Using SCBA equipment for this type of procedure, however, is not certified by NIOSH, **violates NFPA, OSHA, and ANSI standards, and is not condoned by most training organizations due to the liability.**

Firefighters must remember to cover their low-pressure hose openings and the regulator opening when neither hose is attached to the regulator (see Figure 9.7). Neglecting to cover the end of the low-pressure hose will allow smoke and toxic gases to enter the facepiece. Using this method is time consuming and requires concentration for both parties involved. Generally, in most house fires, firefighters should be able to exit the structure in less time than required to set up this operation.

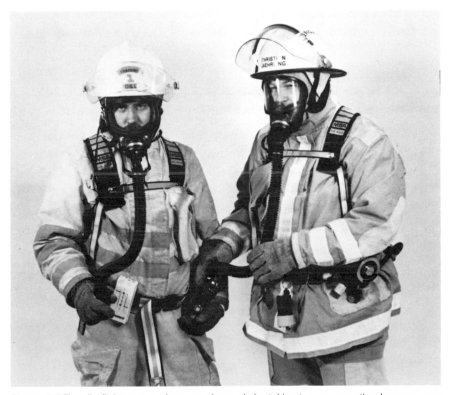

Figure 9.7 Two firefighters can share an air supply by taking turns connecting low-pressure hoses to the functioning regulator.

Using The Low-Pressure Hose-To-Facepiece Method

Another method of team emergency conditions breathing is the low-pressure hose-to-facepiece method. Using this method, a firefighter wearing a harness-mounted regulator can use air from a team member's facepiece. When a firefighter's SCBA malfunctions or runs out of air, the firefighter should hold his or her breath and disconnect the low-pressure hose from the regulator. The other team member should then insert a finger between his or her cheek and lower facepiece strap. The firefighter without air can then insert the low-pressure hose between the cheek and facepiece and can breathe air from the other team member's facepiece. The team member with the adequate air supply may need to slightly open the bypass valve to allow enough air for both of the firefighters.

CAUTION: The metal coupling on the low-pressure hose can become very hot and can cause burns on the firefighter's face.

The facepiece seal of each firefighter is violated when this method is used. Also, using this method violates NIOSH certification of the equipment. Using this type of procedure **violates NFPA, OSHA, and ANSI standards, and is not condoned by most training organizations due to the liability.**

Using The Filter Method

If a firefighter's air supply is depleted and the firefighter does not have a means to share air with another person, the firefighter must practice some life-saving measures. A firefighter should, if possible, immediately exit when the SCBA runs low on air or malfunctions. However, if exiting is not immediately possible, the firefighter must practice individual emergency conditions breathing. One method that can be used by a firefighter using a harness-mounted regulator is the filter method.

To use the filter method, the firefighter disconnects the low-pressure hose from the regulator and places the low-pressure hose end in a pocket, a glove, or inside the turnout coat (Figures 9.8 and 9.9). Doing this procedure helps to filter smoke particles from the breathing air. Because the end of the hose is covered, the filter method also offers the firefighter some degree of protection against inhaling superheated air. Filtering air in this manner *will not*, however, prevent the firefighter from inhaling toxic gases or hazardous substances, nor will it provide any assistance in an oxygen-deficient atmosphere. The firefighter should use the filter method only when it is part of the department's SOPs and when better methods are not possible. Using this type of procedure, however, is not certified by NIOSH, **violates NFPA, OSHA, and ANSI standards, and is not condoned by most training organizations due to the liability.**

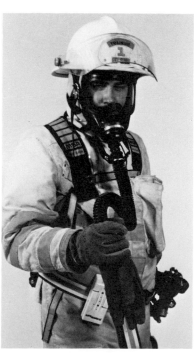

Figure 9.8 When air supply is exhausted or the SCBA is malfunctioning, insert the end of the low-pressure hose into a glove and seal by holding hand tightly around hose to help filter smoke particles from breathing air.

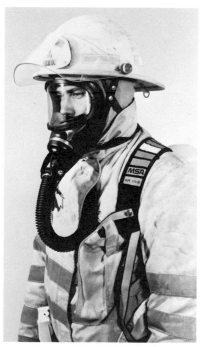

Figure 9.9 Place end of low-pressure hose inside turnout coat to help filter smoke particles and to help prevent inhaling superheated air.

Using A 5-Minute Escape Device

When working in environments containing hazardous materials, firefighters may be connected to an airline. Airlines are also used when firefighters need a greater-than-normal supply of air. The airline, connected to a source of breathing air located away from the hazardous atmosphere or the firefighter's working area, provides the firefighter with a constant flow of breathing air. Emergency procedures for those using airlines should be included in the fire departments' SCBA policies, also.

A 5-minute escape device can be used when the air supply through the airline is interrupted. A typical 5-minute escape device used with airline equipment consists of an auxiliary cylinder filled with a 5-minute supply of air that is connected to the airline unit (Figure 9.10). When needed, the firefighter can open the valve on the auxiliary cylinder. The firefighter can then use this air supply while exiting the area. Normally, these devices are not associated with fire fighting but with other operations involving airlines.

Another type of 5-minute escape device not approved for fire fighting use includes a small air cylinder and a hood or facepiece. This type is more commonly used in industrial situations by individuals not wearing SCBA.

ACCIDENTAL SUBMERSION

NFPA 1404 states that firefighters wearing SCBA must know what to do if they fall into a body of water. SCBA is not SCUBA and is not intended for underwater use. Some firefighters may routinely work near large bodies of water; many others may work near swimming pools, ponds, rivers, lakes, or flooded basements. Therefore, accidental submersion is possible, and the firefighter must know how to react in such situations.

Every fire department should include procedures for accidental submersion in its SCBA program. These procedures should follow the SCBA manufacturer's recommendations. It is a good idea for the department to test the underwater operation of its SCBA to determine how regulator operation is affected and to determine the buoyancy of a firefighter wearing full protective clothing and SCBA. Department policies for water emergencies should take into account these test results. If SCBA is tested, it is recommended that it be serviced by factory-authorized personnel before putting the equipment back in service.

NOTE: The information presented in the following two sections is from the findings of a test conducted by the Louisiana State University Firemen Training Program.

SCBA Operation

Whether or not the SCBA will offer any flotation assistance depends upon the particular type of SCBA being worn; whether or

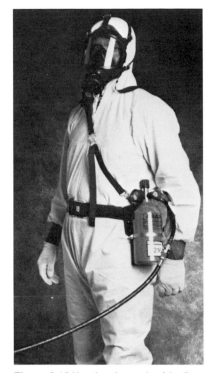

Figure 9.10 Use the air supply of the five-minute-escape device when airline air supply is interrupted. *Courtesy of ISI.*

not the firefighter will be able to use his or her SCBA air supply also depends upon the type of SCBA worn. In a study conducted by Louisiana State University Firemen Training Program, various models of SCBA were tested to determine how each of the models was affected when submerged. Those models tested are listed below:

- MSA™ 401
- MSA Ultralite™ II
- Survivair® Mark I
- Survivair® Mark II
- Scott Air-Pak® II-A
- Scott Air-Pak® 2.2
- Scott Air-Pak® 4.5
- BioPak 45®
- BioPak 60®
- Draeger PA-80-FS-30
- North 816™

The test results revealed that SCBA may experience a complete loss of airflow, a free-flow condition, or no change in operation. Most of the regulators became freeflowing. Only the BioPak 45® experienced complete loss of air, but it worked with the bypass valve. Conversely, only the BioPak 60® experienced no change in airflow. So, only one of the models tested would not provide the firefighter with air. All others continued in some manner to provide air. Those free-flowing regulators continued to provide air to the firefighter until the cylinder was empty.

Whether the firefighter sank (became negatively buoyant) or floated (became positively buoyant) depended upon the buoyancy the firefighter maintained in his or her protective clothing, along with the buoyancy of the SCBA cylinder worn. Air trapped in the firefighter's protective clothing provided some degree of buoyancy. Steel cylinders were negatively buoyant; aluminum cylinders were slightly negatively buoyant. Composite cylinders, conversely, were positively buoyant. Therefore, a firefighter having positive buoyancy (due to air trapped in clothing) and equipped with a steel cylinder will have slightly positive buoyancy and should be able to float. A firefighter equipped with an aluminum cylinder will most likely have positive buoyancy. A firefighter with a composite cylinder will have positive buoyancy; however, the more buoyant composite cylinder will tend to move upward, positioning the firefighter facedown in the water.

Another factor that helps determine a firefighter's buoyancy is the movement of the firefighter while in the water. When submerged, the firefighter must remain calm and control body movement. Exaggerated movements used as an attempt to get out of the water can cause the firefighter to lose buoyancy and sink.

Firefighter Guidelines

There are several guidelines that the firefighter wearing SCBA should observe when immersed in water. Most importantly, the firefighter should remain calm both mentally and physically. By staying calm, the firefighter will more likely be able to maintain buoyancy and exit the water. More guidelines for accidental submersion are listed below:

- Keep the facepiece in place to avoid breathing in water.

- Remain calm; do not try to quickly swim or walk out of the water. Draw knees up to chest to trap air in boots. Air trapped in clothing provides buoyancy, and excessive movement can cause this air to escape.

- Use explosive breathing technique. To perform explosive breathing, hold your breath until you are ready for another one. Then rapidly exhale and rapidly inhale, and hold your breath again.

- Attempt to float in a horizontal position with face up. Then, keeping arms below the water surface, use a gentle back stroke to move to the water's edge. Remaining in a vertical position may force air from the clothing and cause the firefighter to lose buoyancy.

- If you fall into a river or are overcome in a flash-flooded area, attempt to float in a horizontal position with face up and feet pointed in the direction of the current. By doing so, you will be aware of obstacles and will be less likely to catch your feet in downstream obstructions. Do not attempt to stand up. Remain in this position until you reach a point in the river where the current is not so swift such as at an inside bend in the river or at an area where the river is wider. Then, gently swim to the inside river bend or river edge, locate shallow water, and walk out.

- Use proper techniques to control airflow if your regulator free-flows upon submersion. The results of tests performed by the LSU Firemen Training Program showed that freeflow could be controlled by using the following methods:
  - With MSA™ 401, Ultralite™ II, Scott Air-Pak® II-A, and Survivair® Mark I models, close the mainline valve and open the bypass valve periodically to take a breath.
  - With Scott Air-Pak® 2.2 and 4.5 models, hold the facepiece tightly against the face to control freeflow.
  - With Draeger PA-80-FS-30 and Survivair® Mark II models, close the cylinder valve, and then open the cylinder valve periodically to take a breath.

— With North 816™ model, place a hand over the exhalation valve on the facepiece, removing the hand only when exhaling.

SUMMARY

There may be times when the firefighter experiences situations in which SCBA components do not function properly or in which the firefighter no longer has an adequate supply of air. In such situations, the firefighter should follow procedures for individual or team emergency conditions breathing as outlined in the department's policy.

If at any time a firefighter resorts to using emergency breathing techniques, the firefighter has overextended the use of the SCBA. Company officers should investigate and document each such occurrence to determine whether it was caused by equipment malfunction or improper SCBA use.

Chapter 9 Review

Answers on page 352

TRUE-FALSE: Mark each statement true or false. If false, explain why.

1. Some emergency breathing techniques void NIOSH certification of SCBA equipment.

   ☐ T ☐ F _____

   _____

2. Because of the dangers involved in emergency conditions breathing, fire departments should not outline emergency breathing methods in department policy.

   ☐ T ☐ F _____

   _____

3. When performing bypass breathing during an emergency situation, a firefighter only opens the bypass valve periodically to take a breath and then closes the valve after each breath.

   ☐ T ☐ F _____

   _____

4. If a firefighter's facepiece becomes slightly damaged, the firefighter should remove the facepiece immediately.

   ☐ T ☐ F _____

   _____

5. Only some models of SCBA regulators become free-flowing when submerged.

   ☐ T ☐ F _____

   _____

6. One method of team emergency conditions breathing involves using a hose to connect the SCBAs of two firefighters and to transfill air from one SCBA cylinder to another.

   ☐ T ☐ F _____

   _____

7. Skip breathing is a breathing technique that should be used whenever the firefighter is using an SCBA.

   ☐ T ☐ F _____

   _____

8. Placing the end of the low-pressure hose in a glove to filter air for breathing may filter out some of the toxic gases but will provide no assistance in an oxygen-deficient atmosphere.

☐ T ☐ F _____

_____

9. A major advantage of using a transfilling system for team emergency conditions breathing is that the facepiece seal of neither firefighter is violated.

☐ T ☐ F _____

_____

10. Firefighters wearing SCBA should work in teams of two or more.

☐ T ☐ F _____

_____

MULTIPLE CHOICE: Circle the correct answer.

11. When a fire department is planning which emergency breathing methods to include in the department's policy, it should _____.

A. realize that using some methods may void the equipment's NIOSH certification

B. consider the type of SCBA used

C. consider recommendations of the SCBA manufacturer

D. all of the above should be considered

12. It is very important for the firefighter to remain calm during emergencies. Staying calm allows the firefighter to do all of the following **except** _____.

A. work more efficiently

B. use air supply more efficiently

C. prevent the SCBA from malfunctioning

D. communicate more clearly

13. After individual and team emergency conditions breathing procedures have failed or after the available air supply has been exhausted, a firefighter can attempt to filter air for breathing by disconnecting the low-pressure hose from the regulator, _____.

A. placing the hose end in pocket, and holding pocket as tightly as possible around the low-pressure hose

B. placing the hose end in glove, and holding glove as tightly as possible around the low-pressure hose

C. placing the hose end inside the turnout coat, and underneath the arm

D. all of the above can be done

14. Firefighters A and B are discussing the use of the bypass valve for emergency breathing. Firefighter A says that the mainline valve should remain closed when using the bypass valve. Firefighter B says that the bypass valve should be opened periodically for the firefighter to take a breath. Who is correct?

A. Firefighter A

B. Firefighter B

C. Both A and B

D. Neither A nor B

15. Firefighter A says that if a firefighter wearing SCBA accidentally falls into the water, the firefighter should immediately swim to the edge of the water and get out. Firefighter B disagrees and says that the firefighter should attempt to float in a horizontal position and use a gentle back stroke to reach the edge of the water. Who is correct?

A. Firefighter A

B. Firefighter B

C. Both A and B

D. Neither A nor B

SHORT ANSWER: Answer each item briefly.

16. What method of individual emergency conditions breathing can a firefighter use if his or her regulator malfunctions?

_____

17. If a victim or fellow firefighter is pinned and cannot be freed by the firefighter, should the firefighter practice team emergency conditions breathing procedures or leave to get assistance? Why?

_____

_____

_____

_____

18. What are some of the disadvantages of using the low-pressure hose-to-facepiece method?

_____

_____

19. One method of team emergency conditions breathing is using a common regulator. Explain how the team members share a nonfacepiece-mounted regulator.

_____

_____

_____

20. Define skip breathing.

_____

_____

_____

_____

_____

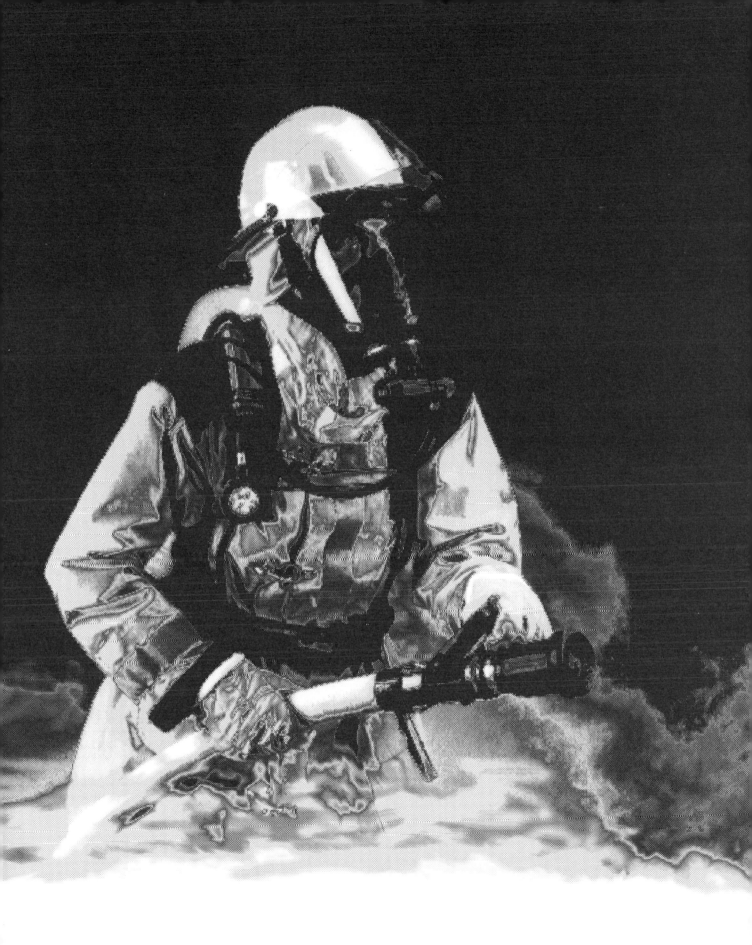

Appendices

Appendix A
SCBA — PAST, PRESENT, AND FUTURE

Recognition of the need for respiratory protection is not new. The Romans realized the need for respiratory protection as early as 50 A.D. when Pliny, a Roman writer, made reference to the use of animal bladders to protect Roman miners against inhalation of red oxides of lead. Later, the need for respiratory protection against hazardous atmospheres was recognized by Leonardo da Vinci (1452-1519) in his analysis of human anatomy, and by Bernardino Ramazzini (1633-1714), who recognized the need for respiratory protection in such occupations as mining, stone cutting, and milling.

Concerns about hazardous atmospheres helped bring about the development of respiratory protection in Europe. The first known SCBA was developed by Alexander V. Humboldt in Germany in 1795 (Figure A.1). An air bag of oiled taffeta was inflated with bellows. About 1830, the Vienna Fire Brigade used a container made of sheet iron that carried atmospheric air; the purpose of the air bag in front of the face is unknown (Figure A.2). This device also had an exhaust valve for expired air.

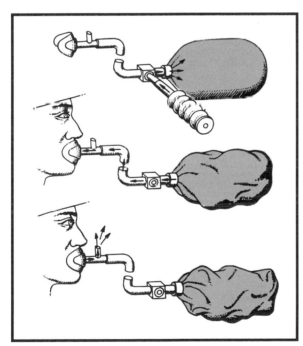

Figure A.1 Alexander V. Humboldt developed the first known SCBA in 1795. *Courtesy of The International Fire Chief.*

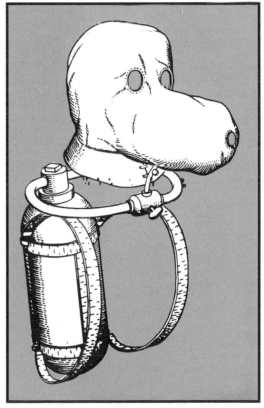

Figure A.2 The SCBA used by the Vienna Fire Brigade in 1830. *Courtesy of The International Fire Chief.*

Galibert's SCBA, developed in 1864, had no exhalation valve and used the principle of rebreathing the air. The user alternated his tongue from one tube to another, blocking off the exhalation duct leading to the bottom of the bag where the "heavier carbon collected" (Figure A.3 on next page).

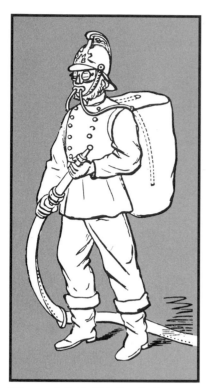

Figure A.3 Galibert's device was developed in 1864. *Courtesy of The International Fire Chief.*

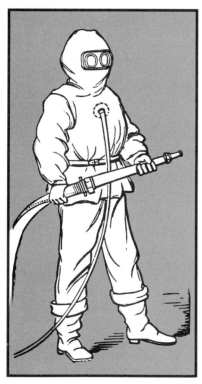

Figure A.5 The Chief of the Paris Fire Department, Paulin, developed this smoke jacket in 1830. *Courtesy of The International Fire Chief.*

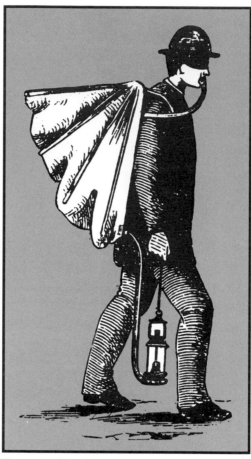

Figure A.4 Fayol, an Englishman, developed what may have been the first pressure-demand apparatus. *Courtesy of The International Fire Chief.*

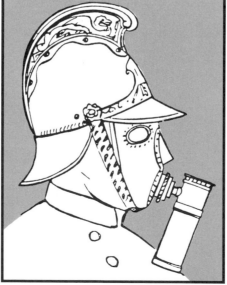

Figure A.6 British inventors Shaw and Tyndall developed this smoke cap with canister in 1890. *Courtesy of The International Fire Chief.*

An apparatus from England may have been the first pressure-demand device. Fayol developed an apparatus that had a lead-lidded, bellows-type air bag filled with clean air. The weight of the lid forced air to the user's mouthpiece for breathing and also supplied air to the lamp to keep it burning in an oxygen-deficient atmosphere (Figure A.4).

An example of another type of breathing apparatus was Paulin's smoke jacket, developed by the Chief of the Paris Fire Department in 1830. A fire engine pump supplied air to the cowhide blouse. The air was discharged at the wrists and waist. An attachment to provide air to a lamp was also provided (Figure A.5).

The canister is another type of breathing apparatus. A facepiece designed by Captain E. M. Shaw with a canister designed by Professor John Tyndall in 1890 is shown in Figure A.6. The inventors were British, and the device was used by the London Fire Brigade for several years. The canister had inhalation and exhalation valves and various layers of materials to remove several types of gases and vapors, as well as particles. The canister was the forerunner of the Type N, Universal gas mask canister used by many fire departments until the 1970s.

The United States had very few, if any, dependable

manufacturers of protective breathing devices before World War I. As late as 1910, many cities required firefighters to have beards at least 6 inches (150 mm) long. Firefighters would dip the beard into a bucket of water, fold it into the mouth, and use it as a smoke filter for breathing.

The earliest known American-made SCBA was the 1877 LaCour's device (Figure A.7). This apparatus was similar to Galibert's device. This device used a leather air bag containing two tubes leading from the bag to the mouth. One tube went into the top of the bag for inhaling oxygen and the other tube went into the bottom of the bag for exhaling carbon dioxide. Smoke hoods containing compressed air or oxygen were also manufactured.

Supplied air equipment was developed for the fire service and saw limited use for some time. For instance, in 1892, Merriman's Smoke Mask featured an air hose located inside a water hose (Figure A.8). Moistened-sponge devices for cooling and filtering inhaled air were also commonly used. The Nealy Smoke Mask of 1877 had sponges that were kept moist from water contained in the "boat" on the user's chest (Figure A.9).

The oxygen-generating canister was developed through a Navy contract during World War II. The moisture from the wearer's exhaled breath reacted with the chemicals in the canister, which produced oxygen and absorbed the carbon dioxide. The product of exchange was mixed well in the breathing bag, then inhaled by the wearer. A collapsible breathing bag connected to the canister served as a reservoir to store the oxygen as it was generated. Since pure oxygen was involved, firefighters were warned to keep oil, grease, or open flame from entering the canister, otherwise, rapid oxidation or explosion of the canister could result. Oxygen-generating canisters were designed to last for 45 to 60 minutes, but once the chemical process started there was no way to turn it off.

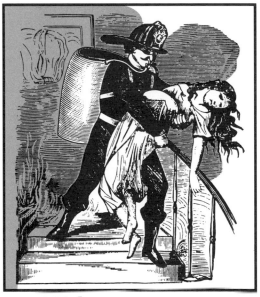

Figure A.7 LaCour developed the earliest known American apparatus in 1877. *Courtesy of The International Fire Chief.*

The first SCBA to be approved in the United States was the Gibbs closed-circuit oxygen breathing apparatus developed by the Mine Safety Appliances Company. The device was approved by the Bureau of Mines (now known as the Mine Safety and Health

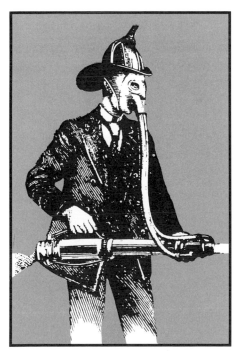

Figure A.8 Merriman, a Denver firefighter, developed his smoke mask in 1892. *Courtesy of The International Fire Chief.*

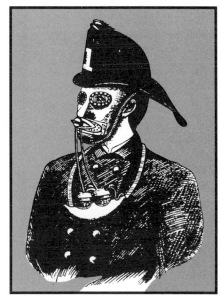

Figure A.9 The Nealy Smoke Mask of 1877 used moistened-sponge devices as part of its design. *Courtesy of The International Fire Chief.*

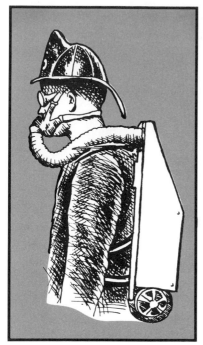

Figure A.10 The first closed-circuit SCBA approved by the Bureau of Mines was the Mine Safety Appliances Company's Gibbs apparatus used in the 1920s. *Courtesy of The International Fire Chief.*

Administration). This device, the forerunner of today's equipment, was the first to use a completely lung-governed principle of operation. The Gibbs apparatus was widely used in the early 1920s (Figure A.10).

Self-contained breathing apparatus have undergone many improvements that have reduced problems such as weight, bulkiness, facepiece leakage, and short duration of air. Although today's SCBA represents a great improvement over earlier respiratory protection devices, there is still room for more improvement. The ideal SCBA of the future would be lighter in weight, provide longer air duration, provide better communications systems, and be easier to don and doff.

Changes occur rapidly in SCBA technology. It was not too long ago that firefighters changed from the widespread use of Type N, Universal gas masks to the lighter weight, positive-pressure SCBA. Because changes inevitably make the SCBA safer and easier to use, the fire service must take an active interest in making certain that their equipment is state of the art — capable of ensuring user safety and performing effectively under the rigorous conditions in which firefighters are required to work.

Appendix B
REGULATING AGENCIES, ORGANIZATIONS, AND OTHER
SOURCES OF INFORMATION

INTRODUCTION

Several government and private agencies recognize the need for regulations and standards regarding respiratory protection in a world of constant technological growth. Because of this growth and the need to maintain the health and safety of all citizens, information and help are available to all industries that require respiratory protection — both now and in the future. The organizations and agencies discussed in the following section were instrumental in providing material necessary to cover the variety of SCBA referred to in this manual and will be continuing sources of information in the future. Other sources of information pertinent to SCBA users cover monitoring systems and emergency command training.

REGULATING AGENCIES AND ORGANIZATIONS
American National Standards Institute (ANSI)

The American National Standards Institute (ANSI) identifies public requirements for national standards and coordinates voluntary standardization activities of concerned organizations. Their activities lead to the publishing of standards and documents that often are adopted by the authority having jurisdiction to provide standardized enforcement.

For more information call (212) 642-4948 or write to ANSI, 1430 Broadway, New York, NY 10018.

Compressed Gas Association (CGA)

The Compressed Gas Association (CGA) represents all facets of industry in the development and promotion of safety standards and safe practices as related to compressed gases.

For more information call (703) 979-4341 or write to CGA, 1235 Jefferson Davis Highway, Arlington, VA 22202.

Canadian Standards Association (CSA)

The Canadian Standards Association (CSA) conducts consensus standards development through the assistance of over 7,000 volunteers with a wide range of backgrounds. Through their efforts, they are able to test, certify, and provide follow-up services for products and product/service designs.

For more information call (416) 747-4000 or write to CSA, 178 Rexdale Boulevard, Rexdale, Ontario M9W 1R3.

Department of Transportation (DOT)

The Department of Transportation (DOT) is responsible for the regulations and enforcement of hazardous materials during transportation.

For more information call (202) 366-4000 or write to DOT, 400 7th Street, S.W., Washington D.C. 20590.

Louisiana State University (LSU)

Louisiana State University (LSU) conducted tests on several different types of self-contained breathing apparatus to determine their behavioral characteristics during a sudden, unexpected water immersion.

For more information call (800) 256-3473 or write to LSU, Fireman Training Program, 6868 Nicholson Drive, Baton Rouge, LA 70820.

Mine Safety and Health Administration (MSHA)

The Mine Safety and Health Administration (MSHA) was created in 1978 when the 1977 Act transferred the Federal mine safety program from the Department of the Interior to the Department of Labor.

MSHA works cooperatively with industry, labor, and other federal and state agencies and others to improve safety and health conditions for all miners.

For more information call (703) 235-1452 or write to MSHA, 4015 Wilson Boulevard, Arlington, VA 22203-1984.

National Fire Protection Association (NFPA)

The National Fire Protection Association (NFPA) is an organization concerned with fire safety standards development, technical advisory services, education, research, and other related services. Its members come from all sectors of the fire protection field, both private and public. There are numerous committees that provide information and develop new standards. The NFPA was organized in 1896.

For more information call (617) 770-3000 or write to NFPA, Batterymarch Park, Quincy, MA 02269.

National Institute for Occupational Safety and Health (NIOSH)

The National Institute for Occupational Safety and Health (NIOSH) is a division of the Department of Health and Human Services. NIOSH is the principal agency responsible for approving self-contained breathing apparatus for use. NIOSH has five major responsibilities:

- Investigate potential hazards in the work place.
- Research effects of hazardous chemicals.
- Perform tests and certify personal protective equipment.
- Devise methods to sample hazardous chemicals.
- Provide educational training for personnel involved in occupational health and safety.

Manufacturers must submit SCBA for testing by NIOSH. If the apparatus passes all tests, it is certified for use. All approved SCBA bear a NIOSH/MSHA label.

For more information call (800) 35-NIOSH or write to NIOSH, 4676 Columbia Avenue, Cincinnati, OH 45226.

Occupational Safety and Health Administration (OSHA)

The Occupational Safety and Health Administration (OSHA) is a division of the Department of Labor. While OSHA and NIOSH are located in different cabinet departments, they coordinate their functions. OSHA has the congressional authority to enforce safety and health standards through citations and fines. OSHA was established by the Occupational Safety and Health Act of 1970.

For more information call (202) 523-8017 or write to OSHA, 200 Constitution Avenue, Washington D.C. 20210.

Underwriters Laboratory (UL)

The goal of Underwriters Laboratory (UL) is to promote public safety through scientific investigation of various materials in regard to the hazard they present by their use. The organization, after testing, then lists and marks the material as having passed its rigorous tests. The nonprofit organization was founded in 1894.

For more information call (312) 272-8800 or write to UL, 333 Pfingsten Road, Northbrook, IL 60062.

OTHER SOURCES OF INFORMATION

The following sections give sources of detailed information about monitoring systems and incident command systems used by various fire departments or countries at the fireground or emergency incident.

Air Quality Monitoring

TRI, Environmental, Inc. is a private company that provides compressed-air sampling kits. These kits can be customized to fit the specific needs of an organization. TRI analyzes returned air samples and then provides a detailed written report to the organization submitting the air samples. The report can then be reviewed and included in the organization's breathing-air records.

For more information call (512) 263-2101 or (800) 880-TEST, or write to TRI, Environmental, Inc., 9063 Bee Caves Road, Austin, TX 78733-6201.

Fireground Command System (FGC)

Chief Alan V. Brunacini's book, *Fire Command* is considered the definitive text on FGC and can be obtained from NFPA, Batterymarch Park, Quincy, MA 02269 (617) 770-3000. Chief Brunacini can be contacted through the Phoenix Fire Department, 520 West VanBuren, Phoenix, AZ 85003.

Incident Command System (ICS)

Fire Protection Publications' book, *Incident Command System (ICS)* contains both the operational system description and the field operations guide for the ICS. Write to Fire Protection Publications, Oklahoma State University, Stillwater, OK 74078-0118.

Entry Control and Guide Line Systems

For information on entry control and guide line systems, write to the following:

- South Australian Country Fire Services
  20 Richmond Road
  P.O. Box 758
  Cowandila, South Australia 5033

- Director of Training
  New Zealand Fire Service College
  P.O. Box 7237
  Wellington 2, New Zealand

- H.M. Inspector of Fire Services
  Home Office Fire Department
  50 Queen Anne's Gate
  London, England SW1H9AT

Appendix C

TULSA FIRE DEPARTMENT
SELF-CONTAINED BREATHING APPARATUS PROGRAM

(Final Revision 11/1/89)

SELF-CONTAINED BREATHING APPARATUS PROGRAM
INDEX

Prefix	Section I
Program Administration	Section II
SCBA Selection	Section III
Use of SCBA	Section IV
Maintenance of SCBA	Section V
Facepiece Fitting	Section VI
Training and Education	Section VII
Special Programs	Section VIII
Program Evaluation	Section IX

SECTION I
PREFIX

1. It is the policy of the Tulsa Fire Department that all personnel who respond and function in areas of hazardous atmospheric contamination will be equipped with self-contained breathing apparatus (SCBA) and trained in its use, care, inspection, and maintenance.

2. The intent of this SCBA program is to avoid any respiratory contact with products of combustion, superheated gases, toxic products, or other hazardous contaminants. SCBA use, care, inspection, and maintenance is in accordance with OSHA 1910.134, "Respiratory Protection"; ANSI Z88.5-1981, "Practices for Respiratory Protection, Respirator Use, Physical Qualifications for Personnel"; NFPA 1500, *Standard for Fire Department Occupational Safety and Health Program;* and NFPA 1404, *Standard for a Fire Department Self-Contained Breathing Apparatus Program.*

SECTION II
PROGRAM ADMINISTRATION

1. The Safety and Health Section is responsible for this SCBA program.

2. Human Resource Development, Physical Resource Management, and Emergency Services are responsible for the implementation of this SCBA program.

3. All members of the Tulsa Fire Department within these Sections and Divisions have a responsibility, whether training, maintenance, inspection, care, or use, in the effectiveness of this program and the health of Tulsa Fire Department members.

SECTION III
SCBA SELECTION

1. Only positive-pressure SCBA approved by the National Institute for Occupational Safety and Health (NIOSH) and Mine Safety and Health Administration (MSHA) will be used by department members.

2. Approved SCBA are as follows:

   .01 SURVIVAIR® "XL-30"

   .02 SCOTT® "PRESSURE-PAK IIA®" (Reserve Apparatus)

   .03 MSA "401™" (Hazardous Materials Response Team)

3. The Survivair® XL-30 must have the regulator switch in the "USE" position to be positive pressure and the Scott® Pressure-Pak IIA® must be in the "ON" position to be positive pressure. The MSA 401™ is constantly in a positive-pressure mode.

SECTION IV
USE OF SCBA

1. All department members using SCBA will be medically certified by the city physician annually.

2. Don the SCBA using one of the following methods:

   .01 OVER THE HEAD METHOD

Step 1	Stand facing the cylinder opposite the valve.
Step 2	Remove facepiece from case or compartment and lay it down with the lens up.
Step 3	Grasp backplate with both hands and lift upward above head.
Step 4	Permit elbows to find respective shoulder strap loops.
Step 5	Lower the cylinder over your head, and allow it to rest on the back.
Step 6	Fasten chest snap (only on Scott® and MSA™).
Step 7	Lean forward at the waist and adjust cylinder on back while adjusting shoulder straps.
Step 8	Snap and adjust waist strap.
Step 9	Check to make sure the regulator is in the "DON" (demand) mode. The mainline valve should be open all the way and locked. The bypass valve should be closed.
Step 10	Fully open cylinder valve.
Step 11	Loosen the helmet strap and slide helmet off the head to the back or side, leaving the chin strap around the neck. Slide hood down around the neck.
Step 12	Don facepiece by gripping between the thumb and fingers, insert the chin well into the lower part of the facepiece and pull the head straps back over the head.
Step 13	Adjust the chin straps, the temple straps, and then the straps for the forehead. (Straps should be pulled straight back, not outward.)
Step 14	Check the seal on the facepiece before entering a contaminated atmosphere. Do this by covering the end of the breathing tube with one hand while inhaling. If there are no leaks, the facepiece will collapse against the face. Continue holding hand over end of breathing tube and exhale to check the exhalation valve.

Step 15 Connect the breathing tube to the regulator and tighten the coupling firmly with the fingers.

Step 16 Pull hood over head and in place. Place helmet on top of head and tighten chin strap.

Step 17 Put regulator in "USE" mode (positive pressure).

.02 OVER THE SHOULDER METHOD

Step 1 Remove facepiece and lay it down with lens shield up.

Step 2 With the right hand, grasp the shoulder strap that supports the regulator.

Step 3 Slip left arm through shoulder strap supported by right hand.

Step 4 Slip right arm through right shoulder strap.

Step 5 Fasten chest strap (if so equipped).

Step 6 Lean over at the waist and adjust the cylinder up on the back while adjusting the shoulder straps.

Step 7 Snap and adjust waist strap.

Step 8 Check to make sure the regulator is in the "DON" (demand) mode. The mainline valve should be opened all the way and locked. The bypass valve should be closed.

Step 9 Fully open the cylinder valve.

Step 10 Loosen the helmet strap and slide the helmet off the head to the back or side, leaving the chin strap around the neck. Slide the hood around the neck.

Step 11 Don facepiece by gripping between the thumb and fingers, insert the chin well into the lower part of the facepiece, and pull the head straps back over the head.

Step 12 Adjust the chin straps, the temple straps, and then the straps for the forehead. (Straps should be pulled straight back, not outward.)

Step 13 Check the seal on the facepiece before entering a contaminated atmosphere. Do this by covering the end of the breathing tube with one hand while inhaling. If there are no leaks, the facepiece will collapse against the face. Continue holding hand over end of breathing tube and exhale to check the exhalation valve.

Step 14 Connect the breathing tube to the regulator and tighten the coupling firmly with the fingers.

Step 15 Pull hood over head and in place. Place helmet on top of head and tighten chin strap.

Step 16 Put regulator in "USE" mode (positive pressure).

.03 SEAT METHOD

Step 1 Sit or stand with back to cylinder.

Step 2 Locate shoulder straps and place in position on shoulders.

Step 3 Fasten chest snap (if so equipped).

Step 4 Adjust shoulder straps.

Step 5 Snap and adjust waist strap.

Step 6   Move forward to remove cylinder from Ziamatic™.

Step 7   Check to make sure that the regulator is in the "DON" (demand) mode. The mainline valve should be opened all the way and locked. The bypass valve should be closed.

Step 8   Fully open the cylinder valve.

Step 9   Loosen the helmet strap and slide the helmet off the head to the back or side, leaving the chin strap around the neck. Slide the hood around the neck.

Step 10   Don facepiece by gripping between the thumb and fingers, insert the chin well into the lower part of the facepiece and pull the head straps back over the head.

Step 11   Adjust the chin straps, the temple straps, and then the straps for the forehead. (Straps should be pulled straight back, not outward.)

Step 12   Check the seal on the facepiece before entering a contaminated atmosphere. Do this by covering the end of the breathing tube with one hand while inhaling. If there are no leaks, the facepiece will collapse against the face. Continue holding hand over end of breathing tube and exhale to check the exhalation valve.

Step 13   Connect the breathing tube to the regulator and tighten the coupling firmly with the fingers.

Step 14   Pull hood over head and in place. Place helmet on top of head and tighten chin strap.

Step 15   Put regulator in "USE" mode (positive pressure).

.04 If cylinder is stored in a compartment, the only difference in donning is that the person dons the shoulder straps and steps away from the apparatus and then snaps the other straps.

.05 On the Survivair® regulator, the mainline valve is silver and the bypass red. On the Scott®, the mainline is yellow and the bypass is red. On the MSA™, the mainline valve is gold and the bypass valve is red.

.06 The seal of the facepiece is to the skin of the face, not the flashover hood. The facepiece is to be donned first, and then the flashover hood pulled up over the head.

.07 It is recommended that the helmet remain on the member during the entire donning procedures. If the member has the Philadelphia chin strap, however, it may be necessary to remove the helmet while donning the mask and then thread the chin strap under the chin after the facepiece is donned. In all cases, the chin strap should be under the chin and not under the facepiece when ready for operations.

3. When using SCBA, personnel will have facepieces in place, breathing air from the supply provided, with the regulator switch in the positive-pressure position. At least two firefighters, both using SCBA will work together and will maintain visual, audible, or physical communications at all times.

4. Self-contained breathing apparatus will be *used* by all personnel in the following circumstances:

.01 In a contaminated atmosphere

.02 In an atmosphere that may suddenly become contaminated

.03 In an atmosphere that is oxygen deficient

.04 In an atmosphere that is suspected of becoming contaminated or oxygen deficient

5. The circumstances include:

 .01 In the active fire area

 .02 Directly above the active fire area

 .03 In a potential explosive or fire area, including gas leaks and fuel spills

 .04 Where products of combustion are visible in an atmosphere, including vehicle fires and dumpster fires

 .05 Where invisible contaminants are suspected of being present (i.e., carbon monoxide during overhaul)

 .06 Where toxic products are present, suspected to be present, or may be released without warning

 .07 In an active chemical spill area where the chemical presents an inhalation hazard

 .08 In any confined space that has not been tested to establish respiratory safety

6. The incident commander will respond the bottle van to any incident where the need for spare cylinders is necessary.

7. Premature removal of SCBA must be avoided at all times. This is particularly significant during overhaul when smoldering materials may produce increased quantities of carbon monoxide and other toxic products. *In these cases SCBA must be used or the atmosphere must be removed.*

8. The decision to remove SCBA will be made by company officers with approval of the Incident Commander, *based on an evaluation of conditions.* Prior to removal, fire areas will be thoroughly ventilated, and where necessary continuous ventilation will be provided.

9. If there is any doubt about respiratory safety, SCBA use will be maintained until the atmosphere is established to be safe by testing. Safety and Health Section personnel will be responsible for this determination. This is required in complex situations, particularly when toxic materials may be involved.

SECTION V
MAINTENANCE OF SCBA

1. All SCBA presently on an Apparatus are permanently assigned to that vehicle. Each SCBA harness must be stenciled with the Apparatus assignment and which unit it is (#1, #2, etc.). The suggested method is to mark the harness as follows: E-8-1, E-8-2, L-11-1, L-11-2, 6-11-1, 6-11-2, etc. Facepieces will also be marked by the SCBA technician. Facepieces will not be exchanged from one unit to another. Number 1 will stay with #1, etc.

2. Company Officers are accountable for each SCBA on their apparatus. After each use, inspection, or maintenance, Company Officers will ensure that all SCBA are in their proper location. Each member will check the condition of the SCBA at the beginning of each shift, after each use, and after any repairs or maintenance.

3. If an SCBA is found to be malfunctioning or is damaged, it will be taken out of service, red tagged "OUT OF SERVICE - DO NOT USE," and replaced immediately. The "out of service" SCBA will be reported immediately and sent in as a complete assembly with facepiece (keep the cylinder). This will be sent to Physical Resource Management, or the District Chief when Supply is closed, in order that a "loaner" unit can be obtained. A tracking form will be sent along with the loaner unit and requires completion by the Company Officer.

4. SCBA will be inspected as follows:

.01 Check cylinder gauge (1,800 to 2,200 is acceptable).

.02 Turn cylinder valve fully on.

.03 Check cylinder and cylinder valve for leaks.

.04 Check high-pressure hose and couplings for wear and leaks (use soapy water if necessary).

.05 Check harness for wear.

.06 Check the regulator by donning the SCBA.

.07 Check facepiece and low-pressure hose for cracks and leaks. (Gently stretch the low-pressure hose and check.)

.08 Put facepiece on; check seal.

.09 Connect low-pressure hose to the regulator and open mainline valve *all the way*. On Survivair® and Scott®, place regulator switch in positive-pressure position.

.10 Close mainline valve on regulator; crack open bypass valve on regulator; check operations; close bypass valve.

.11 Take SCBA off; turn cylinder valve off.

.12 On Survivair® and Scott®, breathe pressure off regulator. On MSA™, the mainline valve will have to be opened.

.13 Close the bypass and open the mainline valve on the Survivair® and Scott®; leave the regulator switch in the negative-pressure position. On the MSA™, close both the bypass and the mainline valves when not in use.

.14 Note low-air alarm as air is breathed off the high-pressure line.

.15 Clean and disinfect facepiece.

.16 Place facepiece in cover.

.17 Place SCBA in ready condition on proper place on apparatus.

5. Each SCBA will be cleaned and sanitized as follows:

.01 Remove cylinder, regulator, and high-pressure hose from harness. Scrub cylinder with a solution of hot, soapy water and rinse with tap water.

.02 Wipe off the outside of the regulator and high-pressure hose with a clean moist cloth or rag, and then dry with a towel; no water is to enter the regulator.

.03 The harness assembly and straps can be scrubbed with a solution of hot, soapy water and rinsed with tap water.

.04 Remove the low-pressure hose from the facepiece. Immerse the hose in a solution of hot, soapy water, and rinse with tap water. Then immerse the low-pressure hose in a disinfecting solution and rinse with tap water. After rinsing, the hose will be stretched and shaken to remove moisture inside and hung up to air dry.

.05 Immerse the facepiece in a solution of hot, soapy water. Use a sponge or cloth to thoroughly clean the inside and outside of the facepiece. Rinse with tap water, making sure to run water through the exhalation valve until all soap residue is removed. Place the facepiece in the disinfecting solution for at least one minute and then rinse thoroughly. Shake out water and hang up to dry.

.06 Disinfectant solution: Quaternary Ammonium Solution obtained through Physical Resources Management Section.

6. After each inspection and use, SCBA and spare cylinders (one per SCBA) will be properly secured in cases or mounting brackets to prevent damage. Survivair® and Scott® SCBA will be stored with the regulator switch in the negative-pressure position.

7. After *all* inspections, cleanings, and repairs of SCBA, the Company Officer will record the condition and function of the SCBA in the Company Log Book. Those items to be recorded for each SCBA include:

.01 SCBA Apparatus Assignment and Unit Number

.02 Cylinder

.03 High-Pressure Hose

.04 Harness Assembly

.05 Backpack

.06 Regulator, Diaphragm, and Valves

.07 Alarm Bell

.08 Facepiece

.09 Low-Pressure Hose

.10 Air Flow

8. Repairs to SCBA will be made only by authorized Tulsa Fire Department personnel and manufacturer's representative.

9. Preventative maintenance on SCBA will be performed by SCBA technician every three months. Maintenance by the SCBA technician will include:

.01 Disassembling the SCBA into major components

.02 Flow testing the regulator

.03 Disassembling and cleaning the regulator

.04 Replacement of worn parts, or those suggested by manufacturer, in regulator assemblies

.05 Disassembling the low-air alarm, cleaning, and replacement of necessary components

.06 Cleaning and replacement of needed components of the facepiece and harness assembly, and replacement of components as needed or scheduled

.07 Reassembling of entire SCBA and testing for proper operation of all components

.08 Proper recording of all maintenance performed on forms provided, and return of SCBA to service

10. Repairs and preventative maintenance records will be kept on each SCBA and cylinder by the department SCBA technician. These records will permit the tracking of each unit from the time it is put in service until it is retired.

11. Breathing air compressors will be operated and maintained to provide breathing air that meets or exceeds the standards of Grade D Air (Compressed Gas Association Commodity Specification G-7.1-1989). Safety and Health Section will run quarterly tests to assure compliance of the breathing air.

12. Breathing air compressors found to be malfunctioning or damaged will be taken out of service, red tagged "OUT OF SERVICE - DO NOT USE," and reported immediately to Physical Resources Management.

13. The following stations are designated as SCBA cylinder satellite stations and are the *ONLY STATIONS TO STORE CYLINDERS*:

STATION 4   (DISTRICT 1)

STATION 27   (DISTRICT 5)

STATION 24   (DISTRICT 4)

STATION 11   (DISTRICT 2)

STATION 18   (DISTRICT 3)

Stations 4 and 27 are also designated "fill stations" and have delivery vans for cylinders. All cylinders are to be stored at the satellite stations only. Damaged cylinders are to be red tagged and sent to Physical Resources for repairs.

SECTION VI
FACEPIECE FITTING

1. All personnel required to use SCBA will demonstrate annually, through facepiece fit testing, that they can achieve a satisfactory facepiece-to-face seal with each type of SCBA facepiece they may be required to wear.

2. Only personnel with a properly fitting facepiece will be permitted to function in a hazardous atmosphere with SCBA.

3. The Safety and Health Section is responsible for facepiece fit testing of all members. The facepiece fit test includes:

.01 Negative-Pressure Test

.02 Positive-Pressure Test

.03 Qualitative Test

4. Excessive facial hair (beard, long sideburns, etc.) and eyeglass temples will prevent a good seal of the SCBA facepiece, and will not be permitted.

5. Records of SCBA facepiece fit testing will be kept on each member. These records indicate:

.01 Name of individual tested

.02 Type of fitting test performed

.03 Specific make and model of facepieces tested

.04 Results of tests

SECTION VII
TRAINING AND EDUCATION

1. All new fire department members expected to use SCBA will be trained in its use, inspection, and cleaning. The Human Resource Development Section will provide at least sixteen (16) hours of training that will include:

.01 Human physiology and respiratory problems

.02 Hazardous environments and special problems that may be encountered

.03 Construction details, safety features, and limitations of each type of SCBA used by the Tulsa Fire Department

.04 Care, inspection, and maintenance of SCBA

.05 Tulsa Fire Department procedures for using SCBA

.06 Practical application

2. An evaluation of all personnel who respond and function in SCBA will be conducted annually by the Human Resources Development Section. Each member will receive at least four (4) hours of retraining on SCBA and will demonstrate a high level of proficiency utilizing the SCBA under simulated conditions. Members will also demonstrate their proficiency on SCBA care, inspection, and SCBA cleaning.

SECTION VIII
SPECIAL PROBLEMS

1. Personnel may encounter a variety of problems associated with the use of SCBA. These problems include, but are not limited to:

.01 Low temperature

.02 High temperature

.03 Rapidly changing temperature

.04 Communications

.05 Confined spaces

.06 Vision

.07 Facepiece-to-face sealing

.08 Absorption through or irradiation of the skin

.09 Effects of ionizing radiation on the skin and whole body

.10 Punctured or ruptured eardrums

.11 Use around water

2. Problems that are encountered when using SCBA must be recognized in order that proper corrective action can be taken to prevent harmful personnel exposure and injury.

SECTION IX
PROGRAM EVALUATION

1. A Quality Assurance Program will be conducted by the Safety and Health Section and Physical Resource Management Section monthly.

2. The Safety and Health Section will annually evaluate the Tulsa Fire Department SCBA program to ensure the health of Tulsa Fire Department members and the continued effectiveness of the program.

Appendix D

EXAMPLE OF A STANDARD OPERATING PROCEDURE (SOP)

	PHOENIX FIRE DEPARTMENT
Safety Procedures	**STANDARD OPERATING PROCEDURES**
CONFINED SPACE OPERATIONS	M.P. 205.09
	4/85-N Page 1 of 3

Incidents that require Fire Department personnel to enter confined spaces to fight fires or to rescue and remove persons in need of assistance present very serious potential dangers. In order to operate safely in these situations, special precautions must be taken and rigidly enforced.

Confined spaces include caverns, tunnels, pipes, tanks, and any other locations where ventilation and access are restricted by the configuration of the space. These factors may also apply to basements. Confined space incidents may involve injured persons, persons asphyxiated or overcome by toxic substances, cave-ins, or fires occurring within the space. Pre-incident planning is an important factor in dealing with these situations.

Operations within confined spaces shall be approached with extreme caution. Direct supervision is required and all safety precautions and procedures shall be rigidly enforced. Operations shall be conducted in a manner that avoids premature commitment to unknown risks.

In order to provide adequate support for confined space incidents, Command shall provide a minimum 2:1 ratio of personnel outside the confined space to support personnel working within. This shall include a stand-by rescue team with a 1:1 ratio to provide emergency assistance to the personnel in the confined space. This team shall be equipped with breathing apparatus and standing by to enter if needed. A Treatment Sector with ALS capability shall also be provided near the entrance/exit point.

In order to provide this capability, Alarm shall dispatch a minimum of a 2-1-Medical assignment on any incident where confined space operations are indicated. The Hazardous Incident Response Team and Safety Officer shall also be dispatched.

Before allowing personnel to enter a confined space, the officer in command must attempt to gather any available information about the nature of the situation or hazard, particularly as it pertains to the atmosphere inside the space. THIS IS CRITICAL WHEN THE SITUATION INVOLVES UNCONSCIOUS VICTIMS OR PERSONS WHO MAY HAVE BEEN OVERCOME BY THE ATMOSPHERE INSIDE THE SPACE. Command must assume that an unsafe atmosphere exists within the confined space until/unless testing establishes it is safe. When test instruments are available, readings of oxygen concentration, explosive gas or vapor concentrations, carbon monoxide, and hydrogen sulfide shall be taken before entering. If these instruments are not immediately available, the Hazardous Incident Response Team shall be requested to respond to evaluate the atmosphere as quickly as possible.

Safety Procedures	**PHOENIX FIRE DEPARTMENT**
	STANDARD OPERATING PROCEDURES
CONFINED SPACE OPERATIONS	M.P. 205.09
	4/85-N Page 2 of 3

ALL PERSONNEL entering confined spaces SHALL use breathing apparatus. Either self-contained or airline supplied breathing apparatus may be used, depending on the nature of the situation. Command must evaluate the need for extended duration breathing apparatus and provide for the response of this equipment when necessary.

Breathing apparatus shall be used without exception in confined spaces until or unless analysis of the atmosphere confirms that it is safe to breathe. Personnel shall not remove facepieces or take any other action to compromise the effectiveness of their breathing apparatus while inside the confined space atmosphere.

Protective clothing shall be worn as required by the situation, depending on an evaluation of the hazards and the products that may be inside the confined space.

When feasible, Command should establish a Ventilation Sector to begin operations directed at providing fresh air and/or exhausting contaminated air from the confined space. Any electrical or mechanical equipment taken inside the confined space, including lighting equipment, shall be explosionproof type, when any flammable hazard is suspected. When ventilating a confined space containing flammable vapors or gases, ventilation must consider the concentration in relation to flammable limits.

The Fire Department Safety Officer will respond to all confined space incidents to consult with Command on the safety measures and precautions to be taken in each case. Command will assign a Safety Sector Officer to assume these responsibilities from the initial stages of the incident until the Safety Officer arrives at the scene. The Safety Sector Officer shall evaluate the risks and enforce all safety requirements associated with the particular situation. If the Safety Sector Officer judges that an operation is unsafe, the operation shall be suspended.

Command shall assure that personnel entering a confined space do not commit themselves to travel within the space beyond a point that provides sufficient air reserve to return and exit safely, with at least a 5-minute safety margin. The time available for operations inside shall be estimated based on air supply and monitored by personnel outside, as well as the entry team. Where feasible, lifelines shall be used by personnel entering the confined space.

A "Lobby Sector" shall be established at the entrance/exit to control access to the confined space. Lobby Sector personnel shall record names, assignments, entry times, and SCBA cylinder pressures of all personnel entering the confined space. The Lobby Sector will

	PHOENIX FIRE DEPARTMENT
Safety Procedures	**STANDARD OPERATING PROCEDURES**
CONFINED SPACE OPERATIONS	M.P. 205.09
	4/85-N Page 3 of 3

maintain a time awareness of the expected exit time for each individual based on air supply at the time of entry and provide a warning at the predetermined time to begin exit procedures. Warning will be provided by radio or other communications system.

When working in confined spaces with very restricted access, personnel shall wear rescue harnesses or wrist straps to provide for extrication by rope.

A primary function of the Lobby Sector is to control the number of personnel and prevent crowding at the entrance to the confined space.

Appendix E
MANUFACTURERS OF SCBA

INTRODUCTION

This appendix provides an overview of the major manufacturers of self-contained breathing apparatus. Departments must decide for themselves what brand best suits their needs. Self-contained breathing apparatus is an important part of a firefighter's equipment, and its purchase must be taken seriously. The operating procedures for self-contained breathing apparatus may vary slightly, depending upon the brand. *Always* follow the manufacturer's operating instructions for care and use of SCBA.

The following information was taken directly from instruction/operating manuals and bulletins furnished by the various manufacturers and is presented for informational purposes only. It is not presented as an endorsement of any particular product nor is it intended to replace a comprehensive training program in care and use of SCBA.

BIOMARINE, INC.

Biomarine, located at 45 Great Valley Parkway in Malvern, PA, 19355, 215-647-7200, has been a leader in closed-circuit technology since 1969.

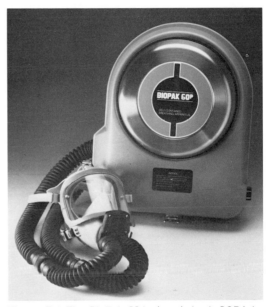

Figure E.1 The BioPak 60® closed-circuit SCBA by Biomarine. *Courtesy of Biomarine, Inc.*

SCBA FEATURES

Biomarine's BioPak 60® is the first NIOSH/MSHA approved closed-circuit SCBA that maintains a positive pressure in the mask (Figure E.1). With a true 1-hour duration, the BioPak 60® is designed for fire fighting and entry into toxic or oxygen-deficient environments. It has proven especially useful in confined-space, long-duration situations like high-rise fire fighting, as well as in refineries, chemical processing, mine rescue, and hazmat use. The gear and facepiece are NIOSH/MSHA approved for any toxic, oxygen-deficient, or immediately dangerous to life or health (IDLH) atmospheres.

The BioPak 60® provides a full hour of protection in a unit weighing 25 pounds. From front to back, the BioPak 60® measures 6⅝ inches, making it convenient for entry through small spaces that can prohibit the use of bulkier equipment. The unit is designed so that its weight is carried on the user's hips instead of the shoulders (Figure E.2).

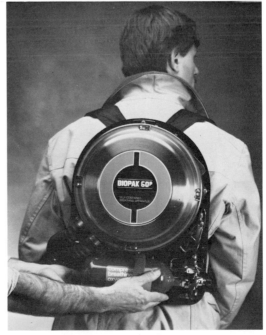

Figure E.2 The BioPak 60® supplies one hour of air with an oxygen bottle one-fifth the size of open-circuit cylinders. *Courtesy of Biomarine, Inc.*

Oxygen bottles for a closed-circuit SCBA are approximately one-fifth the size of open-circuit bottles, permitting easier storage and transport. Turnaround is fast since the absorbent can be changed and a new oxygen bottle inserted in 60 seconds.

The BioPak 240® is a 4-hour, closed-circuit, positive-pressure SCBA (Figure E.3). BioPak 240® is the only 4-hour positive-pressure unit that meets all NIOSH and MSHA approvals. This unit is designed for mine rescue teams, hazardous materials teams, and industrial workers who have to be in potentially dangerous atmospheres for extended periods of time (Figure E.4).

The BioPak 60® and BioPak 240® are American-made closed-circuit SCBA. They recirculate the major portion of the user's exhaled gas. A small oxygen cylinder provides makeup gas to a breathing chamber. The user inhales the gas into a silicone facepiece. The user's exhaled breath passes through a carbon dioxide absorbent and back into the breathing chamber, where fresh oxygen is added. The replenished gas is then available for the next inhalation. In the BioPak 240®, a "blue ice" coolant canister is added to the inhalation side of the breathing circuit to cool the breathing gas on the way to the mask.

A spring-loaded diaphragm in the breathing chamber maintains the positive pressure in the system. If the user's inhalation fully depletes the breathing chamber, the demand/free-flow valve automatically supplies the additional oxygen required. If the user's exhalation causes the diaphragm to fully expand, excess gas is vented out the relief valve.

A loud, high-pitched, pressure-activated whistle alarm sounds when approximately 20 to 25 percent of the service life remains. A manual bypass is provided to override the supply system in an emergency.

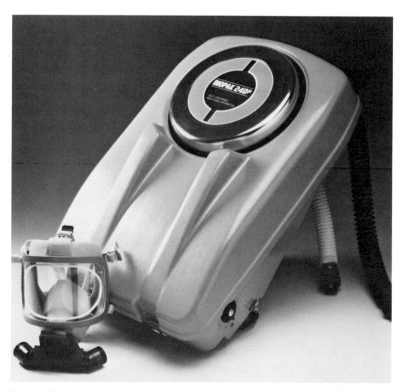

Figure E.3 The BioPak 240® closed-circuit SCBA by Biomarine. *Courtesy of Biomarine, Inc.*

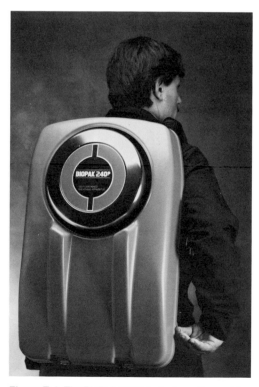

Figure E.4 The BioPak 240® is designed for working in dangerous atmospheres for up to four hours. *Courtesy of Biomarine, Inc.*

ACCESSORIES

BioShield™. The BioShield™ is used for additional head, face, and neck protection against flashovers or other extreme hazards.

Monitors. Biomarine provides triple atmospheric monitors for safe confined space entry. Model 903 simultaneously detects oxygen deficiency, combustible gas and carbon monoxide. Model 904 monitors oxygen deficiency, combustible gas, and hydrogen sulfide. Both instruments may be used for spot checks and continuous monitoring. Both models also feature audiovisual alarms for all three gases, low battery, and flow interruption.

Testing and Training. Most repairs and testing can be done in the field for the BioPak 60® and the BioPak 240®. Optional training videotapes describing tests and procedures necessary to keep the BioPak 60® and BioPak 240® in perfect operating condition are available. If a disaster occurs, Biomarine maintains an emergency supply of units, parts, and accessories to adequately supply the rescue effort.

Others. Other accessories available include wall mounting brackets and protective covers, spectacle kit, antifogging agent, cool sleeve kit, leak-test fixture and Leak-Tec compound, Therma-Clear lens insert, and microphone assemblies.

DONNING AND DOFFING PROCEDURES
Donning The BioPak 60®

Before placing a BioPak into service, be certain that turnaround maintenance has been performed and that an inspection tag is attached to the bottle valve.

Step 1: Place the BioPak face down and lengthen the lower shoulder straps so that the free ends extend 2 or 3 inches.

Step 2: Grasp the body of the BioPak with its back toward you and the top down. Hold the body approximately 6 inches from its bottom. Raise the unit over your head and allow it to slide slowly down your back.

Step 3: Lean forward and tighten the shoulder straps

Step 4: Tighten the chest strap. Take care not to restrict breathing.

Step 5: Fasten the waist strap and tighten.

Step 6: Disengage the facepiece from the harness.

Step 7: Hold the facepiece snugly against the chin, tighten chin straps, temple strap, and top head strap by pulling straight back. Check to be certain that the nosecup fits properly over your nose and mouth.

Step 8: Quickly reach back with your right hand and open the bottle valve. Listen for a short chirp from the alarm whistle.

Step 9: Check the chest-mounted pressure gauge. It should read at least 2,250 psi. Then reach back and tear off the maintenance tag.

When the alarm whistle sounds, the time remaining is 20 to 25 percent of the service life. The user must allow sufficient time to complete work and exit the contaminated area.

The bypass valve is used manually to supply oxygen to the breathing chamber if the demand/free-flow valve should fail. If inhalation resistance increases due to the depletion of breathing oxygen supply in the breathing chamber, add a 2-second burst of the oxygen by pushing the bypass valve button. Add additional bursts of oxygen as required to maintain an adequate oxygen supply in the breathing chamber. It is important for the user to make sure that the bypass valve is functioning properly before operating the unit.

WARNING
The bypass valve button is for emergencies only and WILL NOT clear facepiece fogging.
WASTEFUL use seriously reduces duration of any SCBA.

Doffing The BioPack 60®

WARNING
Most breathing device malfunctions are directly traceable to careless handling after use. Many years of trouble-free operation are possible if reasonable care is given to the BioPak.

When it is time to doff the BioPak, perform the following steps:

Step 1: Reach back with your right hand and close the bottle valve.

Step 2: Loosen the facepiece straps by pushing the release tabs forward. Remove the facepiece and clip the mask "D" ring to the harness.

Step 3: Lean forward slightly and release the chest strap and waist strap. Loosen the right harness strap. Grasp the left shoulder strap and allow the right shoulder strap to fall from the shoulder. Swing the BioPak around to your front and grasp the other shoulder strap. Loosen the left harness strap after the unit has been doffed.

Step 4: Perform turnaround maintenance before reuse. Store in carrying case or other safe location. Do not store in an excessively warm environment.

INTERNATIONAL SAFETY INSTRUMENTS, INC. (ISI)

International Safety Instruments (ISI) creates, designs, manufactures, and markets life support respiratory protection equipment for industrial and commercial customers and applications. Their products are distributed throughout the United States, Canada, Puerto Rico, and several foreign countries. ISI products fall into three major categories: products for entry, work, and rescue in environments that are immediately dangerous to life and health; products for escape from work areas that have suddenly been exposed to dangerous toxic gases or vapors, fumes, smoke, or fire; products for work in areas that endanger a person's health on a long-term basis. ISI is located at 922 Hurricane Shoals Road, Lawrenceville, GA, 30243, 404-962-2552.

SCBA FEATURES

ISI manufactures the Ranger and Magnum SCBAs for use in hazardous atmospheres. The Ranger is a 30-minute duration, positive-pressure SCBA. Ranger's single-stage, pressure-demand regulator reduces cylinder air pressure to a breathable level with only two moving parts. Airflow originates in the cylinder and exits through a manually opened cylinder valve. Two high-pressure stainless steel hoses connect to the cylinder valve. One brings air to the pressure gauge and whistle alarm. The other delivers air to the demand valve mounted on the facemask.

Design of the Magnum was a direct response to NFPA Standard 1981 (Figure E.5). Instead of upgrading existing products, ISI created the Magnum specifically to comply with the new standard. Both 2,216 psi (with three 30-minute cylinders) and 4,500 psi models (with 30-, 45-, and 60-minute cylinders) are available.

ACCESSORIES

Airline Pigtail / Buddy Breathing. By disconnecting a second person's demand valve hose and plugging it into the first person's pigtail, air is supplied to both facemasks while both escape to a safe atmosphere in an emergency. The airline connection is used with a haz mat passthrough. The haz mat passthrough is available for any Class A haz mat suit. It is quick and simple to switch between airline and buddy breathing or to use both options (Figure E.6).

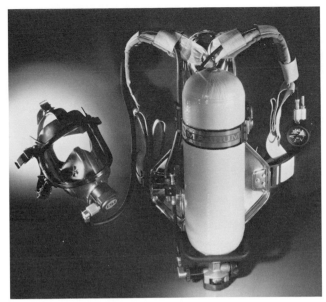

Figure E.5 The Magnum SCBA by International Safety Instruments (ISI) is available in both 2,216 or 4,500 psi models. *Courtesy of ISI.*

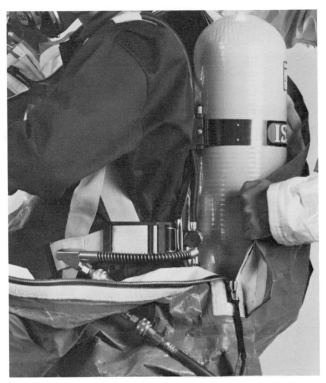

Figure E.6 A haz mat passthrough connection is available for use with the ISI Magnum. The airline pigtail is a versatile attachment that can also be used for buddy breathing. *Courtesy of ISI.*

Voice Communication Systems. The Voice Amplification System (VAS) allows the user to speak normally into a facemask-mounted microphone that broadcasts from a powerful voice amplifier (Figure E.7). The Comm 1 is a two-way radio interface device that supplies clear voice communications through a speaker mounted at the ear and a mask-mounted microphone (Figure E.8).

Others. Flow/Go test kits, bench test kits, conversion kits, and tool kits are available with the Magnum SCBA. A silicone facemask that adapts to a wider range of facial types is also available.

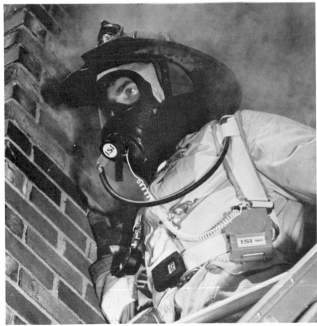

Figure E.7 The Voice Amplification System (VAS) allows the user to speak normally into a facemask-mounted microphone, which then broadcasts from a voice amplifier. *Courtesy of ISI.*

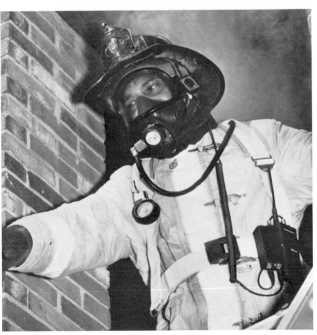

Figure E.8 The Comm 1 is a two-way radio interface that supplies voice communications through a speaker mounted at the ear and a mask-mounted microphone. *Courtesy of ISI.*

DONNING AND DOFFING PROCEDURES
Donning The ISI Magnum

> # WARNING
> All personnel using this apparatus shall be thoroughly trained by qualified instructors in donning, operation, and emergency procedures.

Step 1: Position the Magnum on the ground with the cylinder valve facing away from the wearer.

Step 2: Spread the shoulder straps and fold open the side arms. Ensure that all strap assemblies, side and waist, are fully extended and the waist belt buckle assembly is not connected. Reach inside the harness assembly to grasp the frame with both hands.

Step 3: Swing the unit up and over the head, making sure that elbows extend through the loops formed by the shoulder straps. Allow the unit to slide down the back.

Step 4: Pull directly down on the shoulder strap "D" rings to adjust position of unit on back.

Step 5: Connect the waist belt buckle and adjust waist belt to a comfortable fit. Tuck the excess shoulder strap pull-downs inside the waist belt.

Step 6: Ensure the on/off lever on the bottom of the demand valve is in the OFF position (toward the bypass) and that the bypass is closed.

Step 7: Open the cylinder valve knob slowly by turning it counterclockwise several turns to the fully open position. The whistle alarm should sound momentarily and then shut off. There should be no flow of air from the demand valve.

Step 8: Remove the facemask from the bag and adjust all head straps to a fully slackened position.

Step 9: With one hand on the head harness straps, put your chin into the facemask first and pull the straps over your head. Position the facemask so that your chin fits snugly into the chin cup.

Step 10: Pull straight back on the five strap ends to adjust facemask tightness. Begin with the bottom straps, then tighten the middle straps, and the top head strap last. **Important:** Pull straps straight back to tighten. Do not overtighten the facemask, which may cause discomfort or deform the facemask, thus causing leakage.

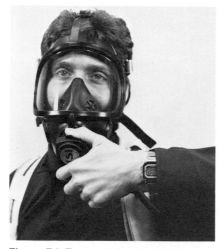

Figure E.9 To attach the demand valve to the facemask, firmly position the demand valve into the facemask fitting with the red bypass at the bottom. *Courtesy of ISI.*

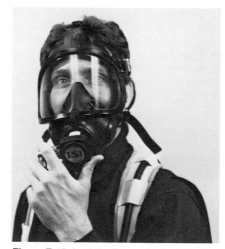

Figure E.10 Lock the demand valve into place by turning it one-quarter. *Courtesy of ISI.*

Step 11: Attach the demand valve to the facemask by firmly positioning the demand valve into the facemask fitting with the red bypass at the bottom (6 o'clock) (Figure E.9).

Step 12: Lock the demand valve into place by turning it one-quarter turn counterclockwise (to the 3 o'clock position). There should be no audible outward flow of air from the facemask (Figure E.10). (**CAUTION:** Ensure that the demand valve is securely locked into the facemask fitting. When securely attached, the demand valve will not rotate in the facemask.)

Safety Checks

> # WARNING
> These safety checks must be performed before entering a hazardous area. Failure to perform these checks may result in respiratory injury or death.

The following procedures assume the SCBA has been completely donned:

Step 1: *Facemask Fit Test and Whistle Check.* Close the cylinder valve. Continue to breathe normally while monitoring the pressure gauge. Listen for the whistle alarm to sound as the gauge drops into the RED zone. Continue breathing until the facemask collapses slightly against your face. Inhale gently and hold your breath. If the seal holds and no leaks can be heard, then fully reopen the cylinder valve.

Step 2: If the facemask pulls away from your face while you are holding your breath, a correct seal has not been achieved. Turn the cylinder valve ON, and readjust the facemask and/or tighten the head harness straps. Repeat the previous procedure until a no-leak condition is achieved. Be sure face or head hair is not interfering with the seal. When a correct seal has been confirmed, turn the cylinder valve fully ON.

Step 3: *Positive-Pressure Check.* Insert two fingers at the side of the facemask between the face and facemask. Gently lift the facemask seal away from the face, and ensure a good outward flow of air, showing that the facemask pressure is positive. Reseal facemask and stop breathing. There should be no sound of air leaking from the demand valve (Figure E.11).

Step 4: *Bypass Check.* The *red* bypass knob is located to the right of the demand valve. Turn the bypass knob counterclockwise (toward the wearer) to the ON position. A constant flow of air should pass into the facemask. Turn the knob to the OFF position.

> # WARNING
> If any of the above checks fail, do not proceed. Remove the apparatus from service, tag, and return it for repair by authorized personnel.

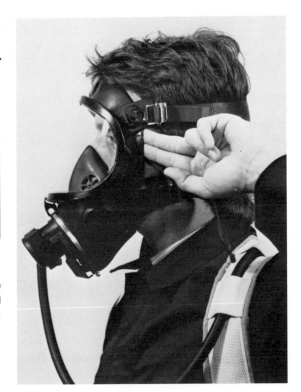

Figure E.11 Check for positive pressure by inserting two fingers at the side of the facemask between the face and facemask and gently lift the facemask seal away from the face. An outward flow of air shows that the pressure is positive. *Courtesy of ISI.*

Step 5: *Recheck Cylinder Pressure.* Check the chest-mounted pressure gauge on the right harness shoulder strap. The gauge should read FULL. Breathe normally and proceed (Figure E.12).

Monitor Cylinder Pressure. Check the pressure gauge during use for remaining air supply and allow sufficient time for egress from irrespirable area.

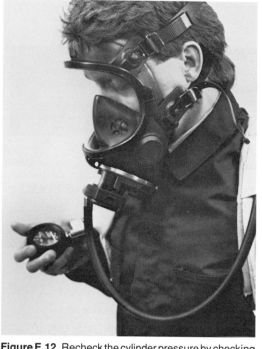

Figure E.12 Recheck the cylinder pressure by checking the chest-mounted pressure gauge on the right shoulder strap—the gauge should read FULL. *Courtesy of ISI.*

> # WARNING
> Immediately egress from contaminated area when whistle alarm starts to sound. It warns the user when approximately 23 to 27 percent of the air supply remains in the cylinder. In high noise areas or where more than one apparatus is being used, the whistle manifold may be lifted to the ear to confirm its operation.

Doffing The ISI Magnum

Important: Do not remove any equipment until you are clear of the irrespirable area.

Step 1: Remove the demand valve from the facemask. Release the safety lock located on the left side of the demand valve by pulling the catch toward the front of the demand valve and simultaneously turning the demand valve one-quarter turn clockwise so that the bypass knob points down (6 o'clock).

Step 2: Remove the demand valve from the facemask connection by pulling it outward. There should be no airflow from the demand valve.

Step 3: Close the cylinder valve by turning it fully clockwise to the OFF position.

Step 4: Release air pressure in the system by turning the bypass ON until the airflow stops, then to the OFF position.

Step 5: Loosen the head harness straps, and remove the facemask.

Step 6: Unfasten the waist belt and loosen the shoulder straps. Extend the adjusting straps and waist belt to the donning position.

Step 7: Remove the apparatus.

Step 8: Remove the cylinder, and tag it for refilling.

Step 9: Do not store or place apparatus in the ready position until after performing the cleaning and testing procedures.

INTERSPIRO USA, INC.

Interspiro manufactures and markets breathing protection for use under toxic conditions, diving systems for professional and military underwater work, and custom-designed equipment for experimental and training projects. Interspiro USA, Inc., is located at 11 Business Park Drive, Branford, CT, 06405, 203-481-3899.

SCBA FEATURES

Interspiro's current line of Spiromatic HPBAs™—High Performance Breathing Apparatus—provides capabilities to put together customized systems to suit specific requirements in fire fighting as well as haz mat applications.

The Spiromatic is a positive-pressure breathing apparatus that consists of a face mask with a breathing valve (Spiromatic Mask), an air supply cylinder, a regulator unit, and a backpack/harness assembly (Figure E.13). The Spiromatic uses clean, dry air compressed in a cylinder. The air is fed to a pressure regulator that reduces the cylinder air pressure to a secondary pressure of approximately 110 psi. The air is then supplied to the breathing valve and facepiece through a low-pressure breathing hose.

The breathing valve is of the pressure-demand type that releases air on inhalation. The Spiromatic operates with positive pressure that keeps toxic gases from leaking into the facepiece. The positive pressure is automatically turned on as soon as the user starts breathing within the mask. In this way there is no risk of forgetting to turn on the positive pressure or for it to be accidentally turned off.

The compressed air supply for the Spiromatic is contained in lightweight, aluminum cylinders fully wrapped in glass fiber. The cylinders are fitted with a valve that includes a built-in pressure gauge. The cylinder valve is also

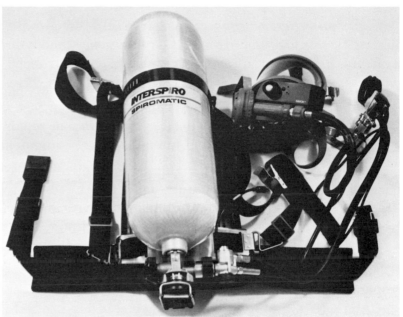

Figure E.13 The Spiromatic HPBA™—High Performance Breathing Apparatus — by Interspiro is available with air cylinders of 30, 45, and 60 minutes' duration.

equipped with a burst disc, designed to rupture and let air out should the cylinder be inadvertently overcharged.

The regulator unit consists of a pressure regulator, a high-pressure hose, and a pressure gauge manifold. The manifold consists of a pressure gauge, a warning whistle, and a quick coupling connection. The pressure regulator used in the Spiromatic is of the piston type with an extremely high flow capacity. In order to keep it small and light, the regulator has been pressure balanced. This balancing ensures a stable secondary pressure, which maintains an effective positive pressure in the mask even at low cylinder pressure.

Rebreathing of exhaled air heavy with carbon dioxide must be eliminated as much as possible by minimizing "dead space." On the Spiromatic, dead space has been minimized by the inner mask and by separate inhalation and exhalation channels that match channels in the breathing valve. The facepiece with an inner mask is made of a natural rubber compound (silicone rubber is optional). It is equipped with a large, easily replaceable lens. The facepiece also has provisions for fitting eyeglasses.

A speech diaphragm is mounted in the connection piece inside the inner mask in order to obtain best possible communication. An external speech cone on the outside improves the communication and locks at the same time as the breathing valve.

ACCESSORIES

Savox Radio Attachment. The Savox radio interface can be operated in automatic VOX (speech-activated) or in PTT (push-to-talk) modes at the flick of a switch. It can also be used with most portable radios.

Spiromatic Escape Device. This device is a lightweight, self-rescue device that requires little training. It features automatic positive pressure and is simple to use and operate. Duration times can be varied depending on tank choice.

Revitox Mask. The Revitox is an auxiliary second mask that can be quick-connected to the Spiromatics to give immediate fresh air to a victim in a toxic environment. A manual control can be used for administering artificial respiration or for beginning CPR.

Spiromatic Rescue Hose. The Spiromatic rescue hose with quick couplings can link two Spiromatic sets together in seconds for emergency "buddy-breathing" (enabling one user to supply air to another without disconnecting should one be trapped and short of air).

Spiromatic Test Kit. In order to comply with exacting safety requirements, the breathing apparatus should be subject to a complete function test at least once a year and after every dismantling and assembly related to maintenance or repair service. These tests are quickly and easily carried out with the aid of Interspiro's test equipment.

Rescue Regulator. This is a regulator and a piece of hose that can be attached to a cylinder. If a firefighter is trapped or is running out of air, the rescue regulator and an extra cylinder can be attached to a port on the firefighter's regulator with an adapter hose. This eliminates the need for firefighters to share the air remaining in one cylinder.

DONNING AND DOFFING PROCEDURES
Preparing For Use
CAUTION: Training in the donning and before-use test procedure should be given before use in an emergency situation. The user must demonstrate knowledge to a responsible teacher or supervisor.

Step 1: Open the toggle link on the harness and check that the strap loop is big enough for the cylinder to be used. If not, press the small locking hook and enlarge the diameter of the loop.

Step 2: Slide the cylinder into the strap loop, and push it in until the valve snaps into its holder and locks. (The cylinder valve connection thread should be on the same side as the toggle link.) Adjust the strap loop by pushing the strap into the guide plate until it fits snugly around the cylinder, making sure that the hook on the side engages in one of the oblong holes. Close the toggle link.

Step 3: Connect the regulator unit to the cylinder valve, with the black rubber cover pointing down. Tighten the handwheel connector by hand.

Step 4: Connect the pressure gauge manifold to the harness, making sure the hoses are not twisted. The pressure gauge manifold should be slipped into the double strap section of the right shoulder strap (Figure E.14 on next page). Insert the extra loop of the right shoulder strap into the clip of the pressure gauge manifold. Stretch the loop down, and insert it into the top and bottom of the webbing buckle.

Step 5: Connect the breathing valve to the facepiece by pushing the valve into the connection piece and by turning it counterclockwise to engage its bayonet coupling (Figure E.15 on next page).

Step 6: Lock the breathing valve in position with the speech cone or radio attachment, as applicable, by tightening the locking screws (Figure E.16).

Step 7: Connect the Spiromatic Mask hose to the manifold (Figure E.17).

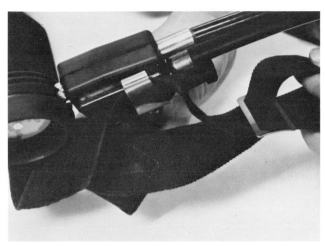

Figure E.14 Connect pressure gauge manifold to the harness. *Courtesy of Interspiro USA, Inc.*

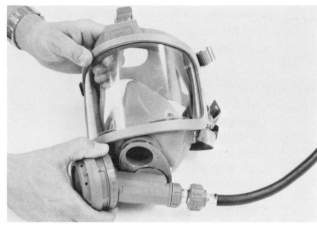

Figure E.15 Connect the breathing valve to the facepiece. *Courtesy of Interspiro USA, Inc.*

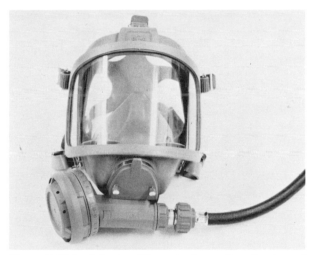

Figure E.16 Lock the breathing valve in position. *Courtesy of Interspiro USA, Inc.*

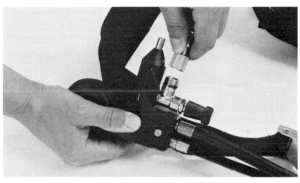

Figure E.17 Connect Spiromatic Mask hose to the manifold. *Courtesy of Interspiro USA, Inc.*

Leakage And Function Test

Step 1: Close the bypass by turning the knob fully counterclockwise (Figure E.18).

Step 2: Ensure that the black lever on the breathing valve is in the OFF position (against the valve housing).

Step 3: Open the cylinder valve carefully. Turn on the positive pressure by slowly lifting the black lever to the ON position, away from the valve housing.

Step 4: A strong flow of air should be heard. Turn off the positive pressure and

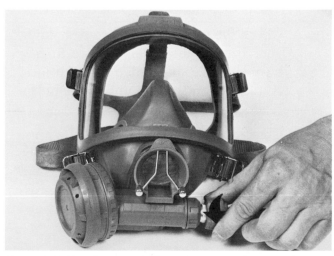

Figure E.18 Close bypass valve by turning counterclockwise. *Courtesy of Interspiro USA, Inc.*

read the pressure gauge. Close the cylinder valve. The needle of the pressure gauge should stay in the green area after one minute. If it does not stay in the green area, leakage repairs should be made by an authorized service representative and the test repeated.

Step 5: With the cylinder closed, open the bypass valve slightly in order to allow the air to slowly evacuate. Read the pressure gauge when the alarm starts to sound. The pressure gauge should read ¼ full. Turn ON the positive pressure to let the system evacuate, then turn OFF the positive pressure. Close the bypass again.

Donning the Spiromatic

Step 1: Open the eccentric side buckles, extend the straps, and put the apparatus on your back with the cylinder valve facing down. Loop the facepiece neck strap over your head.

Step 2: Grip the waist buckle and pull the straps while taking a small jump (or rest the apparatus on a support behind you) so the anatomically designed backplate gets lodged firmly and comfortably on your back.

Step 3: The eccentric side buckles will automatically lock after adjustment.

Step 4: Still holding the waist buckles, press them together in locking position, then move hands to loose ends and tighten.

Step 5: When tightened, press down eccentric levers of both side buckles. Preferably, tuck loose strap ends under the straps.

Step 6: Ensure that the positive pressure is turned OFF; then reach back with your left hand, and open the cylinder valve completely. Put on the Spiromatic Mask and moderately tighten the head harness straps. Inhale to reset the diaphragm assembly in a neutral position. Stop breathing and listen for any leakage. If you hear any leakage, check that your hair is not interfering with the face seal. Readjust the head harness if necessary. Check also that the bypass is closed.

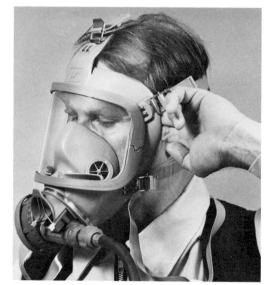

Figure E.19 Check for positive pressure by holding your breath and inserting two fingers between seal and face. *Courtesy of Interspiro USA, Inc.*

Step 7: Check the positive pressure by holding your breath and inserting two fingers between the sealing edge and your face. A strong sound of escaping air should be heard (Figure E.19).

Step 8: Check the pressure shown on the pressure gauge. To make this easier, lower your right shoulder to take the weight of the shoulder strap, and pull the pressure gauge manifold down and outward (Figure E.20).

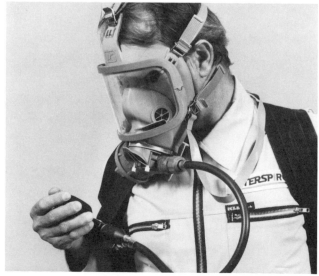

Figure E.20 Check pressure gauge. *Courtesy of Interspiro USA, Inc.*

> # WARNING
> If the cylinder has been charged very quickly, the air is warm and the volume available for breathing is reduced.

Step 9: Slide your left hand up the breathing hose to locate the bypass knob. Check the bypass operation by turning the knob clockwise and listening for the flow of air. Close the bypass by turning the knob counterclockwise against stop. The apparatus is now ready.

Doffing The Spiromatic

Step 1: Loosen the head harness straps, then turn OFF the positive pressure by pressing the black lever toward the valve housing (Figure E.21). Remove the facemask.

Step 2: Open the waist buckle by pressing the male buckle pawl in the center. If necessary, follow the waist strap with thumbs and lift the eccentric side buckles' locking devices. The straps will automatically loosen. Stop when suitable. Take off the apparatus by sliding it under the right arm and forward.

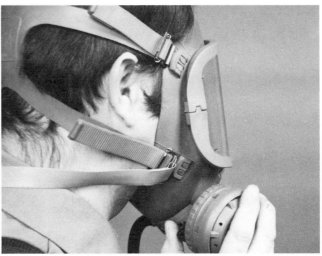

Figure E.21 Turn off positive pressure by pressing black lever toward valve housing. *Courtesy of Interspiro USA, Inc.*

Step 3: Close the cylinder valve.

Step 4: Store the Spiromatic with the positive pressure turned ON (the black lever in the position away from the valve housing).

MINE SAFETY APPLIANCES COMPANY (MSA)

MSA provides more than 4,000 personal protective products and hazard detection instruments for many industries, including fire fighting, haz mat, nuclear, petroleum, chemicals, energy, mining, steel, and more. They also provide product training seminars and audiovisual training aids on product use and applications. MSA also has a network of repair and service centers. Corporate headquarters are at P.O. Box 426 in Pittsburgh, PA, 15230. MSA has 21 stocking locations, the nearest of which can be reached toll free at 1-800-MSA-2222 (internationally call 412-273-5000).

SCBA FEATURES

MSA has developed a variety of open-circuit self-contained breathing apparatus, both low-pressure and high-pressure air masks, and other accessories. MSA air masks include the Ultralite™ II and Ultralite MMR™ Air Masks (30-minute-rated service life) and the Custom 4500™ II and Custom 4500 MMR™ Air Masks (30- or 60-minute-rated service life). Ultralite™ II and Custom 4500™ II models feature a belt-mounted two-stage regulator (Figure E.22 on next page). Ultralite MMR™ and Custom 4500 MMR™ units feature a regulator configuration in which the first stage is mounted on the backplate near the cylinder, and the second stage is mounted on the facepiece (Figure E.23 on next page). All four models are tested for compliance with NFPA 1981. MSA air masks are also available with dual-purpose capability, which combines the features of a

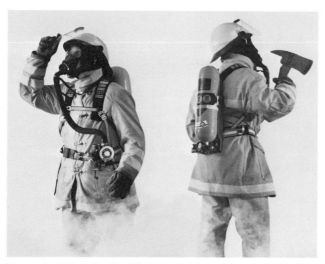

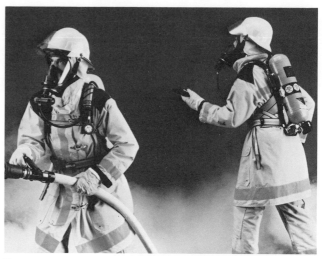

Figure E.22 The Ultralite™ II Air Mask (left) and the Custom 4500™ II Air Mask (right) by MSA feature a new harness and carrier assembly for added durability. *Photo courtesy of MSA.*

Figure E.23 The Ultralite MMR™ Air Mask (left) and Custom 4500 MMR™ Air Mask (right) by MSA feature mask-mounted regulators. *Photo courtesy of MSA.*

self-contained breathing apparatus and an airline respirator in one unit. All MSA air masks, including dual-purpose versions, are pressure-demand apparatus.

Ultralite™ Air Masks are low-pressure self-contained breathing apparatus which accommodate three types of 30-minute-rated cylinders. Ultralite™ Air Masks are available with the fully-wound Composite II Cylinder and can also be used with a conventional steel cylinder. When equipped with the Composite II Cylinder, the Ultralite™ Air Masks weigh approximately 22 pounds. The third cylinder option is the Composite III Cylinder, which is about the same size as the Composite II Cylinder, but holds nearly a third more air to more closely approximate 30 minutes' use under heavier exertion. The Composite III Cylinder has a high-strength Kevlar™/glass outer wrap and is pressurized to 3,000 psig rather than 2,216 psig.

Custom 4500™ Air Masks have a choice of interchangeable 4,500 psig air cylinders that allow the apparatus to be used as a 60-minute or 30-minute-rated unit. With the 30-minute fully-wound composite cylinder, the unit weighs approximately 23 pounds. With the 60-minute fully-wound composite cylinder, the unit weighs approximately 34 pounds.

Ultralite™ II and Custom 4500™ Air Masks are equipped with the Ultravue® facepiece and a breathing tube that connects to the belt-mounted regulator. Ultralite MMR™ and Custom 4500 MMR™ Air Masks are equipped with the Ultra-Elite™ facepiece, which features a conical wide-vision lens. Since the second stage of the regulator is mask-mounted, the MMR units do not use a breathing tube.

MSA facepieces are available in either green or black Hycar™ rubber or black silicone (Figure E.24) and are available in small, medium,

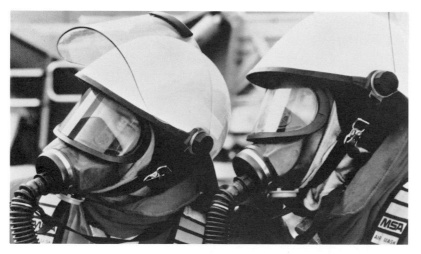

Figure E.24 MSA Air Masks feature Ultravue® facepieces with a glass laminated lens for scratch and chemical resistance. The lens is constructed of glass on the outside and shatter-resistant polyvinyl butyral (PVB) on the inside. *Photo courtesy of MSA.*

and large sizes, color-coded as to size. Five adjustable straps secure the Ultravue® facepiece to the head. Ultra-Elite™ facepieces are equipped with the EZ-Don™ FHR Facepiece Harness, a flame- and heat-resistant (FHR) unit featuring self-adjusting straps. The EZ-Don™ Harness is available as an option on Ultravue® facepieces. MSA also offers optional nosecups in three sizes.

MSA belt-mounted regulators are made of a high-strength aluminum alloy (Figure E.25). The regulator is mounted on the waist strap with a sliding bracket. The aluminum components are

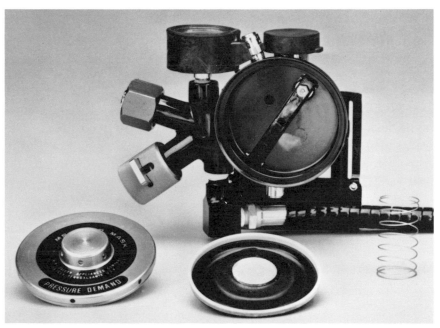

Figure E.25 The MSA belt-mounted pressure-demand regulator maintains positive pressure in the facepiece during inhalation and exhalation. *Photo courtesy of MSA.*

color-coded to make it easy to distinguish high-pressure regulators from low-pressure regulators: Ultralite™ II units are black, and Custom 4500™ II units are gray. Airflow is activated by turning the quick-acting mainline valve.

With MMR units the balanced first-stage regulator provides a constant output of air to the second stage, even as cylinder pressure decreases. Air travels to the second stage via an intermediate-pressure hose that runs through the left shoulder strap. The unusually compact second stage features a unique "pilot-operated" design that responds quickly and accurately to the user's changing breathing requirements. Airflow is initiated by inhaling, and it can be stopped by pushing the mainline shut-off button.

Both types of regulators feature bypass valves that can be activated with a simple twist in the event of a regulator malfunction. With MSA belt-mounted regulators, both the first and second stages are bypassed. MMR units bypass the second stage only.

All MSA air masks are equipped with the Audi-Larm™ low-pressure warning device that signals the user by a loud, clear bell when there is a 20 to 25 percent air supply left in the cylinder.

Standard MSA compressed air cylinders are color-coded to match the cylinder clamp of the apparatus for which they are used — yellow for Ultralite™ Air Mask low-pressure units and green for Custom 4500™ Air Mask high-pressure units. The optional Composite III Cylinder, which is silver, is also for use with low-pressure apparatus (Figure E.26). Cylinders for low-pressure

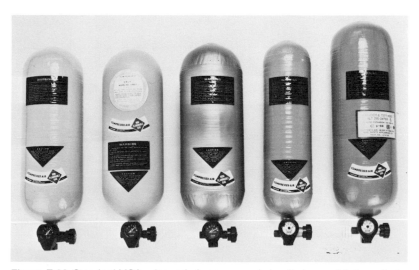

Figure E.26 Standard MSA color-coded compressed air cylinders match the cylinder clamp of the apparatus for which they are used (yellow or green). The optional Composite III cylinder is silver. *Photo courtesy of MSA.*

breathing apparatus have a 30-minute-rated service life. Low-pressure cylinders are available with fully-wound composite or steel construction. High-pressure cylinders are either 60-minute- or 30-minute-rated. High-pressure cylinders are of fully-wound composite construction only.

ACCESSORIES

The Quick-Fill™ System. This system allows MSA air mask users to refill and transfill air cylinders while the mask is worn, without the need to remove the air cylinder. MSA air masks retain their NIOSH certifications during use of the Quick-Fill™ System for two primary reasons: the system does *not* affect the airflow performance of the SCBA regulator during use, and it does *not* require firefighters to be permanently tethered to each other during escape situations. The Quick-Fill™ System has three primary applications:

- Quickly refill the cylinder from a mobile compressor or cascade system without a changeover (Figure E.27).

- Transfill between two cylinders, providing an Emergency Escape Breathing Support System (EEBSS) (Figure E.28).

- Extend the air supply over longer durations when a remote cascade system or other compressed air source is conveniently located in an IDLH work area.

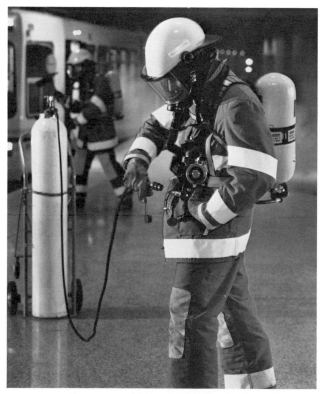

Figure E.27 Quick refilling using MSA's Quick-Fill™ System from a cascade-type fresh air station permits "instant" cylinder refills closer to the fire scene. *Photo courtesy of MSA.*

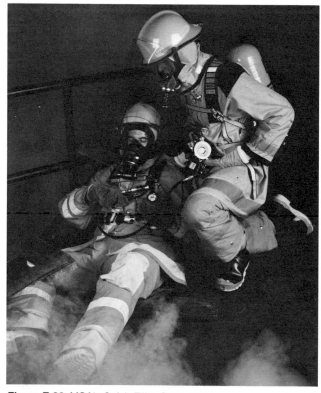

Figure E.28 MSA's Quick-Fill™ System allows emergency transfill of air between air masks, thus providing an Emergency Escape Breathing Support System (EEBSS). The system's compatible adapter assemblies also allow emergency transfilling of air between MSA's mask-mounted units and their waist-mounted units. *Photo courtesy of MSA.*

The Quick-Fill™ option consists of a special inlet, called the male adapter assembly, which is located on the air mask. Any accessory Quick-Fill™ Hose with a "female" quick-disconnect can connect a pressurized air source to the male adapter assembly to achieve air transfer. The pressurized air source can be a compressor truck, a cascade system, or another Quick-Fill™-equipped air mask. The Quick-Fill™ System must be used with Quick-Fill™ Hose.

ClearCom™ Communications Systems. ClearCom™ Communications Systems amplify voice communications, provide two-way radio interface, or both, while maintaining NIOSH extensions of certifications. The ClearCom™ RI system utilizes a high-performance aviation microphone and mounts an extension speaker from a two-way radio close to the wearer's ear for radio reception in high noise areas. It comes with a "Y" cable which permits the simultaneous use of the ClearCom™ V amplifier (Figures E.29 and E.30).

EZ-Don™ FHR Facepiece Harness. This harness is a flame- and heat-resistant facepiece suspension system that is optional with the Ultravue® facepiece and standard with the Ultra-Elite™ facepiece. The top strap and temple straps self-adjust (Figure E.31).

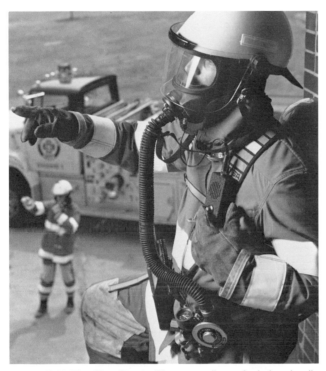

Figure E.29 The ClearCom™ RI system allows single-hand radio communication with other firefighters. A "Y" cable permits simultaneous use with the ClearCom V Amplifier system. *Photo courtesy of MSA.*

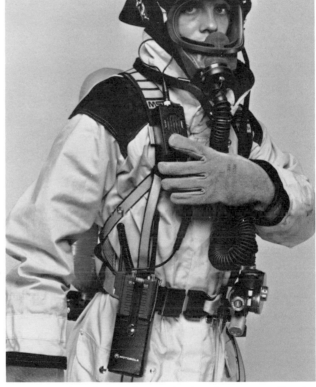

Figure E.30 ClearCom™ Communications Systems amplify voice communications, provide two-way radio communication, or both. *Photo courtesy of MSA.*

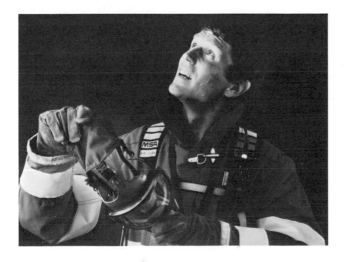

Figure E.31 The glass laminated facepiece lens and EZ-Don™ FHR facepiece harness, constructed of flame- and heat-resistant fabric, are optional with the Ultravue® facepiece, but standard with the Ultra-Elite™ facepiece. *Photo courtesy of MSA.*

Portable Regulator Testers. For regulator maintenance in accordance with MSA's maintenance programs, users can select either the Portable Regulator Tester II (Figure E.32) or PURT™ 1000 System. The Portable Regulator Tester II checks basic regulator functions, and the PURT™ 1000 is a computerized system that runs a more comprehensive battery of tests.

Breathing Air Test Kit. When checking air cylinders or compressed air sources, this kit can simultaneously test for the presence of carbon monoxide, carbon dioxide, water vapor, and oil vapors (Figure E.33). An air sample is released from the test kit regulator into the manifold and into the four detector tubes simultaneously.

Others. MSA supports basic user training in the care and use of air masks through a series of in-depth audiovisual presentations and posters plus inspection and maintenance programs. Maintenance accessories such as spare parts kits, tool kits, paint kits, and overhaul kits are available.

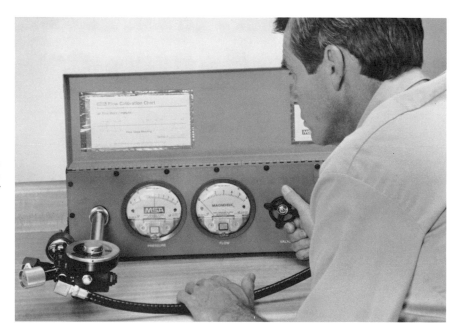

Figure E.32 The Portable Regulator Tester II checks regulator functions with both flow and static pressure tests. *Photo courtesy of MSA.*

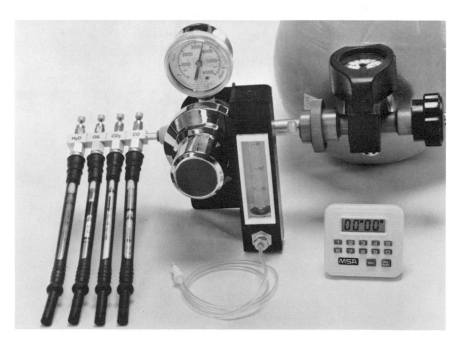

Figure E.33 A breathing-air kit tests for carbon monoxide, carbon dioxide, water vapor, and oil vapors in the compressed air source or cylinder. *Photo courtesy of MSA.*

DONNING AND DOFFING PROCEDURES

NOTE: These procedures are offered as an example, however, the steps may vary between different models of MSA air masks. Refer to the operating instructions supplied with the unit being used.

CAUTION: Always read and follow the instructions furnished with the device. This SCBA is for use by qualified, trained personnel only. Don and remove mask in a safe, nonhazardous, nontoxic atmosphere. Parts must not be interchanged among self-contained breathing devices from different manufacturers.

Donning The Ultralite™ Air Mask

Step 1: Remove the facepiece from case.

Step 2: Check the cylinder gauge — should be on the FULL mark (2,216 psig).

Step 3: Reach inside the shoulder straps and hold the cylinder with both hands.

Step 4: Lift over head and rest on back. Fasten the chest strap to position shoulder straps.

Step 5: Pull the adjusting strap tabs out and straighten up. Hike unit up on your back.

Step 6: Fasten the waist belt and pull tight for snug fit. Position the regulator to reach controls.

Operational Check-Out

Step 1: Close the mainline and bypass valves. Cover the regulator outlet.

Step 2: Open the cylinder valve fully. Audi-Larm™ should ring briefly.

Step 3: Open the quick-acting mainline valve. Check the regulator gauge — should read 2,216 psig, ± 100 psig. Keep the regulator outlet covered, and close the cylinder valve. The regulator gauge must not drop more than 100 psig in 30 seconds.

Step 4: Very slowly uncover the regulator outlet. Watch needle drop. At approximately 540 psig, the Audi-Larm™ should ring. When ringing stops, close mainline valve.

Donning The Facepiece

Step 1: Hold the facepiece by the straps and put your chin in first.

Step 2: Pull the harness back over head.

Step 3: To tighten straps, pull straight back, not out.

Checking The Facepiece Fit

CAUTION: This device may not provide a satisfactory face seal with certain physical characteristics (such as beards or full, heavy sideburns), resulting in leakage in connection with the facepiece, which voids or limits the protection. If such a condition exists, the user assumes all risks of death or serious bodily injury which may possibly result.

Step 1: Block the inlet to breathing tube, and inhale gently (Figure E.34 on next page).

Step 2: Hold breath at least 10 seconds—the facepiece should collapse and stay collapsed against face (Figure E.35 on next page).

Step 3: To test the exhalation valve, block breathing tube and gently exhale. If the valve is stuck, you will feel a heavy rush of air around the facepiece. You may need a sharp exhalation at first to "crack" valve (Figure E.36 on next page).

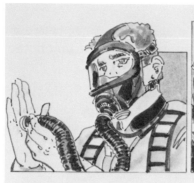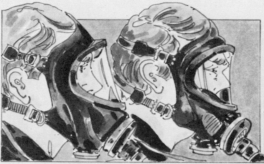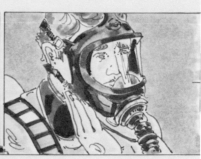

Figure E.34 To check facepiece fit, first block breathing tube and inhale gently. *Photo courtesy of MSA.*

Figure E.35 Second, hold breath at least 10 seconds—facepiece should collapse and stay collapsed against face. *Photo courtesy of MSA.*

Figure E.36 To test exhalation valve, block breathing tube and gently exhale. If valve is stuck, a sharp exhalation may be needed to "crack" valve. *Photo courtesy of MSA.*

Testing Before Entry

CAUTION: If the apparatus does not perform as specified in the instructions furnished with the device, it must not be used until it has been checked by authorized personnel.

Step 1: Open the cylinder valve fully — at least 3 turns.

Step 2: Connect breathing tube to regulator while opening quick-acting mainline valve (Figure E.37).

Step 3: To test the bypass valve, crack it open, then close quickly.

Doffing the Ultralite™ II Air Mask

Step 1: Close the cylinder valve and disconnect breathing tube. The remaining air in the high-pressure hose is released if mainline valve is open.

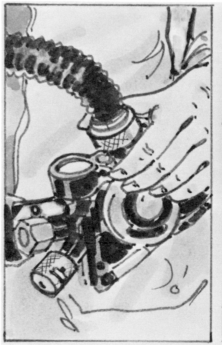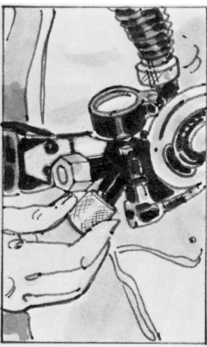

Figure E.37 After opening cylinder valve, connect breathing tube to regulator while fully opening mainline valve. *Photo courtesy of MSA.*

Step 2: When the Audi-Larm™ stops ringing, close the mainline valve.

Step 3: To remove facepiece, put thumb under buckles to loosen headbands. Fully extend headbands. Hold the facepiece by the speaking diaphragm assembly, and pull up and away from face.

NATIONAL DRAEGER, INC.

National Draeger, Inc., is a subsidiary of Draegerwerk A.G., which is headquartered in Lubeck, West Germany. National Draeger, Inc., has its headquarters at P.O. Box 120, Pittsburgh, PA, 15230, 412-787-8383. Draeger Canada Ltd., is located at 5925 Airport Road, Suite 200, Mississauga, ONT L4V1W1, 416-671-0629. Besides SCBA units, Draeger manufactures supplied air respirators, emergency escape breathing apparatus, air purifying respirators, and protection suits.

SCBA FEATURES

The Draeger PA-80 SCBA is an entire multi-function breathing system in that each piece of breathing equipment is compatible with the rest of the Draeger line (Figure E.38). This system gives the ability to work in a variety of industrial and rescue conditions, using the same basic equipment. Exclusive features of the Draeger PA-80 are as follows:

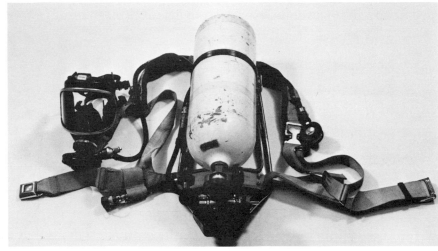

Figure E.38 The Draeger PA-80 SCBA, one of National Draeger's multi-function breathing systems.

- Panorama Nova mask, a panoramic lens, nosecup, and flushing mask with soft, double-sealing edge and adjustable harness.

- Demand regulator that gives more air when needed with a flexible diaphragm and air admission system.

- Stainless steel backplate formed to the shape of a person's back and lined with neoprene padding.

- First stage regulator, a pressure-compensating, piston-type regulator, designed for long service life with minimal maintenance. Placement on the backplate protects the first-stage regulator against damage during use.

- Pressure gauge positioned on the shoulder strap to allow for easy checking of air supply, with a rubber jacket for protection.

The Draeger model PA-80 FS features:

- 30-, 45-, and 60-minute service lightweight cylinders.

- Quick-adjust hardware on straps.

- Quick-release fastener on cylinder straps.

- Cylinder handwheel color-coded for pressure requirements. The low-air warning audible alarm is designed to make it easier to tell whose air is low.

- Pushbutton positive-pressure-only regulator gives air when needed. Design provides low breathing resistance during peak inhalation.

- Aramid straps and backpack padding for comfort.

- Yellow 2,216-psi cylinders, making it easier to identify low- and high-pressure cylinders.

- Wide-angle, Panorama Nova Mask with a facepiece of neoprene or silicone rubber and a built-in speaking diaphragm.

The PA-80 FS is a two-stage compressed air SCBA. The first-stage pressure reducer regulates air pressure from the compressed air cylinder to an intermediate pressure of approximately 100 psi. The second-stage regulator is a positive-pressure-only, lung-demand regulator. The second stage regulates the intermediate pressure to breathing pressure and maintains a slight pressure in the mask.

The unit meets the requirements of NFPA 1981. The PA-80 FS is an open-circuit SCBA, is available in both 2,216 psi and 4,500 psi, and is certified by NIOSH/MSHA for use as respiratory protection in hazardous or oxygen-deficient atmospheres (Figure E.39). Some of its features are

- Aramid harness and webbing
- Abrasion resistant lens
- Automatic lung demand regulator with silicone diaphragm
- Stainless steel backplate and hardware
- Stainless steel speaking diaphragm

ACCESSORIES

4,500-psi/45-Minute Cylinder. The 4,500-psi, 45-minute cylinder offers the user an alternative to the standard 30- and 60-minute cylinders. Where the air supply of a 30-minute cylinder does not meet user demand during work conditions and a 60-minute cylinder is too heavy, the 45-minute cylinder is the recommended choice.

PA-Test 80. The PA-Test 80 is the only portable test kit that provides the ability to check the basic functions of the PA-80 "Multi-Function Family" right at the site or in a fire department's own service department. The complete test kit contains a precision low-pressure gauge, test gauges for high and medium pressures, test head, pump and tubing, plus connection adapters.

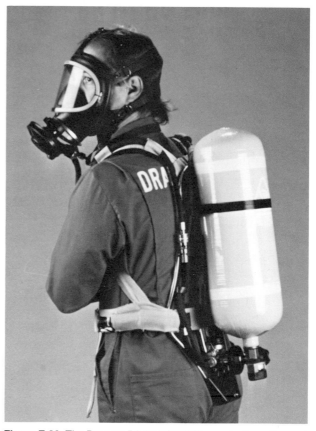

Figure E.39 The Draeger PA-80 FS SCBA was designed to meet the requirements of NFPA 1981. *Courtesy of National Draeger.*

Others. Other accessories available include conversion kits, spectacle frame for mask, welding shield, tinted lens, disinfectant, antifog solution, buddy breather pigtail, backplate pad, and various slide and tape training presentations.

DONNING AND DOFFING PROCEDURES
Donning The Draeger PA-80

Step 1: (Coat Method) Hold the apparatus by the shoulder straps, with the front of the cylinder facing toward you.

Step 2: Swing the apparatus around the left side of your body. Slide your left arm through the harness, then the right arm. The backplate should rest comfortably on your back.

Step 3: (Over the Head Method) Grasp the rubber side of the backplate with the cylinder valve pointing upward.

Step 4: Swing the apparatus over the head making sure that the elbows extend through the loops of webbing.

Step 5: Pull the shoulder straps until the apparatus fits the contour of your back. The apparatus is designed to be worn low on the back.

Step 6: Fasten the waist belt around your waist, and adjust for comfort. Tuck the loose shoulder strap ends under your waist belt.

Donning The Mask

Step 1: Using the long neck strap, hang the mask around your neck. Then fasten the mask in the "ready" position. (The center forehead strap is attached to the neck strap.)

Step 2: Spread the head harness, and place your chin in the mask.

Step 3: Secure the mask to your face, then pull the straps over the top of your head. (Make sure that the mask seal is free of any hair.)

Step 4: Tighten the lower straps.

Step 5: Tighten the temple straps. Then tighten the top strap, if necessary.

Adjusting The Regulator

Step 1: With the regulator in the donning mode, turn on the apparatus at the cylinder valve (Figure E.40).

Step 2: Insert the demand regulator into the connection on the front of the mask (Figure E.41).

Step 3: The positive-pressure lung demand is breath activated (Figure E.42). For selector switch lung demand regulator, turn selector knob to positive-pressure mode.

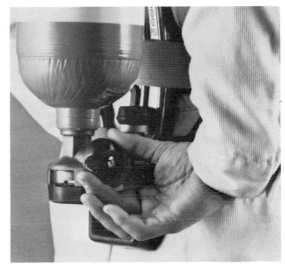

Figure E.40 Turn on the apparatus at the cylinder valve. *Courtesy of National Draeger.*

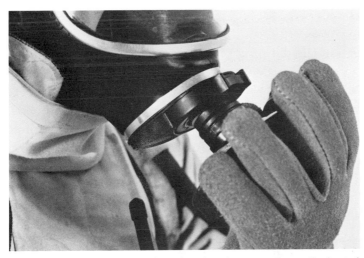

Figure E.41 Insert the demand regulator into the connection on the front of the mask.

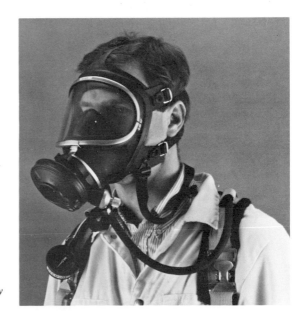

Figure E.42 The positive-pressure lung demand is breath activated. *Courtesy of National Draeger.*

Step 4: The bypass valve operates simply by depressing the silver knob to the left side of the demand regulator and can be locked in place (Figure E.43).

Step 5: Check the pressure gauge (Figure E.44).

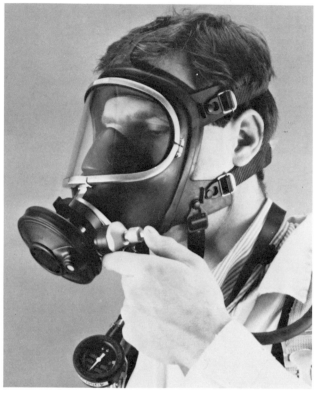

Figure E.43 Operate the bypass valve by depressing the silver knob to the left side of the demand regulator. *Courtesy of National Draeger.*

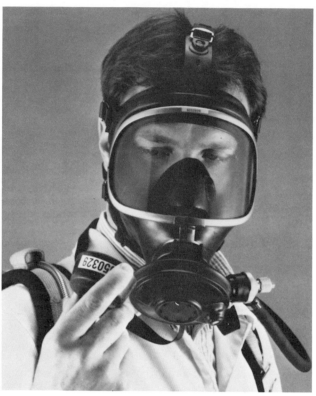

Figure E.44 Check the pressure gauge. *Courtesy of National Draeger.*

Doffing The Draeger PA-80

The doffing procedure is simply the reverse of the donning process.

SCBA TRAINING CENTERS

National Draeger, Inc., provides SCBA training centers to accommodate SCBA training needs. This system can be either installed in a building or incorporated as part of a mobile training trailer. The mobile unit consists of a 45-foot trailer or a 26-foot truck body. An example of Draeger's fixed system is housed at their headquarters in Pittsburgh, PA. The design of the training center permits the users to learn about their SCBA and their ability to perform under stressful but controlled conditions.

NORTH SAFETY EQUIPMENT

North Safety Equipment is a division of Siebe North, Inc., located at 2000 Plainfield Pike, Cranston, RI, 02921. For more information, call 401-943-4400. In Canada, the company is North Safety Products.

SCBA FEATURES

The North 800 Series™ SCBA is an open-circuit self-contained pressure-demand-type compressed air breathing apparatus. This series includes units having a 30-minute duration rating and a 60-

minute duration rating. Major components of the North 800 include the pressurized air cylinder, high-pressure reducer/regulator, full facepiece with speaker diaphragm, valve, backplate with integral harness (with straps and hoses), pressure gauges, and a warning whistle (Figure E.45). A special buddy breathing/test fitting is provided. The full facepiece is made of silicone. The silicone oral/nasal cup and speaking diaphragm are standard equipment along with a fully padded harness, luminous pressure gauge, locking quick-connects, and fail-open design.

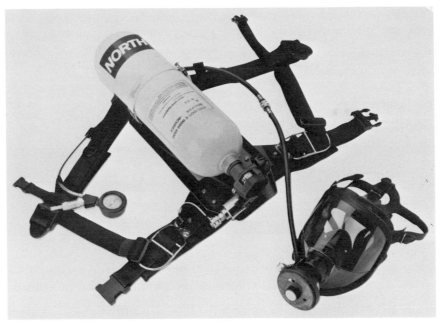

Figure E.45 The North 800 Series™ SCBA by North Safety Equipment includes both 30- and 60-minute duration air cylinders. *Courtesy of North Safety Equipment.*

The fail-open design assures the user a supply of air (if air is in the cylinder) if a malfunction occurs, thus eliminating the need for a bypass valve. The reducer/regulator incorporates a dual spring-loaded pressure balancing piston. High-pressure cylinder air flows through a sized orifice in the piston stem. The spring tension prevents the piston from moving until the desired back pressure of approximately 80 psi is achieved. Thus the flow of air through the device is not stopped by an internal part malfunction.

The North 800 has a quick-connect fitting for rapid rescue procedures using a buddy breathing fitting or airline accessory fitting. This fitting eliminates the need for the rescuer to dislodge his or her facepiece.

The demand valve is either fixed positive pressure or positive pressure with donning feature. The donning feature eliminates the loss of air with cylinder valve on during donning and doffing of the facepiece. The demand valve is facepiece mounted.

However, when a high flow of air is desired to purge the facepiece of contaminants which may have leaked in or to clear severe facepiece lens fogging, a supplemental airflow purge button is provided on the demand valve. When depressed, the purge button overrides the pressure-balancing mechanism in the demand valve and allows large quantities of air to flow through the facepiece. Since that reduces the amount of air available for subsequent use, the purge button should be used only when absolutely necessary.

ACCESSORIES

Airline Accessory Fitting. This quick-connect fitting can be used for buddy breathing rescue because it eliminates the need to remove the facepiece.

Antifog Cloth. This cloth is suggested for use in temperatures below 32°F.

Spectacle Assembly. Either plastic or glass lens glasses with temples or straps can be inserted into a special frame for use in the facepiece. The frame assembly can be attached to the inside of the full facepiece.

Others. Other accessories include cylinder valving tool, fit testing probe, maintenance accessory kit, leak detection solution, cleaner/sanitizer powder, tool and test kit, backpressure reducer/regulator test gauge, carrying case, and wall/truck mounting brackets. A slide training program with audio cassette is also available.

DONNING AND DOFFING PROCEDURES
Donning And Use Of North 800 Series™

WARNING
All personnel using the 800 Series™ SCBA shall be fully trained by qualified personnel in the proper donning, operation, and emergency operation of the unit.

Step 1: Visually check the unit to make certain that all major components are in place and in good condition. Check that all components on the facepiece and backplate are secure.

Step 2: Check to ensure that all straps are fully extended, buckles are not connected, and hoses are not tangled.

Step 3: Check that all fingertight connections are secure: cylinder valve to reducer/regulator, demand valve to facepiece (Figure E.46), and facepiece air supply line quick-connect (Figure E.47). Ensure that the exhalation valve assembly is secure in the facepiece.

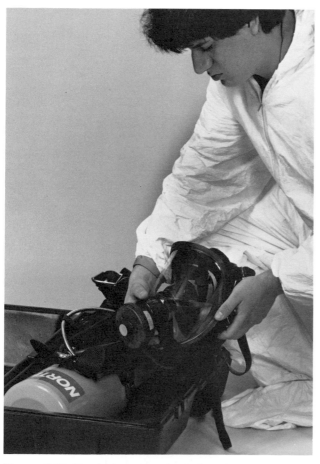

Figure E.46 Check demand valve-to-facepiece connection. *Courtesy of North Safety Equipment.*

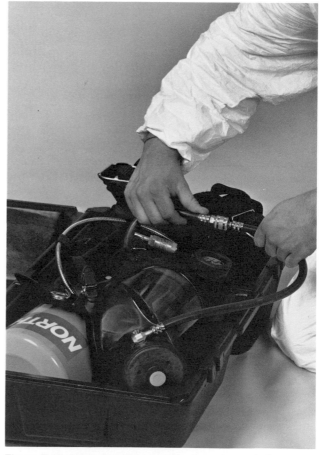

Figure E.47 Check facepiece low-pressure air supply line quick-connect connection. *Courtesy of North Safety Equipment.*

Step 4: Check that the air cylinder gauge registers full. If not *full*, replace with a full air cylinder (Figure E.48).

Step 5: Stand facing the unit and make sure that the air cylinder valve is at the top. Lean forward and use both hands to grasp the edges of the backplate and cylinder between the waist harness and the shoulder harness.

Step 6: Bending over, swing the unit straight up and over the head, keeping elbows close to body. Rest unit on your back while still bent over, and allow the shoulder harness straps to slide along arms and into place on the shoulders. Be sure that the elbows are through the shoulder harness and its side strap loops. Check to ensure the straps are not twisted.

Step 7: Pull down the shoulder adjusting straps while slowly rising to an erect standing position. Position the cylinder and backplate to your comfort.

Step 8: Grasp waist belt buckles; extend right hand male buckle to fit waist. Snap two buckles together. Pull waist belt from right to a snug fit.

Step 9: Connect and adjust the chest strap assembly. (**NOTE:** Do not lay the chest strap over the air supply line or the chest-mounted pressure gauge.)

Step 10: Adjust the five facepiece head straps to their full outward position.

Step 11: Place the neck strap around the collar as shown (Figure E.49).

NOTE: For units having the demand valve with fixed positive pressure, proceed to Step 19. For units having the demand valve with the donning feature, continue with Steps 12 through 18.

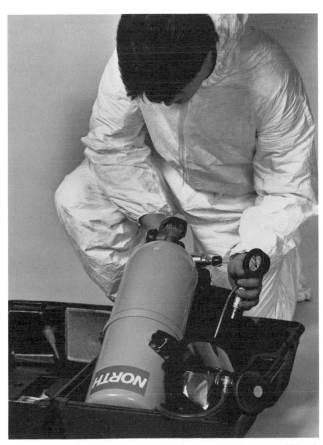

Figure E.48 Check air cylinder pressure gauge. *Courtesy of North Safety Equipment.*

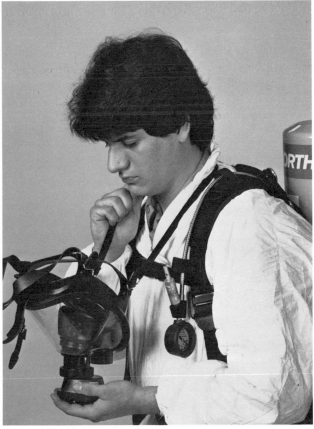

Figure E.49 Place neck strap around collar. *Courtesy of North Safety Equipment.*

Step 12: If equipped with donning feature, grasp knob gently outward and turn into locking position. Unit is temporarily set into demand-air donning mode (Figure E.50).

Step 13: Open the cylinder valve by rotating counterclockwise at least two turns. The alarm should whistle briefly as the system pressure builds.

Step 14: Grasp the head strap harness with thumbs through the straps; spread outward.

Step 15: Push the harness top up the forehead, brushing hair upward from the face seal area. Continue up and over the head until the harness is centered at the rear of the head and the chin is fitted into the chin cup.

Step 16: Pull both lower straps at the same time toward the rear. Tighten the two temple straps.

Step 17: Tighten the top head strap.

Step 18: Set the mask for positive pressure (Figure E.51).

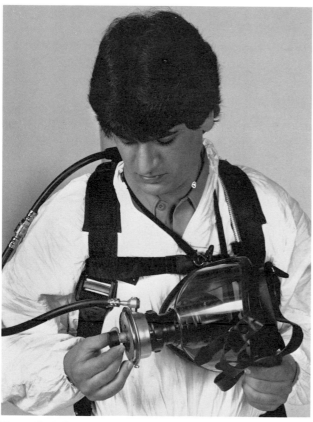

Figure E.50 Set donning feature by grasping knob outward and turning into locking position. *Courtesy of North Safety Equipment.*

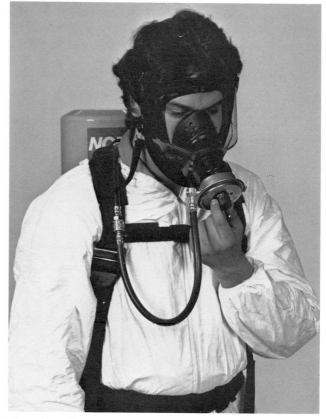

Figure E.51 Set the demand valve for positive pressure. Be sure to release knob on donning feature. *Courtesy of North Safety Equipment.*

WARNING
Release the knob on the donning feature to ensure that the breathing apparatus is in the positive-pressure mode. Failure to do this will then allow the contaminants in the facepiece during inhalation.

NOTE: For units having the demand valve with the donning feature, now proceed to Step 25.

Step 19: Grasp the head strap harness with thumbs through the straps from the inside and spread gently.

Step 20: Push the harness top up the forehead, brushing hair upward from the face seal area. Continue up and over the head until the harness is centered at the rear of the head, and the chin is fitted into the chin cup.

Step 21: Pull the lower straps both at the same time towards the rear.

Step 22: Tighten the two temple head straps.

Step 23: Tighten the top head strap.

Step 24: Immediately open the cylinder valve by rotating at least two turns in the counterclockwise direction. As you draw your first breath from the facepiece, listen for the alarm whistle to momentarily sound as the system pressure builds.

Step 25: Read the chest-mounted pressure gauge. It should read full cylinder pressure. If the gauge does not read full, remove the unit and obtain a full cylinder (Figure E.52).

Step 26: Test for positive pressure in the facepiece by gently breaking the seal at the cheek. Airflow should be heard and felt. If you feel it, release the flange to allow the facepiece to reseal. If you do not hear the airflow, you do not have positive pressure. Return the facepiece and demand valve assembly to the service area, and replace it with a new unit (Figure E.53).

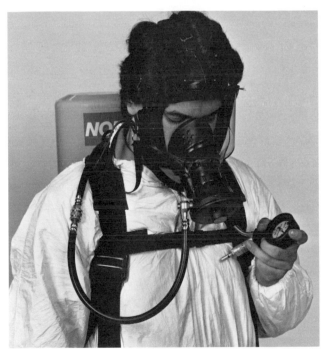

Figure E.52 Check the chest-mounted pressure gauge for full cylinder pressure. *Courtesy of North Safety Equipment.*

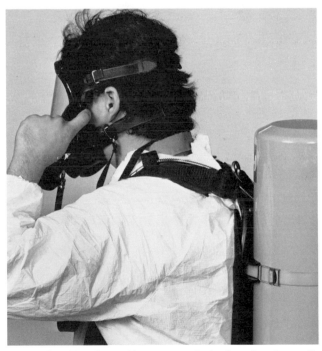

Figure E.53 Test for positive pressure in the facepiece by gently breaking the seal at the cheek. Airflow should be heard and felt. *Courtesy of North Safety Equipment.*

Step 27: Test the facepiece seal by holding your breath and listening for airflow through the demand valve control. There should be no sound and no outward leakage through the exhalation valve or around the facepiece. If you detect any leakage, the head straps should be readjusted until a no-leakage condition is achieved. If leakage is still present, remove the facepiece, and take the SCBA out of service.

Step 28: Test the purge button. Hold your breath, as in Step 27, and briefly push the purge button (located in the center of the cover of the demand valve). Air should flow into the facepiece.

If it does, release the button and breathe normally. If air does not flow into the facepiece, remove the facepiece and return it to the service area (Figure E.54).

Step 29: After you are assured that the unit is functioning properly, close the air cylinder valve. Inhale/exhale very slowly, watch the air pressure gauge, and listen for the warning whistle. The warning whistle should sound when the dial on the pressure gauge drops to the red band (Figure E.55).

WARNING
If whistle does not sound at proper setting, remove unit from service, and have it repaired by authorized personnel.

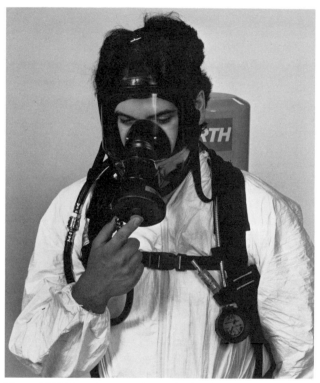

Figure E.54 Test the purge button by holding breath and briefly pushing the button. *Courtesy of North Safety Equipment.*

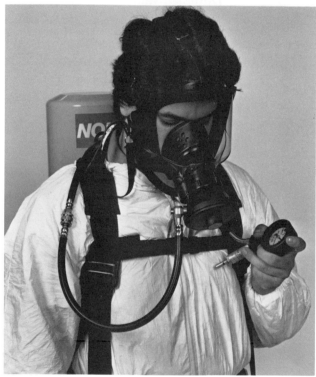

Figure E.55 Check the warning whistle. It should sound when dial on pressure gauge drops to the red band. *Courtesy of North Safety Equipment.*

Step 30: Reopen the cylinder valve. You are now ready to use the 800 Series™ SCBA.

WARNING
You must have air in your cylinder to sustain life. Be sure to check the air pressure gauge during use for remaining air supply to allow sufficient time for exit from a contaminated area.

Doffing The North 800 Series™

Step 1: Exit to a clear air area.

Step 2: Shut off the air cylinder by rotating the valve knob clockwise (frontward).

Step 3: Remove facepiece by flicking the head strap quick-release tabs forward. Lift the mask from under the chin upward and out. Return the head straps to their full outward position.

Step 4: Release the chest strap and then the waist strap buckles by pinching the release mechanisms on the top and bottom of the buckles.

Step 5: Loosen the shoulder straps by lifting up on the shoulder strap buckles. The weight of the unit will then do the job. Remove the unit in a fashion similar to removing a jacket. Be careful not to drop the unit.

Step 6: Prior to storage, ensure that the units equipped with the donning feature are set in the positive-pressure mode.

Step 7: Return the used unit to the service area for "Turnaround Maintenance."

RACAL PANORAMA, INC.

What began in 1976 as Racal Airstream exists today as Racal Health and Safety, Inc. The company name changed to Racal Health and Safety in 1988 to reflect the market areas reached by such new products as the Classic hearing protectors and the Ally personal-alert system. The Globe Safety line of self-contained breathing apparatus became part of Racal and is now a division named Racal Panorama, Inc. Racal Panorama, Inc., makers of the Racal Guardsman™ SCBA and the Buddy Pak™ ESCBA/SAR, is located at 109 Webb Street, Dayton, Ohio 45403, 800-336-7222 or in Ohio 513-254-2312.

SCBA FEATURES

Racal Guardsman™ units are available with 30-, 45-, and 60-minute-duration cylinders, with 30-minute units generally weighing less than 24 pounds (Figure E.56). The backpack is fully adjustable, and quick-release buckles are used to aid the user in getting in and out of the backpack quickly. The pack is balanced to ride on the user's hips.

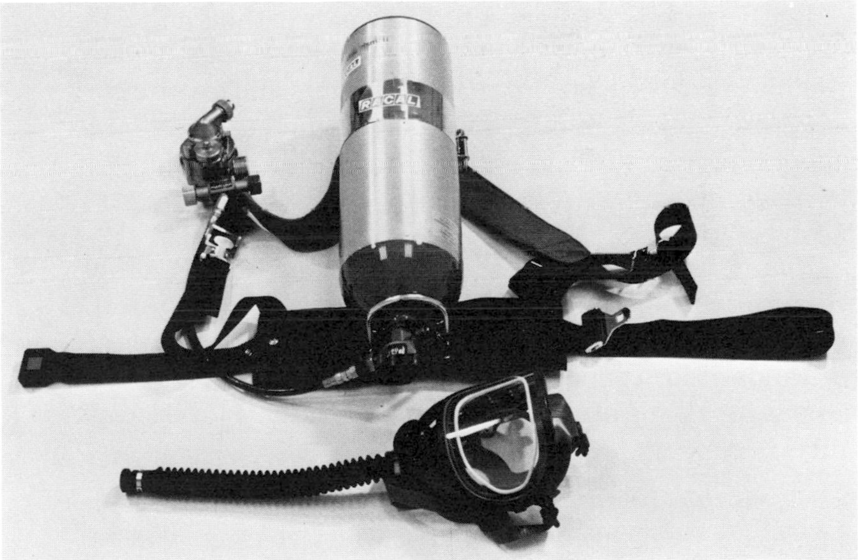

The Guardsman™ uses a pressure-demand breathing valve that maintains a positive pressure in the facemask at all times. This positive pressure keeps the smoke or toxic atmosphere from entering the face mask accidentally.

Figure E.56 The Racal Guardsman™ SCBA from Racal Panorama, Inc., features 30-, 45-, and 60-minute duration cylinders.

A shrill, piercing whistle sounds when the Guardsman's™ mainline valve is first opened, confirming that air pressure is available. The same whistle alerts the wearer when there is approximately 20 percent of the air supply remaining, allowing enough time to leave the hazardous area and replace the spent cylinder.

The Guardsman's™ pressure demand valve allows air into the facemask only when the wearer demands it and maintains a positive pressure in the mask. However, in an emergency or when the face mask needs to be flushed, the demand valve and regulator can be manually bypassed to provide a steady stream of air to the facemask.

Guardsman™ is provided with the Racal Resculator Quick Connect—an exclusive feature for use with the Racal escape hood or Racal buddy hose (Figure E.57). In an emergency, the hood permits a second person to escape from toxic atmospheres along with the wearer of the Guardsman™ mask. The buddy breathing hose can be used with two Guardsman™ units having Resculator Quick Connects. The hose is sealed on both ends by mechanical check valves to prevent entry of dirt or moisture. The hose has sufficient length to allow two users to move relatively independently.

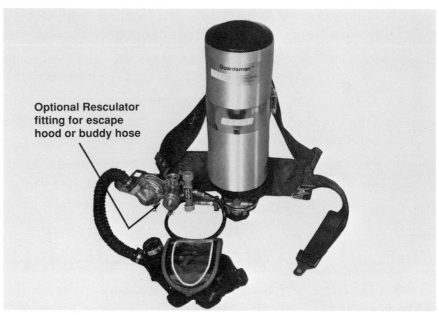

Figure E.57 The Racal Guardsman™ with optional Resculator fitting for escape hood or buddy hose. *Courtesy of Racal Panorama, Inc.*

Racal Panorama offers a full line of breathing air cylinders for Guardsman™ SCBA. The cylinders are made of aluminum or fiberglass-wrapped aluminum and feature horizontal handwheels, a built-in protected gauge, and a large, rubber bumper.

ACCESSORIES

Buddy Pak™ ESCBA/SAR. Five- and fifteen-minute pressure demand Buddy Paks™ are available for entry, work, and emergency egress situations. An airline fitting is included as standard for connection to an external compressor or a cascade breathing air system to provide the entry/work capability.

Respirator Communication System (RCS). The RCS comes complete with speaker/amplifier, battery charger, and surface-activated microphone (Figure E.58).

Escape Hood Kit or Buddy Breathing Hose. The escape hood with continuous flow orifice and hoseline is used with the Resculator connection. The buddy breathing hose is used to connect two Guardsman™ units in an emergency escape situation. Each comes in a cordura nylon pouch with a loop for the waist belt.

Facemask/Nosecup. The facemask and antifog nosecup are available in neoprene as well as silicone. Facemask disinfecting systems and lens cleaning kits are also available.

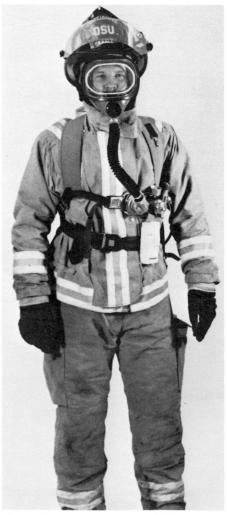

Figure E.58 Racal Guardsman™ unit with Respirator Communication System (RCS).

Others. Other accessories include Therma-clear antifog facemask lens insert, eyeglass frames and temple bars kit, neck strap for facemask with clips, wall-mount bracket and cover, and carrying/wall case.

DONNING AND DOFFING PROCEDURES
Predonning System Checks

Step 1: Carefully remove the apparatus from the case. Check the gauge on the cylinder. It should register 2,216 psi if fully charged to the maximum permissible pressure.

Step 2: With the yellow "mainline" valve closed, open the cylinder valve to pressurize the system up to this valve. Check for signs of air leaks at all threaded joints, paying particular attention to the connection between the high-pressure cylinder and the high-pressure hose.

Step 3: Put on the facepiece by placing your chin in first. Adjust the straps by tightening the lower chin straps first, the center straps second, and the top strap last.

Step 4: Test the facepiece for leaks by closing the bottom of the breathing tube hose with your hand and inhaling. The facepiece will collapse and remain collapsed while the breath is held if there are no leaks.

Step 5: With the facepiece secure on your face, thread the nut on the demand valve outlet onto the breathing tube coupling, and tighten firmly with your fingers.

Step 6: Open the "mainline" valve slowly. Listen for the whistle alarm to sound and then stop. The regulator gauge should show the same pressure as the gauge on the cylinder. (**NOTE:** The facemask must be secure on the face whenever the cylinder is turned on in order to prevent loss of air.)

Step 7: Close the cylinder valve, observe the regulator gauge, and if pressure remains constant while breath is held, the remaining pressure system is free of leaks. If pressure drops, check for leaks with soap suds, tighten connections, or have the equipment repaired as necessary.

Step 8: Turn the cylinder valve handwheel clockwise to close the valve. Inhale on the facemask, and breathe down the residual air pressure. The whistle alarm should sound as the pressure drops below 600 psi.

WARNING
If the whistle alarm does not sound, remove the equipment from service and tag for repair.

Donning The Racal Guardsman™

Step 1: Put on the apparatus as you would a coat with the cylinder valve pointing down and the flat portion of the backpack resting against your back. Inserting left arm first into harness is recommended.

Step 2: The breast plate on which the regulator and valves are mounted should now be adjusted so that the flat sole of plate rests against your chest. Snap the chest buckle onto the tang of breast plate (Figure E.59 on next page). Adjust by pulling tab end of strap. Pull the two remaining narrow straps down and back to tighten shoulder straps. The backpack should be positioned high on your back for the most comfortable fit. It is easier to adjust the harness by leaning forward so that the backback rests directly on your hips rather than hanging from the straps. Tighten waist belt last.

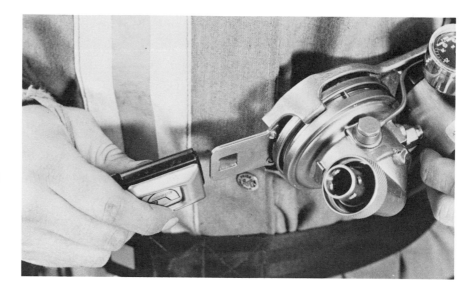

Figure E.59 Snap chest buckle onto tang of breast plate and adjust straps.

Step 3: When using the pressure-demand SCBA, the facemask must be secure on the user's face and the breathing tube connected to demand valve before unit is turned on to prevent loss of air. After donning backpack, check that the *mainline* knob (yellow) is in OFF position. Turn on cylinder valve approximately two turns.

Step 4: Check facemask for proper seal by putting the palm of your hand over quick-connect coupling at end of breathing tube. Inhale. Mask should collapse and remain collapsed while breath is held.

Step 5: Thread quick-connect coupling into demand valve outlet, and tighten firmly with fingers. At that instant, turn ON *mainline* knob (yellow) fully (approximately 2 turns). Begin breathing.

Step 6: Open red *bypass* valve momentarily at this time to be sure that it operates properly, and then close. Adjust head straps on facepiece as necessary to eliminate air leaks between face and facemask. There should be no noticeable airflow while holding breath.

Step 7: Inhale and exhale in facepiece to make sure that the mask is functioning properly. You are now ready to enter the danger area.

Step 8: To conserve cylinder contents, close mainline valve and do not wear facepiece until ready to enter the danger area. In the meantime, the facepiece may be attached through its "D" ring to snap on shoulder strap.

Step 9: Read pressure gauge at frequent intervals. The low-pressure warning alarm will begin to sound as soon as the cylinder pressure is reduced below approximately 600 psi.

Step 10: After use, close the cylinder valve and mainline valve (yellow knob).

Step 11: Replace used cylinder with cylinder fully charged with breathing-quality air.

Doffing The Racal Guardsman™
Step 1: Close the mainline valve.

Step 2: Uncouple facemask breathing tube from pressure-demand valve.

Step 3: Remove facemask by flipping tabs forward on head strap buckle. Leave head strap in fully extended position.

Step 4: Close cylinder valve.

Step 5: Open yellow mainline valve to relieve system pressure. When all pressure is released, close mainline valve.

Step 6: Release waist belt, and fully extend strap.

Step 7: Release chest buckle, and fully extend strap.

Step 8: Loosen shoulder adjusting straps, and extend fully. Swing backpack assembly off right shoulder first, and place in carrying case (if provided).

Step 9: Follow manufacturer's instructions for cleaning, disinfecting, and storage.

SCOTT AVIATION

Scott Aviation, a Figgie International Company, provides health and safety products for fire departments, industrial applications, and workers in potentially hazardous or emergency situations. Scott's Field Service and Technical Support Program coordinates and implements training, technical assistance, and other service and support activities for distributors and end users of Scott products. Scott is headquartered at 225 Erie Street, Lancaster, NY, 14086, 716-683-5100.

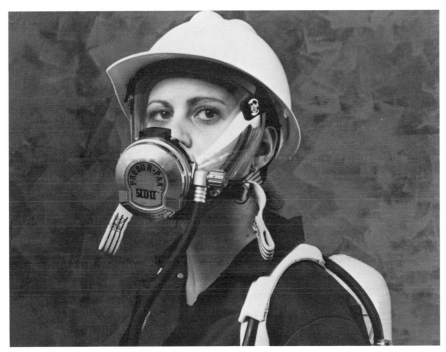

Figure E.60 The Scott Air-Pak® 4.5 SCBA features a facepiece-mounted regulator. The Vibralert® alarm vibrates, using both sound and feel to alert the user of low air supply. *Courtesy of Scott Aviation.*

SCBA FEATURES

The Scott Air-Pak® 4.5 SCBA provides breathable air in a choice of 30-minute, 45-minute, or 1-hour rated duration, when charged to 4,500 psi (Figure E.60). Features included are the cone-shaped Scott-O-Vista® facepieces in three color-coded sizes. The facepiece-mounted regulator has a quick-connect, ¼-turn capability. The Vibralert® alarm, pressure reducer, cylinder and valve assembly, Kevlar® harness and backframe assembly complete the list of performance features. The Vibralert® alarm vibrates to warn the user of diminishing air supply by both sound and feel.

An air-saving donning switch that stops airflow during donning and doffing is also available. The breathing regulator is also equipped with a Vibralert® end-of-service alarm. The pressure reducing regulator has no manual bypass control. Instead it uses a redundant dual path reducing system. The secondary system automatically supplies air if the primary system fails. When the secondary system is in operation, the Vibralert® alarm is also actuated to warn the user that the primary system has malfunctioned.

The Scott Air-Pak® 2.2 SCBA has similar features in a choice of 15-minute aluminum cylinders or 30-minute cylinders in either standard aluminum or lightweight construction when charged to

2,216 psi (Figure E.61). Features included with the Air-Pak® 2.2 are the Scott-O-Vista® facepiece and facepiece-mounted regulator with Vibralert® alarm, pressure reducer, cylinder and valve assembly. The donning switch is also available (Figure E.62).

Since most of the performance levels required by NFPA standard 1981 were already built into the Air-Pak® 2.2 and 4.5 SCBA, upgrading was easily accomplished by Scott. Scott was confident that their Air-Paks® would outperform the minimum acceptable requirements stipulated in NFPA 1981 and chose to test the units under conditions even more severe than required for compliance. Scott engineers learned that most units only required a new Scott-O-Vista® facepiece and regulator cover/diaphragm retaining ring. Others also needed new lubricants, O-rings, diaphragm, and Scott's flame-resistant harness assembly for extended temperature operation. Once upgraded at a Scott authorized facility, all Air-Pak® equipment will receive a new five-year warranty.

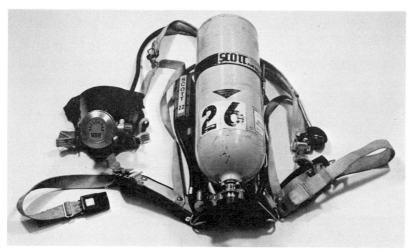

Figure E.61 The Scott Air-Pak 2.2® SCBA is available in 15- or 30-minute cylinders.

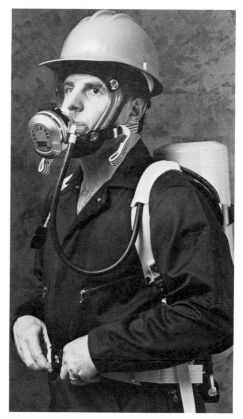

Figure E.62 The Scott Air-Pak 2.2® SCBA. *Courtesy of Scott Aviation.*

ACCESSORIES

Cascade Installation Systems. These systems are for cylinder recharge or extended duration applications and provide all the hardware necessary for installation. Available are 300-cubic-foot cylinders, cylinder interconnect pigtails, "T" blocks, manifolds, pressure reducers, high-performance quick-connect couplings, gauges, and other hose and accessory items.

Monitoring Instruments. Scott's Instruments and Control Group provides portable and continuous monitoring instruments for determining the presence and levels of combustible and toxic gases and vapors.

Speak-Ezee® Voice Amplification System. Models C and CP are battery-powered, personal voice amplification systems designed to improve voice communication for individuals wearing SCBA. They are also compatible with 2-way radios. The Model CP has a Personal Alert Safety System (PASS) and a low-battery warning signal.

All-Pro Voice Amplification and Radio Interface System. The Scott All-Pro Voice Amplification and two-way radio interface is a compact, battery-powered communication system designed to provide communication between personnel wearing Scott Air-Paks® 2.2 and 4.5, while maintaining the respirator certification, whether voice amplification or two-way radio communication is required.

Antifog Applique and/or Nosecup Assembly. Both accessories are used to minimize facepiece fogging, and one or the other is required for operation below 32°F.

Others. Other accessories include airline manifold, carrying and storage cases, neck strap, prescription and welding lens kits, and testing equipment.

DONNING AND DOFFING PROCEDURES
Preparing Scott Air-Pak® 4.5 For Use

> # WARNING
> The information below is meant to supplement, not replace, the instructions, training, supervision, maintenance, and other elements of your organized respiratory protection program.

Step 1: Place carrying case on ground or level surface, open lid, and check cylinder gauge for FULL indication. If not full, replace cylinder before use. Ensure that cylinder is firmly locked in position by the cylinder band and toggle strap.

> # WARNING
> A gauge indication of other than FULL may indicate an air leak in the cylinder and valve assembly or a malfunction of the gauge assembly.

Step 2: Stand to the right (top of cylinder end) of the open case, lean forward, position and spread out the shoulder straps, grasp the backframe with both hands, one on each side of the cylinder. Do not grasp the pressure reducer. Swing the respirator straight up and over the head, keeping elbows close to body.

Step 3: Rest the respirator on the back while slightly bent over. The shoulder straps will slide along the arms and into place on the shoulders. Straighten up as you pull down on the side straps to adjust the harness to fit the body.

Step 4: Connect the waist belt buckle and adjust by pulling forward on the two side-mounted belt ends.

Step 5: Readjust shoulder straps to ensure the weight is carried on the hips.

Step 6: Fully depress center of the donning switch on top of regulator and release.

Step 7: Slowly open cylinder valve fully. The user will both hear and feel the Vibralert® alarm in the facepiece start and stop. There will be no freeflow of air from the facepiece at this time.

> # WARNING
> If the Vibralert® alarm fails to actuate or does not stop after a brief interval, do not use the respirator. Remove it from service, and tag for repair by authorized personnel.

NOTE: If the donning switch has not been depressed prior to opening the cylinder valve, the alarm will not actuate due to the air flowing freely from the facepiece.

The user is now in "stand-by" condition. The respirator is in place but not in use.

Donning The Respirator

To begin use of respirator, don the facepiece (i.e., place facepiece on face and obtain a proper seal) as follows:

Step 1: With neck strap adjusted to the fully outward position, hold the head harness out of the way with one hand, or fold it back over the viewing area of the lens.

Step 2: Place the facepiece on the face with the chin properly located in the chin pocket.

Step 3: Pull the head harness over your head, and tighten the neck straps by pulling on the two strap ends.

Step 4: Stroke the head harness down the back of the head using one or both hands. Retighten neck strap.

Step 5: When the facepiece is sealed to the face, inhale sharply to actuate respirator. Air will then be supplied during inhalation.

Step 6: Ensure that the purge valve knob is rotated to the fully closed position (pointer on knob upward). Fully depress and hold the center of the donning switch on the top of the regulator. Inhale slowly and hold your breath momentarily. No leakage of air should be detected, and the facepiece will be drawn slightly to your face. (**NOTE:** If the purge valve is adjusted to produce a flow, it will not be possible to perform this check.)

WARNING
Do not use respirator if leakage of air into the facepiece is detected or if flow of air cannot be started automatically by inhaling. Repeat donning procedure, and stroke head harness strongly down the back of the head. In the event the facepiece cannot be adjusted to eliminate these conditions, a different size facepiece may be required to obtain proper facial fit.

Step 7: Remove your finger from the donning switch, and inhale sharply. The respirator shall function normally and supply air during the user's inhalation. (**NOTE:** If the purge valve is adjusted to produce a flow, it may not be possible to reset the donning switch by inhaling.)

Step 8: Proceed with use of respirator in accordance with your respiratory protection program.

WARNING
Entry into hazardous, potentially hazardous or unknown conditions is to be made using a full cylinder whenever possible.

NOTE: Every entry into a contaminated or unknown atmosphere should be planned to ensure that there is sufficient air supply to enter, carry out the tasks required, and return to a safe breathing area. The user should check the remote reading pressure gauge on the shoulder strap periodically to determine the rate of air consumption. In any event, the user must be certain to allow sufficient air for egress from the contaminated area. If entry is attempted after the air has been partially consumed (cylinder less than full), the user must be certain that the remaining air will be sufficient for safety.

Step 9: Leave the contaminated or unknown atmosphere immediately if the Vibralert® alarm actuates and, in a safe area, determine cause of alarm. When air supply has been depleted, replace cylinder.

> # WARNING
> When the Vibralert® alarm actuates, it warns the user that approximately 20 to 25 percent of the full pressure remains in the air cylinder (that is, approximately ¾ of the total air supply has been used) or that there is a malfunction in the primary breathing circuit. In either event, leave the contaminated area at once. In areas where more than one respirator is being used, you can identify your own alarm by sensing the vibrations through your facepiece.

Doffing

To doff the facepiece (i.e., remove the facepiece and terminate respiratory protection), proceed as follows:

Step 1: Leave the contaminated area or be certain that respiratory protection is no longer required.

Step 2: Loosen the neck strap by simultaneously lifting buckle-release levers outward (away from the head) and lifting the facepiece away from the face. The buckle-release levers are U-shaped extensions of the facepiece buckle assemblies.

Step 3: To stop the flow of air from the facepiece, fully depress the donning switch on top of the regulator and release.

> # WARNING
> If airflow from the regulator cannot be stopped by depressing the donning switch, immediately close the cylinder valve to prevent depletion of the air remaining in the cylinder.

NOTE: Operation of the donning switch is intended to prevent a freeflow of air and the depletion of the air supply when the facepiece is doffed. With the donning switch activated, the purge valve and Vibralert® will function normally. If the purge valve has been adjusted to produce a flow or if the Vibralert® is in operation, the air supply will continue to be depleted.

Step 4: Remove the facepiece by pulling it up and over the head.

Step 5: To prepare the facepiece for quick "re-donning," fold the head harness over the facepiece lens.

CAUTION: Any impact to the regulator while the cylinder valve is open and the donning switch is activated may cause air to flow from the regulator and deplete the air remaining in the cylinder.

NOTE: If the respirator is not going to be used for a period of time, close the cylinder valve. Leaving the donning switch activated and the cylinder valve open for an extended period of time may result in intermittent activation of the Vibralert® even when more than 25 percent of the air supply remains.

Step 6: To resume use of the respirator, repeat the facepiece donning procedure.

> # WARNING
> If respirator use is resumed after the air has been partially consumed (cylinder less than full), you must be certain that the remaining air will be sufficient for your safety.

WARNING

The flow of air may not start automatically when you inhale if the facepiece is not properly donned and sealed to the face. Redon facepiece or open purge valve.

Step 7: When respirator operations are completed and only when in a safe breathing area, remove unit from service. Replace the cylinder with a fully charged cylinder, and carry out the instructions for inspection, cleaning, and storage.

SURVIVAIR

Survivair®, located in Santa Ana, California, designs and manufactures a complete line of respiratory protection and life support equipment for industrial and fire fighting applications. Survivair, established in 1961, is a division of Comasec, Inc., a manufacturer and U.S. distributor of safety products. For more information about Survivair products, contact them at 3001 S. Susan St., Santa Ana, California, 92704, 800-821-7236 or 714-545-0410 in California.

SCBA FEATURES

Survivair introduced a new Mark 2™ SCBA in 1988 that was redesigned to meet and exceed all NFPA performance requirements (Figure E.63). Among the changes that were made to the Mark 2™ were the following:

- Increased airflow capacity to provide easier breathing and added respiratory protection
- New abrasion-resistant mask lens
- New Nomex® exterior and Kevlar® interior harness straps
- New placement of the second-stage regulator on the shoulder strap
- New cylinder band that allows 60-minute cylinders to be quickly changed to 30-minute cylinders, or vice versa

Standard features of the Mark 2™ include the following:

- Automatic, truly redundant backup for the first stage regulator
- Quick-connect facemask-to-regulator hose fittings
- Speaking diaphragm for clear communication with nearby firefighters
- Wide-view lens
- Mask molded from silicone

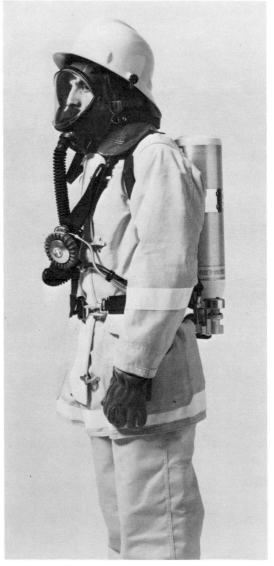

Figure E.63 Survivair's new Mark 2™ SCBA has been redesigned to meet and exceed NFPA performance requirements. *Courtesy of Survivair.*

- Four-point mask head strap
- Hinged backpack that bends with the wearer and transfers equipment weight from shoulders to hips

Currently, Survivair has introduced two new Mark 2™ breathing apparatus: a 60-minute Mark 2™ high-performance SCBA and a 30-minute Mark 2™ SCBA with hoop-wrapped cylinders (Figure E.64).

The 60-minute Mark 2™ breathing apparatus is available in the same performance configurations as the 30-minute NFPA Mark 2™ (Figure E.65). While the new Mark 2™ does not meet the NFPA 1981 standards if used as a 60-minute SCBA, it does meet the standards if used in a 30-minute configuration. Also available is a 30-minute Mark 2™ with hoop-wrapped cylinders.

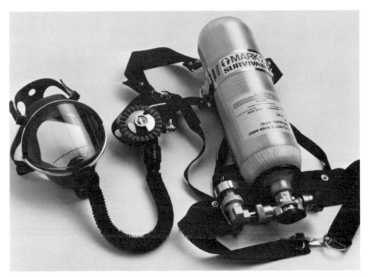

Figure E.65 The Mark 2™ features a truly redundant backup for the first-stage regulator and a cylinder band that allows 60-minute cylinders to be changed to 30-minute cylinders in seconds. *Courtesy of Survivair.*

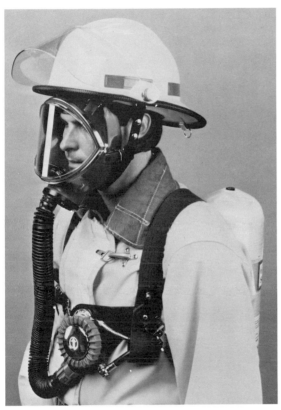

Figure E.64 The Mark 2™ includes a 60-minute and a 30-minute SCBA with hoop-wrapped cylinders. *Courtesy of Survivair.*

The Mark 2™ is being upgraded by introducing a new gauge. The new gauge line travels up the side of the air cylinder and over the wearer's right shoulder to where the gauge can be read more easily. Two kits are also available to upgrade the existing Survivair® XL-30 SCBA to the NFPA 1981 standard (Figure E.66). The flow kit provides all parts necessary to upgrade the mask and regulator, while the harness kit upgrades the unit's straps.

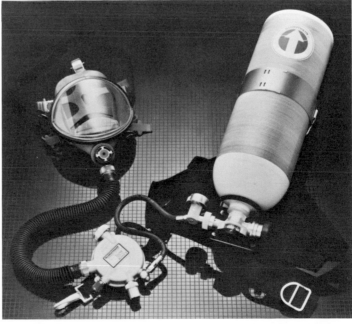

Figure E.66 Survivair offers XL-40 Self-Contained Breathing Apparatus NFPA approval upgrade kits. *Courtesy of Survivair.*

To assist in the training process, Survivair offers a four-color wall poster demonstrating how to don the Mark 2™ SCBA (Figure E.67). The poster is for display on job sites where workers will be using the Mark 2™ SCBA. The poster details, step to step, how to ready the Mark 2™ for use,

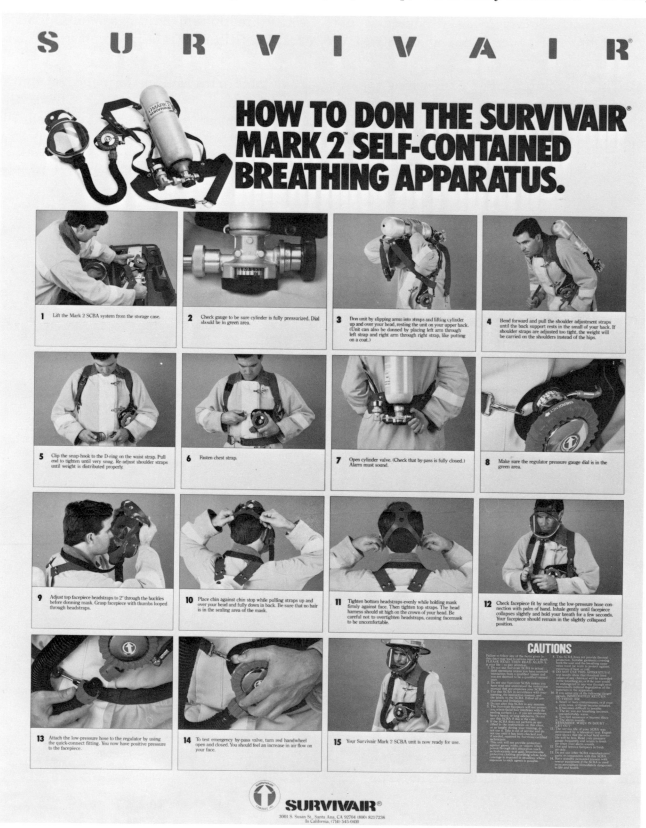

Figure E.67 This four-color wall poster by Survivair details donning procedures. *Courtesy of Survivair.*

remove the SCBA from the storage case, check the gauge to be sure the cylinder is fully pressurized, don the unit and facepiece, and check the emergency bypass valve.

ACCESSORIES

Small-Size Facepieces. Two small-sized facepieces are available for use with both the Mark 2™ SCBA and their full-face air-purifying respirators (Figure E.68). All components of the mask, such as lens, rims, and nozzle, are interchangeable.

Radio Communication System. Another accessory from Survivair is a radio communication system that enables workers wearing full-face masks to communicate with each other or with a base station by two-way radio (Figure E.69). A small bidirectional microphone is installed inside a prepunched facepiece lens, and a speaker on an adjustable boom is attached to either side of the lens rim assembly. The system allows the wearer to hear sounds in the environment in addition to radio transmissions. The radio communication system kit includes all necessary mounting hardware for factory-trained technicians to assemble the system.

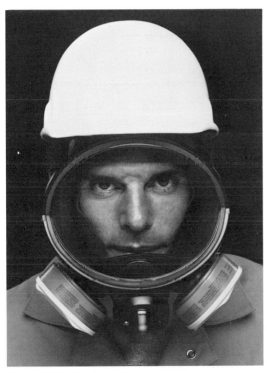

Figure E.68 Survivair offers two small facepieces for use in conjunction with both the Mark 2™ SCBA and their full-face air purifying respirators (shown). *Courtesy of Survivair.*

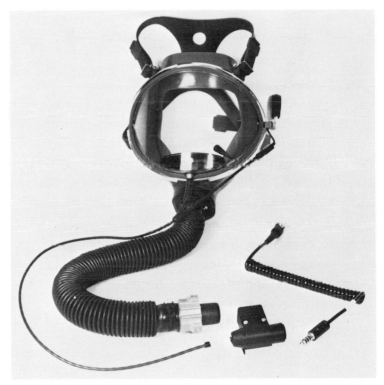

Figure E.69 Survivair's Radio Communication System enables workers wearing full-face masks to communicate with each other or with a base station via two-way radio. *Courtesy of Survivair.*

Mask Cleaners and Fit Test Ampules. Survivair respirator mask cleaners are individually wrapped pads designed to quickly clean respirator masks.

The respirator fit test ampules are individual packets of banana oil (amyl acetate) used to determine the proper fit of a respirator. Each Survivair respiratory fit test ampule box contains ten individual ampules.

High Temperature Harness. An upgrade to both the Mark 2™ and XL-30 offers a high temperature harness, which is coated with a dual fire retardant, aluminum/polyester resin for both flame and abrasion resistance.

Others. Survivair offers a full line of respirator accessories, including shower cap, nose cup kit, antifog solution, elastic headband set, spectacle kit, mask bag, probed full mask lens, and lens cover.

DONNING AND DOFFING PROCEDURES

Donning The Survivair® Mark 2™

CAUTION: Do not use Survivair SCBA in actual field operations unless you have received instruction from a qualified trainer and you are deemed to be a qualified, trained user.

Step 1: Lift the Mark 2™ SCBA system from the storage case.

Step 2: Check the gauge to be sure the cylinder is fully pressurized. The dial should be in the green area (Figure E.70).

Step 3: Don the unit by slipping your arms into straps and lifting the cylinder up and over your head, resting the unit on your upper back. (The unit can also be donned coat-fashion, by placing the left arm through the left strap and the right arm through the right strap.)

Step 4: Bend forward and pull the shoulder adjustment straps until the back support rests in the small of your back. If shoulder straps are adjusted too tight, the weight will be carried on the shoulders instead of the hips.

Step 5: Clip the snap-hook to the D-ring on the waist strap. Pull end to tighten until very snug. Readjust shoulder straps until weight is distributed properly.

Step 6: Fasten the chest strap.

Step 7: Open the cylinder valve. (Check that bypass is fully closed.) Alarm must sound (Figure E.71).

Step 8: Make sure the regulator pressure gauge dial is in the green area (Figure E.72).

Step 9: Adjust top facepiece head straps to 2 inches through the buckles before donning the mask. Grasp the facepiece with your thumbs looped through the head straps.

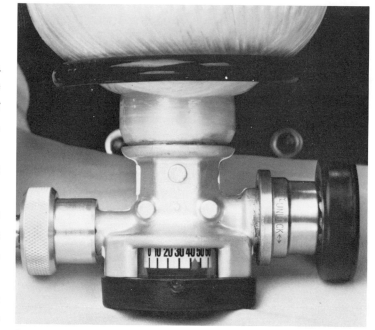

Figure E.70 Check the gauge to be sure the cylinder is fully pressurized. The dial should be in the green area. *Courtesy of Survivair.*

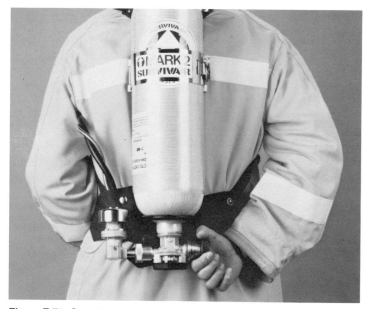

Figure E.71 Open the cylinder valve. Check that bypass is fully closed. Alarm must sound. *Courtesy of Survivair.*

Step 10: Place your chin against the chin stop while pulling the straps up and over your head and fully down in back. Be sure that no hair is in the sealing area of the mask.

Step 11: Tighten the bottom head straps evenly while holding the mask firmly against your face. Then tighten the top straps. The head harness should sit high on the crown of your head. Do not overtighten the head straps or the facemask will be uncomfortable.

Step 12: Check facepiece fit by sealing the low-pressure hose connection with the palm of your hand. Inhale gently until the facepiece collapses slightly, and hold your breath for a few seconds. Your facepiece should remain in the slightly collapsed position (Figure E.73).

Step 13: Attach the low-pressure hose to the regulator by using the quick-connect fitting. You now have positive pressure to the facepiece (Figure E.74).

Step 14: To test the emergency bypass valve, open and close the red handwheel. You should feel an increase in airflow on your face (Figure E.75).

Step 15: Your Survivair® Mark 2™ SCBA unit is now ready for use.

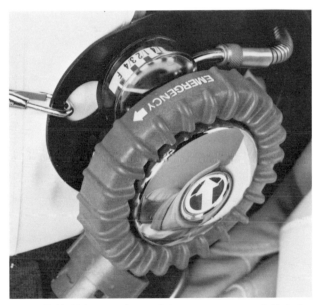

Figure E.72 Make sure the regulator pressure gauge dial is in the green area. *Courtesy of Survivair.*

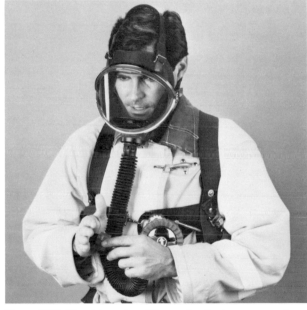

Figure E.73 Check facepiece fit by sealing the low-pressure hose connection with the palm of your hand. Inhale gently until facepiece collapses slightly. *Courtesy of Survivair.*

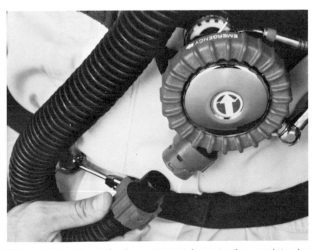

Figure E.74 Attach the low-pressure hose to the regulator by using the quick-connect fitting. *Courtesy of Survivair.*

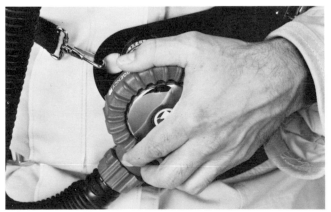

Figure E.75 Test the emergency bypass valve by opening and closing the red handwheel; there will be an increase in airflow to the face. *Courtesy of Survivair.*

Doffing The Survivair® Mark 2™

Step 1: When you are in fresh air, disconnect the low-pressure hose from the second-stage regulator.

Step 2: Remove the facepiece.

Step 3: Push in the locking sleeve on the cylinder valve, and rotate it counterclockwise to disengage it. Close the cylinder valve.

Step 4: Open the bypass valve to vent the high-pressure air from the lines.

Step 5: Unsnap the waist belt, loosen the shoulder straps, and remove the apparatus.

NOTE:

Hycar is a Trademark of B.F. Goodrich Company.

Nomex is a registered trademark of DuPont.

Appendix F

SCBA INSPECTION AND MAINTENANCE CHECKLIST

Serial Number _____ **Identification** _____ **Location** _____

	FACEPIECE ASSEMBLY			CYLINDER ASSEMBLY				REGULATOR ASSEMBLY					HARNESS/BACKPACK	
Date	Low-Pressure Hose OK	Exhalation Valve/Speaking Diaphragm OK	Facepiece, Lens, Harness OK	Cylinder Pressure	Cylinder Valve Closed	High-Pressure Hose OK	Gaskets, Seals, Screens OK	Mainline Valve in Correct Position	Bypass Valve Closed	Regulator Operation OK	Low-Pressure Alarm OK	Diaphragm OK	Straps Adjusted Out	Harness, Backpack OK

DAILY/WEEKLY MAINTENANCE CHECKLIST

INSPECTION AFTER EACH USE

Date Used	Date Inspected	Facepiece Assembly Cleaned	Harness Cleaned	Entire SCBA Cleaned	Case/Mounting Area Cleaned	Daily/Weekly Inspection Performed	SCBA Operation Checked	Remarks	Inspected By

MONTHLY INSPECTION

Date	Daily/Weekly Inspection Performed	Tested Bypass Valve for Leaks	Tested Mainline Valve for Leaks	Tested Regulator*	Hydrostatic Test Date Checked	Tested Cylinder Connections	SCBA Operation Checked	Remarks	Inspected By

*Regulator should be tested by qualified technician or as recommended by manufacturer.

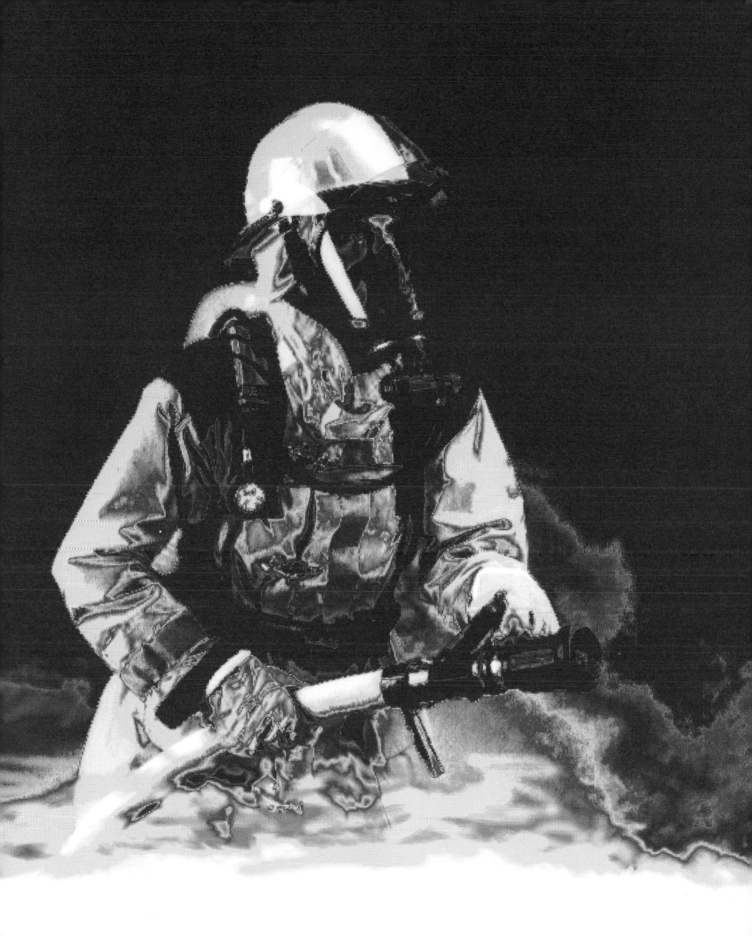

Answers

Review Answers

Chapter 1

1. True
2. False. The epiglottis is a muscle that closes off the trachea when a person swallows. The trachea and esophagus are the two air passages.
3. True
4. False. Arteries carry oxygenated blood away from the heart, and veins carry deoxygenated blood to the heart.
5. False. A tense or fearful firefighter will use more air than a calm firefighter in the same period of time.
6. False. Duration testing does not consider the additional amount that will be needed by persons that are physically unfit.
7. A. Deliver oxygen to body cells
   B. Remove carbon dioxide from body cells
8. A. Nose
   B. Pharynx
   C. Larynx
   D. Trachea
   E. Bronchi
   F. Lungs
9. A. Being overweight
   B. Smoking cigarettes
10. A. Arteries
    B. Veins
    C. Capillaries

11. Pressure
12. Atrium, ventricle
13. Heart rate, breathing rate
14. Hemoglobin
15. External respiration is the transfer of oxygen and carbon dioxide in the lungs.
16. Internal respiration is the exchange of oxygen and carbon dioxide between the blood and body cells and the use of oxygen by the body cells.
17. Controlled breathing is a conscious effort to reduce air consumption by forcing exhalation from the mouth and allowing natural inhalation through the nose.
18. Diffusion is the movement of a substance from an area of higher concentration of the substance to an area of lower concentration.
19. Toxic gases burn lung tissue and can damage the alveoli.
20. Self-contained breathing apparatus will generally cause a 20 percent decrease in physical performance caused in part by the firefighter inhaling previously exhaled air, which contains carbon dioxide, and by the negative pressure created in the mask.

Chapter 2

1. False. Flashover is a condition in which excessive accumulation of heat from a fire raises flammable gases and other combustibles to their ignition temperatures, and the combustibles then ignite simultaneously. Rollover is the movement of flames upward to and across the ceiling.
2. True
3. False. Carbon monoxide levels are extremely high during the overhaul stage due to incomplete combustion.
4. True
5. True

6. False. The effects of asbestos exposure may not show up for many years.
7. B
8. D
9. C
10. A. Black smoke becoming dense gray-yellow
    B. Confinement and excessive heat
    C. Little or no visible flame
    D. Smoke leaving the building in puffs or at intervals
    E. Smoke-stained windows with heat-induced cracking of glass

11. A. By inhalation
    B. By absorption through the skin
    C. By ingestion into the digestive tract
12. A. Nature of the combustible source
    B. Rate of heating
    C. Temperature of the evolved gases
    D. Oxygen (O_2) concentration
13. Lighter, heavier
14. Hydrochloric acid
15. Nitrogen-bearing, nylon, wool
16. Benzene
17. Excessive heat quickly entering the lungs can cause a serious drop in blood pressure, leading to cardiovascular collapse through shock, and it can also burn the respiratory tract.

18. A synergistic effect occurs when the combined effect of inhaling two or more substances is more toxic or irritating than the total effect would be if each were inhaled separately.
19. The chief danger of carbon dioxide exposure is the increased respiratory rate it causes, which in turn increases the amount of smoke and other toxic gases inhaled.
20. The U.S. Department of Transportation defines a hazardous material as "any substance or material in any form which may pose an unreasonable risk to health and safety or property when transported in commerce."

Chapter 3

1. False. Open-circuit is the most commonly used type of self-contained breathing apparatus.
2. True
3. True
4. False. The valve settings should not be changed unless the emergency bypass is needed.
5. A. Backpack
   B. Air cylinder
   C. Regulator
   D. Facepiece
6. A. To reduce the pressure of the cylinder air to a pressure slightly above atmospheric pressure
   B. To regulate the flow of air to meet the respiratory requirements of the wearer
7. A. Releasing cylinder air
   B. Using a nosecup
   C. Applying an antifogging chemical
8. A. Physical condition of the user
   B. Degree of physical exertion
   C. Emotional stability of the user
   D. Condition of the apparatus
   E. Cylinder pressure before use
   F. Amount of training and experience with breathing apparatus

9. Maximum
10. Minimum
11. Less
12. Compressed, liquid, compressed air
13. 45, 1 275, 88, 1 699
14. 100, 700
15. Speaking diaphragms
16. Chemical scrubber
17. With positive-pressure SCBA a slight increase in pressure is maintained in the facepiece. This increase in pressure helps prevent contaminants from entering the facepiece if there is a leak.
18. Interchanging parts is not a recommended practice, voids NIOSH/MSHA certification, may void warranties, and may leave the department or firefighter liable for any injuries incurred.
19. Using an airline enables the firefighter to travel up to 300 ft (90 m) from the air supply and to work for several hours, if necessary, without wearing a backpack.
20. A closed-circuit SCBA is sometimes called a "rebreather" apparatus because when using such as system, the user's exhaled air stays within the system for reuse.

Chapter 4

1. False. SCBA, including the facepiece, should be donned and airflow started in fresh air.
2. True
3. True
4. False. Each firefighter is responsible for determining his or her individual point of no return.
5. False. Qualitative fit testing is subjective, whereas quantitative fit testing, which requires using a special test instrument, is not.
6. B
7. C
8. C
9. B
10. A. Using the provided SCBA in accordance with instructions and training
    B. Protecting the SCBA from damage as appropriate
    C. Reporting any malfunctions or damage
    D. Inspecting and maintaining the SCBA in accordance with department SOPs
11. A. The firefighter's training
    B. The firefighter's physical condition
    C. The firefighter's activity
    D. The firefighter's mental state under the stressful conditions of an emergency
12. A. Before entering a hazardous atmosphere, don the apparatus, start the airflow, and make sure that the equipment is operating properly.
    B. Always work in pairs.
    C. Stay in contact with a wall, hoseline, life line/guide line, or SCBA team member.
    D. Work to control breathing and conserve air.
    E. Be extremely cautious if forced to breathe through the bypass valve and exit immediately.
    F. Do not take off the facepiece if out of breathing air while still in a hazardous atmosphere.
    G. Report any malfunctions or apparent damage and immediately take the unit out of service.
13. 20, 25
14. Least
15. Irritant smoke, odor, taste
16. PASS stands for "personal alert safety systems." A PASS device sounds an audible alarm when the firefighter remains motionless for a predetermined length of time, alerting others that the firefighter is in trouble and may be injured.
17. Yes. SCBA must always be worn during overhaul inside buildings until the buildings are well ventilated with fresh air and it has been established through monitoring or air sampling that toxic gases are removed and the atmosphere is not oxygen deficient.
18. If a firefighter knows his or her air consumption rate, the firefighter can then predict how many minutes of air he or she has available at any given time, can determine the point of no return, and can watch the regulator pressure gauge and pace himself or herself accordingly.
19. Guide lines are used by firefighters to stay together, make searches more methodical and thorough, and provide escape and rescue routes. A guide line is a special rope that may be used either as a main guide line to indicate a route between the entry control point and the scene of operations or as a branch line (personal line) when it is necessary to traverse or search deeply off the main guide line.
20. The Breathing Apparatus Officer is responsible for monitoring the length of time each firefighter spends in the structure; predicting each firefighter's maximum safe operating time; calculating, at intervals, the remaining air available for each firefighter; and recalling the team when a firefighter is low on air.

Chapter 5

1. False. Methods for donning the facepiece differ, depending upon the manufacturer and whether the regulator is harness-mounted or is facepiece-mounted.
2. False. When preparing to don the backpack using the over-the-head method, the firefighter should crouch or kneel at the end opposite the cylinder valve.
3. True
4. True
5. False. Facepiece harness straps should be tightened by pulling them evenly and simultaneously to the rear.
6. True
7. C
8. C
9. D
10. B
11. A
12. A. Lever clamp
    B. Spring clamp
    C. Flat hook
13. Either
14. Fastened
15. After
16. The firefighter can press the facepiece against his or her face and exhale to free the valve. The firefighter must use caution when doing so in order to prevent discomfort and possible damage to the inner ear from exhaling forcefully.
17. The firefighter should cross arms, left over right, so that the left hand is holding the left strap and the right hand is holding the right strap at the top of the shoulder harness.
18. The two differences in design that affect donning are the number of straps used to tighten the head harness and whether or not the regulator attaches to the facepiece.
19. No. A facepiece tightened too much will be uncomfortable or may cut off circulation to the face. Additionally, a firefighter should be fitted with the type and size of facepiece that fits his or her face properly.
20. The firefighter can check for positive pressure by gently breaking the facepiece seal by inserting two fingers under the edge of the facepiece. The firefighter should be able to feel air moving past his or her fingers if positive pressure is present.

Chapter 6

1. True
2. False. Steel and aluminum cylinders must be checked every five years, and composite cylinders must be checked every three years.
3. True
4. False. Only those disinfecting agents recommended by the manufacturer should be used. Alcohol may damage the rubber.
5. False. SCBA should be thoroughly cleaned and disinfected after every use. Properly stored SCBA may not require cleaning at every inspection.
6. True
7. True
8. False. According to ANSI Z88.5-1981, SCBAs must be reconditioned by authorized personnel whenever necessary and at intervals specified by the manufacturer.
9. C
10. C
11. D
12. A
13. B
14. A. Cylinder assembly
    B. Regulator assembly
    C. Facepiece assembly
    D. Harness and backpack assembly
15. 90
16. Open, closed
17. The low-pressure hose and the exhalation valve should be checked for visible signs of wear, broken parts, hardening, or deterioration. The low-pressure hose should be checked for any cracking by pulling or stretching the hose.
18. This difference in readings indicates that the regulator is not functioning properly and that it should be removed from service and tagged for repair.

19. The inspection of the harness assembly should include checking to see that all straps are adjusted out fully and are untwisted and smooth, checking buckles to see that they readily clasp and unclasp, and checking harness for worn or torn areas.

20. The main difference between the procedures is that certain tests should be performed during monthly inspection.

Chapter 7

1. True
2. True
3. False. Compressors used for breathing air cannot be treated as if they are shop compressors; a department should use its breathing-air compressor only for producing breathing air used to recharge cylinders.
4. True
5. False. The air intake filter on the compressor removes only solid particles and suspended liquids; it does not remove oil vapors, gaseous hydrocarbons, toxic gases, or enough water.
6. D
7. C
8. A
9. C
10. C
11. A. Quantity of air needed by the department
    B. Space availability
    C. Water availability
    D. Air purity at compressor installation
    E. Cost of maintenance
12. A. Mechanical filter
    B. Dryer
    C. Air sweetener
    D. Carbon monoxide converter

13. 300 (149), aftercooler
14. Dryer
15. 25, -64 (-53.3)
16. 300, 600
17. Outside intake pipes should be made of a noncorrodible material such as plastic, copper, or stainless steel. Galvanized pipe should not be used.
18. If sumps or the collector is not drained, the water and oil will be forced through each stage of the compressor, through the components of the air purification system, and probably into the breathing air cylinders.
19. Oil used in compressors is specially formulated to reduce the possibility of toxic air developing during compressor use. Only the type of oil recommended by the manufacturer should be used in a compressor.
20. Dew point is the temperature at which the water vapor in the air begins to condense as droplets of liquid.

Chapter 8

1. True
2. True
3. False. Rescue operations may or may not require breathing apparatus, depending on the situation found by the responding company.
4. True
5. False. Low temperature extremes can adversely affect SCBA performance.
6. False. SCBA will not protect against absorption of chemicals and radiation through the skin.

7. D
8. D
9. B
10. A. Fire or waterflow alarms
    B. Structure fires
    C. Smoke investigations
    D. Gas leaks and spills
    E. Vehicle fires
    F. First response at hazardous materials incidents
11. Effects of heat on the firefighter
12. Level B

13. -25, -31.69
14. Chemical entry
15. 300, 100
16. Atmosphere that is hazardous, that is suspected of being hazardous, or that may rapidly become hazardous
17. Failure to use a nosecup can result in facepiece fogging and severely impaired vision.
18. By using a remote-type fill station connected to an air unit, it is not necessary to carry SCBA cylinders from street level to an interior staging area on an upper floor, thereby saving manpower for fire fighting tasks.
19. The firefighter in a fully encapsulated suit first has to leave the hazardous area, undergo primary decontamination, partially remove the suit, have the cylinder changed, and put the suit back on before the firefighter can resume work.
20. A confined space is an enclosure that has limited openings for entry and exit, has unfavorable natural ventilation that may contain or produce contaminants, and is not intended for continuous occupation.

Chapter 9

1. True
2. False. According to NFPA standards, emergency breathing methods should be outlined in a department's policy.
3. True
4. False. A damaged facepiece offers some protection. The firefighter should keep the facepiece on so that he or she will still have the benefit of positive pressure to the face.
5. True
6. True
7. False. Skip breathing is an emergency breathing technique and should be used only in emergencies.
8. False. Using a glove to filter air for breathing may filter out some of the smoke particles but none of the toxic gases and will provide no assistance in an oxygen-deficient atmosphere.
9. True
10. True
11. D
12. C
13. D
14. C
15. B
16. Bypass breathing
17. If a victim or another firefighter is pinned and cannot be freed by the firefighter, it is recommended that the firefighter leave to get assistance rather than stay and attempt to share air with the victim and possibly become a victim.
18. Some of the disadvantages of using the low-pressure hose-to-facepiece method are that using the procedure may void NIOSH certification of the equipment, that the firefighter with the available air can be burned by the hot metal coupling on the other firefighter's low-pressure hose, and that the facepiece seal of each firefighter is violated.
19. The team members share the same regulator by alternately pressing each team member's low-pressure hose against the regulator of the SCBA having the adequate air supply.
20. Skip breathing is an emergency breathing technique used to extend the remaining air supply. The firefighter inhales, as during regular breathing, holds the breath as long as it would take to exhale, and then inhales once again before exhaling.

Index

A

Accidental submersion, 267
   firefighter guidelines, 269-270
   SCBA operation in, 267-269
   training for, 85
Acrolein (CH_2CHCHO), 40-41
Activated carbon, 208
Adrenaline, 15-16
Adsorbents, 207-208
Aerobic exercises, 18-19
Aftercooler, 205
Air consumption
   caused by various activities, 17
   individual rate of, determining, 89-90
   records, 115
   see also Air supply, duration of
Air cylinders
   assembly, 58
   inspection, 177-178
   changing
   closed-circuit SCBA, 162-163
   during hazardous materials incident, 243
   open-circuit SCBA, 160
   moisture in, 237
   rapid refilling, while wearing SCBA, 221-222
   recharging systems, 199-223
Airline system, 242
   equipment, 66-67
   procedures for, 247
Air purification cartridge
   replacement, 211
   service life of, 210-212
Air purification systems, 207-212
   four basic components of, 207-208
   overloading, 204
Air purifier, 208
Air quality
   standards, 210
   testing, 212-215
Air supply
   components of system, 199
   duration of, 54-55, 88, 241-242
   problems, handling of, 199
   variables affecting, 54
Air sweetener, in air purification system, 208
Alveoli, 9-11
  damage to, 12
  effect of smoke on, 30
American National Standards Institute (ANSI), 2, 17, 53
ANSI. *See* American National Standards Institute
Antifogging chemicals, 64, 66

Anxiety, 103-104
Aorta, 10, 13
Arteries, 13-14
Asbestos, 42, 236
Asphyxiant, 38
Asphyxiation, 41
Atmosphere(s)
   hazardous, 32-34, 88, 97
   oxygen-deficient, 38, 42-43
   toxic, 32-34
Audible alarm, 86, 126, 129, 132, 137

B

Backdraft, 29-30
   indications of, 30
Backpack and harness assembly, 58
   inspection, 180
Benzene (C_6H_6), 42
Bleed, 179, 221
Brain stem, 10
Branch guide line, 100
Breathing air
   allowable contamination levels, 213-214
   approved, 218
   compressor and purifier guidelines, 222-223
   filtering, 266
   quality of, 212
Breathing-air system, 236
Breathing apparatus (B.A.), 99
Breathing Apparatus Officer, 101, 260
Buddy breathing, 114, 243, 257
Buddy system, 247
Bypass valve, 60, 178
   inspection of, 183-184
   internal fogging, 64
   use of in regulator malfunctions, 261

C

Capillaries, 13-14
Carbon dioxide (CO_2), 11, 38-39
Carbon monoxide (CO), 14, 34-37
   toxic effects of, 36
Carbon monoxide converter, 208
Carbonyl chloride, 39
Carboxyhemoglobin (COHb), 35
Carcinogen, 41-42
Cardiovascular system, 12-14
   improving aerobic capacity, 18
Cascade system, 215-221
   filling from, 218-221
Catalysts, 207
Center for Disease Control, 182

Chemical entry suits, 240-241
Chemical scrubber, 69, 162
Cigarette smoking, 17, 19
Cilia, 12
Claustrophobia, 15
Cleaning and sanitizing guidelines, 95
Climate, as SCBA selection factor, 70
Closed-circuit breathing apparatus, 2, 67-70
    advantages and disadvantages, 70-71
    maintenance, 69-70
    positive pressure in, 69
Clothing, protective, 83, 240-241
Common regulator, sharing, 264-265
Communication devices, 65-66
Communications, 65-66
    improving, 65
    teaching, 259
    training in, 85-86
Composite cylinders, 184, 189
Compressed air, quality of, 212
Compressed Gas Association (CGA), 209-210
Compressed oxygen, 219
Compressor/purifier, filling from, 220-221
Compressors, 200-202
    buying, factors to consider in, 201-202
    location of, 202-204
    maintenance, cost of, 202
    safety factors, 204-207
    shop-built, 207
Condensation, 64
Conditioning program, 55
    points to consider, 19
Confined space, 43
Confined space entry, 243-250
    harnesses and lifelines for, 246
    procedural outline, 244
Contact lenses, 84
Controlled breathing, 15-16, 88, 113-114
Controlled test atmosphere, 93
Corrugated hose, 63
Crash courses, 104
Cyanosis, 39-40
Cylinder gauge, 126, 132
Cylinder pressure, 56
Cylinder pressure gauge, 54, 184
Cylinder testing, 189-190
Cylinder valve, 137, 162
    inspection of, 183, 184

D

Decontamination, 242-243
Defects, SCBA, inspection and testing for, 95
Defense mechanisms, 11-12
Dermatitis (skin rash), 181
Desiccants (drying agents), 207-208
Dew point, 209, 212

recommended levels, 209-210
Diastole, 13
Diffusion, 10-11
Doffing, 86
    closed-circuit SCBA, 158-159
    open-circuit SCBA, 148-152
Donning, 178
    backpack
        compartment or backup mount, 136-137
        cross-armed coat method, 128-132
        over-the-head method, 125-128
        regular coat method, 132-134
        seat mount, 134-136
        side or rear mount, 136
    closed-circuit SCBA, 152-159
    open-circuit SCBA, 125-147
Donning mode, 132, 137, 148, 151
Donning switch, 126, 129, 132, 137, 141, 146, 148, 151
Dryer, in air purification system, 208
Duration rating tests, 17

E

Economics, as SCBA selection factor, 71
Edema, 41-42
Elastomer, 64, 176
Electrolysis, 209
Emergency conditions breathing, 257-269
    department responsibility, 258
    firefighter responsibility, 259
Emergency escape, 243
Emergency escape breathing support system (EEBSS), 262
    using other types of, 264
Emotional stability, 15-16
Engine company operations, 234
Entry Control Officer (E.C.O.), 99
Entry control system, 97-99
Epiglottis, 9
Equipment, interchanging of, 175
Esophagus, 9
Etiologic agents, 43
Exertion, levels of, 16-17
Exhalation valve, 55, 60, 63-64
    checking, 141, 146, 175
    frozen, coping with, 238
Explosion, 204
Explosive breathing technique, 269
Explosive limits, 244
Eyeglasses, 66, 84

F

Facepiece
    checking seal, 146
    cleaning and sanitizing, 95
    donning, 138-139

fit of, 90
fogging, 66
interchanging, 139
proper sealing of, 64, 82-83, 139
records, 94
removal of, 86
seal failures, 94
sharing, 260
testing fit, 91
Facepiece assembly, 63-65
    inspection, 175-177
Facepiece-mounted regulator
    doffing with, 151-152
    donning facepiece with, 143-148
Fight or flight response, 15
Filter, air purification system, 208
Filter breathing, 266
Fire entry suits, 240-241
Fire extinguishment, 234
Fire gases, chart of common, 33
Fireground
    special situations involving operations, 237-240
    uses of SCBA, 234-237
Five-minute escape device, 267
Flashover, 29
Fluorine gas, 205
Fogging, 64, 66
Formaldehyde (HCHO), 41
Free-burning stage, of fire, 29
Fume test, 91

G
Geographical area, as SCBA selection factor, 70
Grade D breathing air, 207
Guide line system, 99-100
Guide ropes, 99-100

H
Hair, facial or long, as safety hazard, 82-83
Hand signals, as communication method, 86
Harness-mounted regulator, 176
    doffing with, 148-150
    donning facepiece with, 139-143
    web-type, 139
Hazardous atmospheres, 32-34, 88, 97
    training in use of SCBA in, 115
Hazardous environments, use of airline respira-
    tors in, 242
Hazardous materials incidents, 43-45, 240
Health risks, 19
Heart, 12-13
    see also Cardiovascular system
Helmets, 83, 141-143, 147-148, 151, 158
Hemoglobin, 14, 35
High-Efficiency Particulate Air (HEPA) filters,
    242

High-pressure hose, 58, 162, 177-178
High-rise buildings, fires in, 239
Hood, protective, 83, 142
Hopcalite™, 208
Horizontal entry, procedures for, 250
Hose advancement, 234
Hydrochloric acid, 37
Hydrogen chloride (HCl), 37
Hydrogen cyanide (HCN), 37-38
Hydrogen sulfide (H₂S), 41
Hydrostatic test, 178, 184, 190
Hypoxia, 28, 35

I
Identification numbers, 186
Immediately Dangerous to Life and Health
    (IDLH), 32
Individual emergency conditions breathing, 257
Information
    other sources of, 283
    tally, 97
Inspection
    after use, procedure for, 181-183
    daily or weekly, 174-175
    external, 190
    internal, 190
    monthly, 183-186
    procedure for, 175
Irritant smoke test, 91-92
Isoamyl acetate (banana oil), 92

L
Laryngospasm, 37
Larynx (voice box), 9
Lawrence Livermore National Laboratory study,
    84
Leak-testing, 183-186
Lens fogging, 66
Level A protection, 240
Level B protection, 240, 243
Lifeline signals, 259
Lift systems, 247
Lipid pneumonia, 30
Lower Explosive Limit (LEL), 244
Low-pressure alarm, 62, 88, 97, 179
Low-pressure hose, 63, 141, 148, 175, 266
Low-pressure hose-to-facepiece method, 265-266

M
Main guide line, 100
Mainline valve, 60, 148, 178
    inspection of, 183-184
    opening, 150, 162
Maintenance
    cylinder testing, 189-190
    preventive, 174

rebuilding, 189
record-keeping, 186
repair and reconditioning, 188-189
SCBA advisories, 190
storage, 187-188
Manufacturer(s)
reliability of, as SCBA selection factor, 71
of self-contained breathing apparatus, 299-344
Manufacturer's warranty, 188
Mask-mounted eyeglasses, 84
Mask-mounted regulator, 61
Mazes, in training firefighters, 107, 110
Mechanical filter, 208
Medium-pressure air compressor, 199
Mental fitness, 15
Mine Safety Appliances Company (MSA), 263
Mine Safety and Health Administration (MSHA), 54
Mobile air supply units, 215-216
Modification, SCBA, 190-191
Moisture conversion data, 211
Molecular sieve, 208
Monitoring systems
in United Kingdom, 97
in United States and Canada, 100-101
MSHA. *See* Mine Safety and Health Administration
Muscle-toning exercises, 18
Myocardium, 13

N
National Fire Protection Association (NFPA), 704
placard, 44
National Fire Protection Association (NFPA), 2, 15, 17, 53, 102
National Institute for Occupational Safety and Health (NIOSH), 2, 42, 54, 190
Negative buoyancy, 268
Negative pressure, 15
Negative-pressure test, 146
NFPA. *See* National Fire Protection Association
NIOSH. *See* National Institute for Occupational Safety and Health
Nitric oxide (NO), 39-40
Nitrogen dioxide (NO$_2$), 39-40
Nonfireground operations, 240-250
Nosecup, 16, 64, 66
freezing temperatures, 237

O
Occupational Safety and Health Administration (OSHA), 2, 53, 84
Odorous vapor test, 92-93
Open-circuit breathing apparatus, 2, 56
four basic components, 56-65
Open-plan buildings, fires in, 239

Operational considerations, in SCBA selection, 71
O-ring, 161-162, 175
Overhaul operations, 236
Overweight, 17, 19
Oxygen, 7, 10-11, 16
concentrations of, and their effects, 43
deficiency, 28, 42-43
rates of consumption, 17
transportation of, 12
Oxygen-deficient atmospheres, 38, 42-43

P
Parts per million (ppm), 31-32, 94, 209
Personal alert safety systems (PASS), 86
Personnel, standby, 247
Pharynx (throat), 8
Phosgene (COCl$_2$), 39
Physical exertion, degree of, 16
Physical fitness, 17-19, 86-87
Piston compressors, 200
Point of no return, 88-90, 113
Polyvinyl chloride (PVC), 37, 39
Portable radio, as method of communication, 85
Posicheck™, 187
Positive buoyancy, 268
Positive pressure, 14, 54, 60, 129, 142
in closed-circuit breathing apparatus, 69
in facepiece-mounted regulator, 147
Positive-pressure switch, 178
Pounds Per Square Inch (PSI; psi), 126, 129, 132, 137
Preventive maintenance, 174
Proper seal, 64
Protection factor, 94
Protection limits, of SCBA, 87
Protective clothing, 83, 240-241
see also specific kind
Proximity suits, 240
Pulmonary edema, 28, 39, 40, 42
Pulse rate
during exercise, 18-19
finding maximum, 18

Q
Qualitative facepiece fit tests, 91-93
Quantitative facepiece fit tests, 93-94
Quick-Fill™ system, 263

R
Rebreather apparatus, 53, 69
Rebuilding, 189
Recharging air cylinders, 199-223
guidelines, 96-97
Reconditioning, 188-189
guidelines, 95
Record keeping, 94-95, 186-187

computerized systems of, 187
Regulating agencies and organizations, 281-283
Regulator assembly, 59-62
    inspection, 178-179
Regulator gauge, 62, 126, 132, 137
Regulator, location of, 138
Relief-valve failure, 204
Remote fill station, 239
Repairs/repairing
    guidelines, 95
    qualified, 188
Rescue company operations, 236-237
Reserve cylinders, 188
Respiration
    external, 9-10
    internal, 10-11
Respiratory hazards, 27-45
    backdrafts, 29-30
    elevated temperatures, 28-29
    flashover, 29
    not associated with fire, 42-45
    oxygen deficiency, 28
    smoke inhalation, 30
    toxic gases, 30-45
Respiratory system, 7-12
    defense mechanisms, 11-12
    hazards, 27-45
    organs of, 8-9
Response hazards, as SCBA selection factor, 70-71
Rollover, 29

S

Safety, 82-87
Safety features, knowledge of, 87
Safety guidelines
    basic, 90
    department's responsibility for following, 95
Safety responsibilities, department's
    at emergency scene, 97-102
    at station, 91-97
Safety responsibilities, firefighter's, 87-90
    air supply duration, knowledge of, 88
    basic safety rules, knowing and applying, 90
    calculating point of no return, 88-90
    facepiece fit, 90
    protection limits of SCBA, 87
Sanitizing guidelines, 95
Search-and-rescue training, 112, 115
Seat-mounted SCBA, 134-136
Self-contained breathing apparatus (SCBA)
    advisories, 190
    body's reaction to wearing, 14-17
    cleaning and disinfecting of, 181-183
    condition of, 55-56
    emotional stability of user, 15
    features and accessories, 71

    inspection and maintenance checklist, 345-346
    malfunctions, 257
    manufacturers of, 299-344
    past, present, and future, 277-280
    record keeping, 94-95
    safety guidelines, general, 95-97
    selection of, 70
    training, 102-116
    types of, 53-72
Short-Term Exposure Limit (STEL), 32
Silo gas, 40
Skip breathing, 261
Smoke, 30
Smoke diver, 113-114
Smoke rooms, 107, 110
Smoldering stage, of fire, 29
Sodium saccharin, 93
Speaking diaphragm, 63, 65, 85, 176
Special protective clothing, potential problems for SCBA users, 240-241
Standard operating procedures (SOPs), 2, 91, 174, 234
    example of, 295-297
Storage
    guidelines, 96
    methods of, 187-188
    procedure for, 181
    proper, 187-188
Structures, handling fire fighting in different types of, 238-240
Submersion, accidental. *See* Accidental submersion
Sulfur dioxide (SO$_2$), 41-42
Sump, 205, 208
Synergistic effect, 31, 38
Systole, 13

T

Target organ, 34
Taste test, 93
Team Emergency Breathing Procedures, 243
Team emergency conditions breathing, 114, 257
Team work, 260
    importance of, 86
Temperatures
    elevated, 28-29
    extreme, 237
    high or low, use of SCBA in, 85
Toxic atmosphere, 32-34
Toxic gases, 30-42
    symptoms of overexposure to, 34
    see also specific gas
Trachea, 9
Trailer-mounted cascade system, 217
Training
    advanced, 113-115

classroom, 104
facilities, 107
makeshift facilities, 110-112
mazes, 110
mobile laboratories, 107-110
permanent centers, 107
preliminary, 102
record-keeping, 115-116
sequence, 104-106
Transfilling system, 261-262
disadvantages of, 262-263
Transportation, Department of (DOT), 43
Truck company operations, 234-236
Tulsa Fire Department, SCBA program, 285-293

Turbinates, 8, 12
Turnaround maintenance tag, 154

V
Vapor density (VD), 32
Veins, 13-14
Ventilation, 235
confined space, 244
negative-pressure, 246
positive-pressure, 246
Vertical entry, procedures for, 249
Voice amplifier, clip-on, 65

W
Web-type harness, 139

IFSTA MANUALS AND FPP PRODUCTS

For a current catalog describing these and other products call or write your local IFSTA distributor or Fire Protection Publications, IFSTA Headquarters, Oklahoma State University, Stillwater, OK 74078-0118.
Phone: 1-800-654-4055

FIRE DEPARTMENT AERIAL APPARATUS

includes information on the driver/operator's qualifications; vehicle operation; types of aerial apparatus; positioning, stabilizing, and operating aerial devices; tactics for aerial devices; and maintaining, testing, and purchasing aerial apparatus. Detailed appendices describe specific manufacturers' aerial devices. 1st Edition (1991), 416 pages, addresses NFPA 1002.

STUDY GUIDE FOR AERIAL APPARATUS

The companion study guide in question and answer format. 1st Edition (1991), 152 pages.

AIRCRAFT RESCUE AND FIRE FIGHTING

comprehensively covers commercial, military, and general aviation. All the information you need is in one place. Subjects covered include: personal protective equipment, apparatus and equipment, extinguishing agents, engines and systems, fire fighting procedures, hazardous materials, and fire prevention. Over 240 photographs and two-color illustrations. It also contains a glossary and review questions with answers. 3rd Edition (1992), 272 pages, addresses NFPA 1003.

BUILDING CONSTRUCTION RELATED TO THE FIRE SERVICE

helps firefighters become aware of the many construction designs and features of buildings found in a typical first alarm district and how these designs serve or hinder the suppression effort. Subjects include construction principles, assemblies and their resistance to fire, building services, door and window assemblies, and special types of structures. 1st Edition (1986), 166 pages, addresses NFPA 1001 and NFPA 1031, levels I & II.

CHIEF OFFICER

lists, explains, and illustrates the skills necessary to plan and maintain an efficient and cost-effective fire department. The combination of an ever-increasing fire problem, spiraling personnel and equipment costs, and the development of new technologies and methods for decision making requires far more than expertise in fire suppression. Today's chief officer must possess the ability to plan and administrate as well as have political expertise. 1st Edition (1985), 211 pages, addresses NFPA 1021, level VI.

SELF-INSTRUCTION FOR CHIEF OFFICER

The companion study guide in question and answer format. 1st Edition, 142 pages.

FIRE DEPARTMENT COMPANY OFFICER

focuses on the basic principles of fire department organization, working relationships, and personnel management. For the firefighter aspiring to become a company officer, or a company officer wishing to improve management skills, this manual helps develop and improve the necessary traits to effectively manage the fire company. 2nd Edition (1990), 278 pages, addresses NFPA 1021, levels I, II, & III.

COMPANY OFFICER STUDY GUIDE

The companion study guide in question and answer format. Includes problem applications and case studies. 1st Edition (1991), 256 pages.

ESSENTIALS OF FIRE FIGHTING

is the "bible" on basic firefighter skills and is used throughout the world. The easy-to-read format is enhanced by 1,500 photographs and illustrations. Step-by-step instructions are provided for many fire fighting tasks. Topics covered include: personal protective equipment, building construction, firefighter safety, fire behavior, portable extinguishers, SCBA, ropes and knots, rescue, forcible entry, ventilation, communications, water supplies, fire streams, hose, fire cause determination, public fire education and prevention, fire suppression techniques, ladders, salvage and overhaul, and automatic sprinkler systems. 3rd Edition (1992), addresses NFPA 1001.

STUDY GUIDE FOR ESSENTIALS OF FIRE FIGHTING

The companion learning tool for the new 3rd edition of the manual. It contains questions and answers to help you learn the important information in the book. 3rd Edition (1992).

PRINCIPLES OF EXTRICATION

leads you step-by-step through the procedures for disentangling victims from cars, buses, trains, farm equipment, and industrial situations. Fully illustrated with color diagrams and more than 500 photographs. It includes rescue company organization, protective clothing, and evaluating resources. Review questions with answers at the end of each chapter. 1st Edition (1990), 400 pages.

FIRE CAUSE DETERMINATION

gives you the information necessary to make on-scene fire cause determinations. You will know when to call for a trained investigator, and you will be able to help the investigator. It includes a profile of firesetters, finding origin and cause, documenting evidence, interviewing witnesses, and courtroom demeanor. 1st Edition (1982), 159 pages, addresses NFPA 1021, Fire Officer I, and NFPA 1031, levels I & II.

FIRE SERVICE FIRST RESPONDER

provides the information needed to evaluate and treat patients with serious injuries or illness. It familiarizes the reader with a wide variety of medical equipment and supplies. **First Responder** applies to safety, security, fire brigade, and law enforcement personnel, as well as fire service personnel, who are required to administer emergency medical care. 1st Edition (1987), 340 pages, addresses NFPA 1001, levels I & II, and DOT First Responder.

FORCIBLE ENTRY

reflects the growing concern for the reduction of property damage as well as firefighter safety. This comprehensive manual contains technical information about forcible entry tactics, tools, and methods, as well as door, window, and wall construction. Tactics discuss the degree of danger to the structure and leaving the building secure after entry. Includes a section on locks and through-the-lock entry. Review questions and answers at the end of each chapter. 7th Edition (1987), 270 pages, helpful for NFPA 1001.

GROUND COVER FIRE FIGHTING PRACTICES

explains the dramatic difference between structural fire fighting and wildland fire fighting. Ground cover fires include fires in weeds, grass, field crops, and brush. It discusses the apparatus, equipment, and extinguishing agents used to combat wildland fires. Outdoor fire behavior and how fuels, weather, and topography affect fire spread are explained. The text also covers personnel safety, management, and suppression methods. It contains a glossary, sample fire operation plan, fire control organization system, fire origin and cause determination, and water expansion pump systems. 2nd Edition (1982), 152 pages.

FIRE SERVICE GROUND LADDER PRACTICES

is a "how to" manual for learning how to handle, raise, and climb ground ladders; it also details maintenance and service testing. Basic information is presented with a variety of methods that allows the readers to select the best method for their locale. The chapter on Special Uses includes: ladders as a stretcher, a slide, a float drag, a water chute, and more. The manual contains a glossary, review questions and answers, and a sample testing and repair form. 8th Edition (1984), 388 pages, addresses NFPA 1001.

HAZARDOUS MATERIALS FOR FIRST RESPONDERS

provides basic information on hazardous materials with sections on site management and decontamination. It includes a description of various types of materials, their characteristics, and containers. The manual covers the effects of weather, topography, and environment on the behavior of hazardous materials and control efforts. Pre-incident planning and post-incident analysis are covered. 1st Edition (1988), 357 pages, addresses NFPA 472, 29 CFR 1910.120 and NFPA 1001.

STUDY GUIDE FOR HAZARDOUS MATERIALS FOR FIRST RESPONDERS

The companion study guide in question and answer format also includes case studies that simulate incidents. 1st Edition (1989), 208 pages.

HAZARDOUS MATERIALS: MANAGING THE INCIDENT

takes you beyond the basic information found in **Hazardous Materials for First Responders**. Directed to the leader/commander, this manual sets forth basic practices clearly and comprehensively. Charts, tables, and checklists guide you through the organization and planning stages to decontamination. This text, along with the accompanying workbook and instructor's guide, provides a comprehensive learning package. 1st Edition (1988), 206 pages, helpful for NFPA 1021.

STUDENT WORKBOOK FOR HAZARDOUS MATERIALS: MANAGING THE INCIDENT

provides questions and answers to enhance the student's comprehension and retention. 1st Edition (1988), 176 pages.

INSTRUCTOR'S GUIDE FOR HAZARDOUS MATERIALS: MANAGING THE INCIDENT

provides lessons based on each chapter, adult learning tips, and appendices of references and suggested audio visuals. 1st Edition (1988), 142 pages.

HAZ MAT RESPONSE TEAM LEAK AND SPILL GUIDE

contains articles by Michael Hildebrand reprinted from *Speaking of Fire's* popular Hazardous Materials Nuts and Bolts series. Two additional articles from *Speaking of Fire* and the hazardous material incident SOP from the Chicago Fire Department are also included. 1st Edition (1984), 57 pages.

EMERGENCY OPERATIONS IN HIGH-RACK STORAGE

is a concise summary of emergency operations in the high-rack storage area of a warehouse. It explains how to develop a pre-emergency plan, what equipment will be necessary to implement the plan, type and amount of training personnel will need to handle an emergency, and interfacing with various agencies. Includes

consideration questions, points not to be overlooked, and t scenarios. 1st Edition (1981), 97 pages.

HOSE PRACTICES

reflects the latest information on modern fire hose and couplin It is the most comprehensive single source about hose and its u The manual details basic methods of handling hose, includ large diameter hose. It is fully illustrated with photographs sho ing loads, evolutions, and techniques. This complete and pra cal book explains the national standards for hose and couplin 7th Edition (1988), 245 pages, addresses NFPA 1001.

FIRE PROTECTION HYDRAULICS AND WATER SUPPLY ANALYSIS

covers the quantity and pressure of water needed to provi adequate fire protection, the ability of existing water sup systems to provide fire protection, the adequacy of a water sup for a sprinkler system, and alternatives for deficient water sup systems. 1st Edition (1990), 340 pages.

INCIDENT COMMAND SYSTEM (ICS)

was developed by a multiagency task force. Using this syste fire, police, and other government groups can operate toget effectively under a single command. The system is modular a can be used to meet the requirements of both day-to-day a large-incident operations. It is the approved basic comma system taught at the National Fire Academy. 1st Edition (198 220 pages, helpful for NFPA 1021.

INDUSTRIAL FIRE PROTECTION

is designed for the person charged with the responsibility developing, implementing, and coordinating fire protection. "must read" for fire service personnel who will coordinate w industry/business for pre-incident planning. The text includ guidelines for establishing a company policy, organization a planning for the emergency, establishing a fire prevention pla incipient fire fighting tactics, an overview of interior structural fi fighting, and fixed fire fighting systems. 1st Edition (1982). 2 pages, written for 29 CFR. 1910, Subpart L, and helpful for NFF 1021 and NFPA 1031.

FIRE INSPECTION AND CODE ENFORCEMENT

provides a comprehensive, state-of-the-art reference and trainir manual for both uniformed and civilian inspectors. It is a compr hensive guide to the principles and techniques of inspection. Te includes information on how fire travels, electrical hazards, ar fire resistance requirements. It covers storage, handling, and us of hazardous materials; fire protection systems; and buildir construction for fire and life safety. 5th Edition (1987), 316 page addresses NFPA 1001 and NFPA 1031, levels I & II.

STUDY GUIDE FOR FIRE INSPECTION AND CODE ENFORCEMENT

The companion study guide in question and answer format wi case studies. 1st Edition (1989), 272 pages.

FIRE SERVICE INSTRUCTOR

explains the characteristics of a good instructor, shows you ho to determine training requirements, and teach to the level of yo class. It discusses the types, principles, and procedures teaching and learning, and covers the use of effective training aic and devices. The purpose and principles of testing as well as te construction are covered. Included are chapters on safety, leg considerations, and computers. 5th Edition (1990), 325 page addresses NFPA 1041, levels I & II.

LEADERSHIP IN THE FIRE SERVICE

was created from the series of lectures given by Robert F. Ham to assist in leadership development. It provides the foundation fc

ting along with others, explains how to gain the confidence of
ir personnel, and covers what is expected of an officer.
luded is information on supervision, evaluations, delegating,
l teaching. Some of the topics include: the successful leader
ay, a look into the past may reveal the future, and self-analysis
officers. 1st Edition (1967), 132 pages.

RE SERVICE ORIENTATION AND INDOCTRINATION

ates the traditions, history, and organization of the fire service.
icludes operation of the fire department, responsibilities and
ies of firefighters, and the function of fire department compa-
s. This exciting and informative text is for anyone dealing with
fire service who needs a basic understanding and overview.
e perfect book for new or prospective members, buffs, your
igressman or council members, fire service sales personnel,
l industrial brigades. 2nd Edition (1984), 187 pages, ad-
sses NFPA 1001.

IVATE FIRE PROTECTION AND DETECTION

oduces the firefighter, inspection personnel, brigade/safety
mber, insurance inspector/investigator, or fire protection stu-
it to fixed systems, extinguishers, and detection. It covers the
ious types of equipment, their installation, maintenance, and
ting. Systems discussed are: wet-pipe, dry-pipe, pre-action,
uge, residential, carbon dioxide, Halogen, dry- and wet-chemi-
, foam, standpipe, and fire extinguishers. 1st Edition (1979),
0 pages, addresses NFPA 1001 and NFPA 1031, levels I & II.

BLIC FIRE EDUCATION

ovides valuable information for ending public apathy and igno-
ice about fire. This manual gives you the knowledge to plan and
olement fire prevention campaigns. It shows you how to tailor
e individual programs to your audience as well as the time of
ar or specific problems. It includes working with the media,
source exchange, and smoke detectors. 1st Edition (1979), 169
ges, helpful for NFPA 1021 and 1031.

RE DEPARTMENT PUMPING APPARATUS

the Driver/Operator's encyclopedia on operating fire pumps
l pumping apparatus. It covers pumpers, tankers (tenders),
ish apparatus, and aerials with pumps. This comprehensive
lume explains safe driving techniques, getting maximum effi-
ncy from the pump, and basic water supply. It includes speci-
ation writing, apparatus testing, and extensive appendices of
mp manufacturers. 7th Edition (1989), 374 pages, addresses
PA 1002.

UDY GUIDE FOR PUMPING APPARATUS

e companion study guide in question and answer format. 1st
lition (1990), 100 pages.

RE SERVICE RESCUE PRACTICES

a comprehensive training text for firefighters and fire brigade
embers that expands proficiency in moving and removing
ctims from hazardous situations. This extensively illustrated
anual includes rescuer safety, effects of rescue work on victims,
scue from hazardous atmospheres, trenching, and outdoor
arches. 5th Edition (1981), 262 pages, addresses NFPA 1001.

ESIDENTIAL SPRINKLERS A PRIMER

tlines United States residential fire experience, system compo-
nts, engineering requirements, and issues concerning auto-
atic and fixed residential sprinkler systems. Written by Gary
ourtney and Scott Kerwood and reprinted from *Speaking of Fire*.
 excellent reference source for any fire service library and an
cellent supplement to **Private Fire Protection.** 1st Edition
986), 16 pages.

FIRE DEPARTMENT OCCUPATIONAL SAFETY

addresses the basic responsibilities and qualifications for a safety
officer and the minimum requirements and procedures for a safety
and health program. Included in this manual is an overview of
establishing and implementing a safety program, physical fitness
and health considerations, safety in training, fire station safety,
tool and equipment safety and maintenance, personal protective
equipment, en route hazards and response, emergency scene
safety, and special hazards. 2nd Edition (1991), 396 pages,
addresses NFPA 1500, 1501.

SALVAGE AND OVERHAUL

covers planning salvage operations, equipment selection and
care, as well as describing methods and techniques for using
salvage equipment to minimize fire damage caused by water,
smoke, heat, and debris. The overhaul section includes methods
for finding hidden fire, protection of fire cause evidence, safety
during overhaul operations, and restoration of property and fire
protection systems after a fire. 7th Edition (1985), 225 pages,
addresses NFPA 1001.

SELF-CONTAINED BREATHING APPARATUS

contains all the basics of SCBA use, care, testing, and operation.
Special attention is given to safety and training. The chapter on
Emergency Conditions Breathing has been completely revised to
incorporate safer emergency methods that can be used with
newer models of SCBA. Also included are appendices describing
regulatory agencies and donning and doffing procedures for nine
types of SCBA. The manual has been thoroughly updated to
cover NFPA, OSHA, ANSI, and NIOSH regulations and standards as they pertain to SCBA. 2nd Edition (1991) 360 pages,
addresses NFPA 1001.

STUDY GUIDE FOR SELF-CONTAINED BREATHING APPARATUS

The companion study guide in question and answer format. 1st
Edition (1991).

FIRE STREAM PRACTICES

brings you an all new approach to calculating friction loss. This
carefully written text covers the physics of fire and water; the
characteristics, requirements, principles of good streams; and fire
fighting foams. **Streams** includes formulas for the application of
fire fighting hydraulics, as well as actions and reactions created by
applying streams under a variety of circumstances. The friction
loss equations and answers are included, and review questions
are located at the end of each chapter. 7th Edition (1989), 464
pages, addresses NFPA 1001 and NFPA 1002.

GASOLINE TANK TRUCK EMERGENCIES

provides emergency response personnel with background information, general procedures, and response guidelines to be
followed when responding to and operating at incidents involving
MC-306/DOT 406 cargo tank trucks. Specific topics include:
incident management procedures, site safety considerations,
methods of product transfer, and vehicle uprighting considerations. 1st Edition (1992) 60 pages, addresses NFPA 472.

FIRE VENTILATION PRACTICES

presents the principles, practices, objectives, and advantages of
ventilation. It includes the factors and phases of combustion,
flammable liquid characteristics, products of combustion,
backdrafts, transmission of heat, and building construction considerations. The manual reflects the new techniques in building
construction and their effects on ventilation procedures. Methods
and procedures are thoroughly explained with numerous photo-

graphs and drawings. The text also includes: vertical (top), horizontal (cross), and forced ventilation; and a glossary. 6th Edition (1980) 131 pages, addresses NFPA 1001.

FIRE SERVICE PRACTICES FOR VOLUNTEER AND SMALL COMMUNITY FIRE DEPARTMENTS

presents those training practices that are most consistent with the activities of smaller fire departments. Consideration is given to the limitations of small community fire department resources. Techniques for performing basic skills are explained, accompanied by detailed illustrations and photographs. 6th Edition (1984), 311 pages.

WATER SUPPLIES FOR FIRE PROTECTION

acquaints you with the principles, requirements, and standards used to provide water for fire fighting. Rural water supplies as well as fixed systems are discussed. Abundant photographs, illustrations, tables, and diagrams make this the most complete text available. It includes requirements for size and carrying capacity of mains, hydrant specifications, maintenance procedures conducted by the fire department, and relevant maps and record keeping procedures. Review questions at the end of each chapter. 4th Edition (1988), 268 pages, addresses NFPA 1001, NFPA 1002, and NFPA 1031, levels I & II.

TEACHING PACKAGES

LEADERSHIP

This teaching package is designed to assist the instructor in teaching leadership and motivational skills. Cause and effect, behavior and consequences, listening and communications are themes throughout the course that stress the reality of the job and the people one deals with daily. Before each lesson is a title page that gives an outline of the subject matter to be covered, the approximate time required to teach the material, the specific learning objectives, and the references for the instructor's preparation. Sources for suggested films and videotapes are included.

CURRICULUM PACKAGE FOR IFSTA COMPANY OFFICER

A competency-based Teaching Package with lesson plans and activities to teach the student the information and skills needed to qualify for the position of Company Officer. Corresponds to **Fire Department Company Officer**, 2nd Edition.

The Package includes the Company Officer Instructor's Guide (the how, what, and when to teach); the Student Guide (a workbook for group instruction or self-study); and 143 full colored overhead Transparencies.

ESSENTIALS CURRICULUM PACKAGE

A competency-based teaching package with lesson plans and activities to teach the student the information and skills needed to qualify for the position of Fire Fighter I or II. Corresponds to **Essentials of Fire Fighting**, 3rd Edition.

TRANSLATIONS

LO ESENCIAL EN EL COMBATE DE INCENDIOS

is a direct translation of **Essentials of Fire Fighting**, 2nd edition. Please contact your distributor or FPP for shipping charges addresses outside U.S. and Canada. 444 pages.

PRACTICAS Y TEORIA PARA BOMBEROS

is a direct translation of **Fire Services Practices for Volunteer and Small Community Fire Departments**, 6th edition. Please contact your distributor or FPP for shipping charges to addresses outside U.S. and Canada. 347 pages.

OTHER ITEMS

TRAINING AIDS

Fire Protection Publications carries a complete line of videos, overhead transparencies, and slides. Call for a current catalog.

NEWSLETTER

The nationally acclaimed and award winning newsletter, *Speaking of Fire*, is published quarterly and available to you free. Call today for your free subscription.

SELF-CONTAINED BREATHING APPARATUS
2nd EDITION
2nd PRINTING, 8/92

COMMENT SHEET

DATE _____ NAME _____

ADDRESS _____

ORGANIZATION REPRESENTED _____

CHAPTER TITLE _____ NUMBER _____

SECTION/PARAGRAPH/FIGURE _____ PAGE _____

1. Proposal (include proposed wording, or identification of wording to be deleted),
   OR PROPOSED FIGURE:

2. Statement of Problem and Substantiation for Proposal:

RETURN TO: IFSTA Editor   SIGNATURE _____
           Fire Protection Publications
           Oklahoma State University
           Stillwater, OK 74078

Use this sheet to make any suggestions, recommendations, or comments. We need your input to make the manuals the most up to date as possible. Your help is appreciated. Use additional pages if necessary.